Epidemiologic Methods

Epidemiologic Methods

Studying the Occurrence of Illness

THOMAS D. KOEPSELL
NOEL S. WEISS

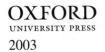

2003

OXFORD
UNIVERSITY PRESS

Oxford   New York
Auckland   Bangkok   Buenos Aires   Cape Town   Chennai
Dar es Salaam   Delhi   Hong Kong   Istanbul   Karachi   Kolkata
Kuala Lumpur   Madrid   Melbourne   Mexico City   Mumbai
Nairobi   São Paulo   Shanghai   Taipei   Tokyo   Toronto

Copyright © 2003 by Thomas D. Koepsell and Noel S. Weiss

Published by Oxford University Press, Inc.
198 Madison Avenue, New York, New York, 10016
http://www.oup-usa.org

Oxford is a registered trademark of Oxford University Press

Library of Congress Cataloging-in-Publication Data
Koepsell, Thomas D.
Epidemiologic methods : studying the occurrence of illness /
Thomas D. Koepsell, Noel S. Weiss.
p. ; cm.
Includes bibliographical references and index.
ISBN-13 978-0-19-515078-0

1. Epidemiology--Methodology.   I. Weiss, Noel S., 1941-   II. Title.
[DNLM: 1. Epidemiologic Methods. WA 950 K78 2003]
RA652.4 .K645 2003
614.4--dc21   2002033763

9 8 7 6

Printed in the United States of America
on acid-free paper

Preface

> Epidemiology at any given time is something more than the total of its established facts. It includes their orderly arrangement into chains of inference which extend more or less beyond the bounds of direct observation. Such of these chains as are well and truly laid guide investigation to the facts of the future.
>
> Wade Hampton Frost[1]

Between us, we have accumulated more than 50 years teaching courses on the principles and methods of epidemiology. We have jointly taught a two-course sequence at the University of Washington since the mid-1980s. During this time, we have listened to the reactions of many students who were being introduced to this field. One came from a woman who said she derived an almost esthetic pleasure from epidemiology: she found both efficiency and beauty in the process of taking raw observations on the occurrence of an illness in humans and weaving them into "chains of inferences" about the causes of that illness, which often had the potential to lead to prevention.

We suspect that not too many of our students would have used the word *esthetic* to describe any of their feelings about our course, even their positive feelings. (Some might have said that *anesthetic* better characterized some of the class sessions!) Nonetheless, we like to think that the first student had internalized what we were trying to convey—that the techniques of structuring observations and analyzing the information gathered (which so much time and effort are expended on in class) are to be used to produce "chains [that] are well and truly laid" in the hope of guiding "investigation to the facts of the future." Having produced extensive classroom materials to achieve our goals, we felt that with a little (!) extra labor we could organize these materials into a book for other students of epidemiology.

The book is aimed at beginning and intermediate students of epidemiologic methods. It is meant to serve as an introduction to the field for people who intend to conduct epidemiologic research themselves, or who need methodologic expertise to interpret and properly synthesize the results of epidemiologic research produced by others. It starts at the beginning, so to speak, but covers much of the material in more detail than would be desired by a reader who wished to have only a general appreciation of epidemiology. Those who have already taken an introductory course in epidemiology may find here a welcome review of basic concepts as well as new, more advanced material.

[1] From his introduction to: Snow: J. Snow on Cholera. New York: The Commonwealth Fund, 1936.

A brief outline of the book may be helpful. Chapter 1 tells the story of a real disease outbreak, introducing epidemiologic concepts and designs along the way that will be covered in depth in later chapters. Chapter 2 sets forth an epidemiologic view of diseases and populations, leading into Chapters 3 and 4 on measuring disease frequency in populations. Chapter 5 paints the "big picture" of research designs in epidemiology, so that their names are familiar when used in chapters that follow. Chapters 6 and 7 highlight several specific sources of numerator and denominator data in epidemiology and provide examples of the person/place/time conceptual framework that underlies many descriptive epidemiologic studies.

As a transition into analytic epidemiology, Chapter 8 discusses the kinds of epidemiologic evidence that bear on an inference that an association may be causal. Chapter 9 also focuses on associations, describing several quantitative measures of excess risk that can be calculated from epidemiologic data. Chapter 10 introduces several quantitative techniques for assessing the reliability and validity of epidemiologic measurements and describes how measurement error affects observed associations. Chapter 11 describes what *confounding* is, how it is assessed, and how it can be controlled.

Chapters 12–15 each focus in depth on a class of epidemiologic study designs: ecologic studies, randomized trials, cohort studies, and case-control studies. Chapter 16 discusses the implications for epidemiologic studies of the temporal relationship between exposure and outcome. Chapter 17 describes ways in which epidemiologic studies can be designed and analyzed to enhance the likelihood that a true association is detected.

Chapters 18–20 cover methodological aspects of several key topics in epidemiology: screening for disease, short-term disease outbreaks, and evaluating the effects of institutional and societal policies on health.

As the book's title indicates, the discussion throughout focuses on the means by which epidemiologic research is conducted and interpreted, not on the substantive knowledge about specific diseases or exposures that has accumulated from specific studies.

Two things that will distinguish this book from others with similar goals are its liberal use of examples from the published medical literature and the sets of questions that appear at the end of most chapters. Most of these questions pertain to actual published studies; our purpose being to emphasize the applicability of the principles and methods to real-life situations.

Each of us drafted about half of the book. There being no better way of deciding the order of the two authors' names on the title page, we flipped a coin to determine whose name would come first. If in a few years' time there is a perceived need for a second edition of this book, and if both of us feel up to the task of preparing one, the order of names will be reversed.

We thank Jane Koehler and Jeffrey Duchin, epidemiologists with Public Health Seattle & King County, for contributing a chapter on outbreak investigation. We also gratefully acknowledge helpful comments on draft chapters from several colleagues and students. Peter Cummings, Sander Greenland, and Bruce Psaty kindly reviewed some of the chapters and made many useful suggestions. Students in our two-quarter course sequence on epidemiologic methods served as "guinea pigs" for several draft chapters, and the final version benefitted from their sharp eyes.

Seattle, Washington   T. D. K.
                                                               N. S. W.

Contents

Epidemiologic Methods

1

INTRODUCTION: AN EPIDEMIC OF BLINDNESS IN YOUNG CHILDREN

DISCOVERY

On February 14, 1941, a Boston pediatrician named Dr. Stewart Clifford was making a routine house call on one of his patients, a baby girl then about three months old. She had been delivered prematurely, weighing about four pounds at birth. Except for some brief early episodes of turning blue (cyanosis), she had done well during her extra days in the hospital and had been discharged.

As he examined her, Dr. Clifford noticed something abnormal about the baby's eyes. Her gaze wandered aimlessly, and her eyes jerked rapidly from side to side. There were prominent gray, opaque bodies in both eyes. He was puzzled and concerned. By all appearances, the baby girl was blind.

Dr. Clifford called in Dr. Paul Chandler, a leading Boston ophthalmologist. Dr. Chandler had not seen this condition before. To permit a fuller evaluation, the baby was hospitalized again and examined under anesthesia. The main abnormality (shown in Figure 1–1) was a gray mass of scar tissue attached to the back of the lens and covered with blood vessels. It later became clear that this tissue was all that remained of a retina that had been so badly damaged by hemorrhage and inflammation that it had delaminated from the back of the eye, become scarred and fibrous, and floated forward to affix itself to the lens. Blindness was profound and irreversible.

This first case proved not to be a bizarre, isolated occurrence. Within a week, Dr. Clifford encountered another blind infant with the condition. Soon a consultant ophthalmologist, Dr. Theodore Terry, had collected information on five such cases in the Boston area, whom he described in an article in the *American Journal of Ophthalmology* (Terry, 1942). Shared pathological features among these early cases led to calling the condition *retrolental fibroplasia* (RLF)—proliferation of fibrous scar tissue behind the lens.

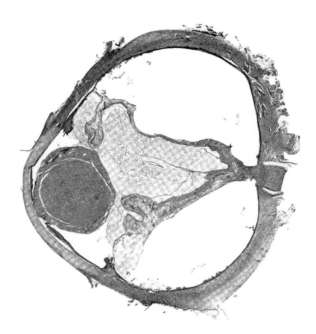

Figure 1-1. Cross-Section of an Eye Showing Retrolental Fibroplasia (courtesy of Arnall Patz, M.D.).

EPIDEMIC

Once Terry's description of RLF appeared in the medical literature, other physicians began to look for it and to find it. In 1945, Terry himself reported on 117 cases, all but five of them babies born prematurely (Terry, 1945). The California School for the Blind found a sharp rise in the number of RLF cases over time in southern California, as shown in Figure 1–2 (Silverman, 1980). During the decade after its discovery, RLF went from being literally unknown to being the most common cause of blindness in preschool children in the U.S. Worldwide, more than 10,000 babies developed the condition.

EARLY SEARCH FOR POSSIBLE CAUSES

The rapid rise in the frequency of RLF and its poor prognosis led to an intensive search for its cause or causes. Early case series suggested that most cases had been born prematurely. Whether the condition was already present at birth or developed after birth remained unclear. One study to help clarify these issues was by Owens

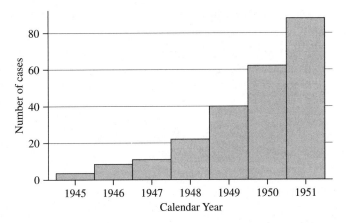

Figure 1-2. Number of Retrolental Fibroplasia Cases by Year in Southern California, Pre-1946 to 1951 (from Silverman, 1980).

and Owens (1949), who performed monthly standardized eye examinations from birth to six months of age on 111 babies born at Johns Hopkins Hospital who weighed 2000 grams (4.5 pounds) or less at birth. To determine whether the degree of prematurity was related to risk of RLF, they grouped study babies according to birth weight (<1360 grams vs. 1360+ grams), a characteristic strongly related to prematurity and often used as a proxy for it. All babies appeared to have normal eyes at birth, but 12.1% of the lowest-birth-weight babies developed RLF, compared to only 1.3% of the higher-birth-weight babies, nearly a tenfold difference.

From the monthly eye examinations, Owens and Owens observed and described the sequence of pathological events that led to RLF among babies who developed it. A typical progression was (*1*) dilation of retinal vessels; (*2*) wild proliferation of vessels throughout the retinal bed, even protruding into the vitreous humor; (*3*) retinal hemorrhage, edema, and inflammation; and finally (*4*) scarring and detachment of the retina. The disease did not always progress inexorably to end in scarring, however; in some cases it seemed to halt at earlier stages.

Both the association with prematurity and the pathological evolution of RLF suggested possible causes. The care of premature infants had advanced in many ways during the 1940s (James and Lanman, 1976). Techniques for giving fluids by vein or subcutaneously had come into widespread use, providing new ways to prevent or treat dehydration and to administer medications. Several vitamin and mineral deficiencies were increasingly recognized and treated with supplements. Incubators made it easier to control temperature and humidity in the baby's local environment and offered a barrier to infection. With immature lungs, many premature babies experienced cyanosis or respiratory distress, which could be treated with supplemental oxygen piped into the incubator or delivered by catheter or face

Table 1–1. Survivorship and Development of Retrolental Fibroplasia by Birth Weight and Calendar Year—Manchester, England, 1947–1951

CALENDAR YEAR	1947	1948	1949	1950	1951
A. Number of surviving infants					
Under 3 lb. at birth	4	7	9	16	13
3–3.5 lb.	11	13	18	21	22
3.5–4 lb.	31	27	30	38	30
Over 4 lb.	72	92	50	75	50
B. Number of surviving infants who developed RLF					
Under 3 lb. at birth	1	0	2	5	12
3–3.5 lb.	0	0	0	2	12
3.5–4 lb.	0	0	0	2	9
Over 4 lb.	0	0	0	2	9
C. Proportion of survivors who developed RLF					
Under 3 lb. at birth	.25	.00	.22	.31	.92
3–3.5 lb.	.00	.00	.00	.10	.55
3.5–4 lb.	.00	.00	.00	.05	.30
Over 4 lb.	.00	.00	.00	.03	.18

[*Source:* Jefferson (1952).]

mask. Penicillin offered a potent new weapon against infectious complications. These and other medical innovations had sharply increased a premature baby's chances of survival.

Improved survival of premature babies raised the possibility that RLF was a complication of prematurity that had escaped notice until enough such babies survived long enough to develop RLF. Table 1–1 presents results from a study by Jefferson (1952) in Manchester, England, that addressed this possibility. Panel A of the table shows the number of surviving babies in each year from 1947 to 1951, by birth weight. Panel B shows the number, and panel C the proportion, of surviving babies who developed RLF, also broken out by birth weight and year. Scanning across panel A, we see that the number of surviving babies increased steadily over time among those weighing under 3 pounds or 3 to 3.5 pounds at birth, while the time trends for babies weighing over 3.5 pounds suggest no parallel increase in births in general. These observations would be compatible with improving survival over time among infants with the lowest birth weights. In panel B, we also see an increasing number of babies with RLF over time in each birth weight category. This simply confirms that the RLF epidemic did not spare Manchester.

Most revealing, however, are the patterns in panel C showing the *proportion* of surviving babies who developed RLF, by birth weight category and year. Each proportion was computed simply by dividing the number of RLF cases in each year and birth weight category by the corresponding number of surviving babies. These data show that (1) within any given year, the proportion developing RLF was generally greatest among babies with the lowest birth weights; and (2) within each birth weight category, the proportion of survivors who developed RLF increased markedly over time. This second observation is direct evidence that, at least in Manchester, the epidemic was due not just to increased survival of premature babies, but also to increased risk of RLF among the survivors.

EARLY TREATMENTS

Early therapies for RLF sought to arrest progression of the disease through the pathological stages described earlier. It was thought that the increase in vessel caliber and vascular density might be a response to hypoxia, to which premature infants were known to be vulnerable. A retinal disease in mice with some RLF-like features appeared to result from experimentally lowered oxygen levels (Ingalls, 1948). This line of thinking seemed to provide still further justification for liberal oxygen supplementation in premature infants, especially those with early signs of RLF.

Another approach to treatment was based on the observations that some premature infants had abnormally low adrenal corticosteroid levels, and that the pathology of RLF was reminiscent of connective-tissue diseases in adults. A group of New York–based physicians tried adrenocorticotropic hormone (ACTH) treatments for babies with early signs of RLF, hoping that it would suppress inflammation and scarring. Of 31 babies who received ACTH, 25 appeared to respond, with reversal of early changes of RLF and preserved eyesight (Blodi et al., 1951). Given the paucity of effective treatments, early reports of success with ACTH were welcome news.

Unfortunately, questions about ACTH soon began to emerge. Some clinicians noted many disturbing treatment failures (Laupus, 1951; Pratt, 1951). They also noted that some early cases *not* treated with ACTH did not progress inexorably to scarring and blindness. Thus, it was not clear how effective ACTH really was.

In an attempt to provide more convincing evidence, Reese et al. (1952) undertook a second study of ACTH treatment using a different research design, as diagrammed in Figure 1–3. This time the study included a second group that did not receive ACTH. Specifically, an equal number of white marbles and blue marbles of similar size were placed in a box. Each time a new baby with early RLF was found to be eligible, a marble was removed from the box without looking. Its color determined whether the baby received ACTH. The investigators sought to keep other forms of treatment similar in both groups, and they monitored all

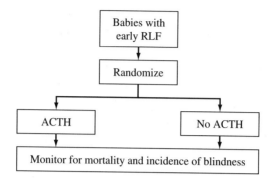

	Treatment received	
Outcome	ACTH	No ACTH
Mortality[a]		
Deaths/babies	6/36	1/49
% deaths	17%	2%
Blindness		
Blind eyes/total eyes	10/30	7/36
% blind	33%	19%

Figure 1–3. Study Design and Results Evaluating ACTH as Treatment for Early Retrolental Fibroplasia (from Reese et al., 1952).
[a]Published report gives only total numbers of deaths and babies, combining randomized-trial results with previous non-randomized comparison.

babies with standardized eye examinations. The results were a rude shock: not only was progression of RLF more common in the ACTH group, but death was more frequent in that group as well, apparently due to increased risk of infection. ACTH had been found to be ineffective and even dangerous as treatment for RLF. It quickly fell out of favor.

NARROWING THE SEARCH FOR CAUSES

A decade after the first reported cases, over 50 factors had been suggested as possible contributors to the rising incidence of RLF (Silverman, 1980). Some had changed little during the period of rising RLF incidence—the gender mix of newborn babies, for example—and thus could hardly explain the epidemic. Other factors were not readily modifiable and hence offered few opportunities for prevention or treatment. Yet the remaining list of plausible and possible contributing causes was lengthy. If each factor had required a randomized trial like the ACTH study to confirm or exclude its role, the process would have been long and costly.

But in 1949 Kinsey and Zacharias showed how other research approaches could be used to narrow the field of plausible hypotheses in order to focus attention on a few prime suspects. Their paper actually reported results from three related studies. The first involved identifying 53 babies weighing four pounds or less at birth who had been born at the Boston Lying-In Hospital over a ten-year period and were known to have developed RLF. They were compared with a second group of 298 babies weighing four pounds or less at birth, born at the same hospital over the same ten-year period, but known not to have developed RLF. The researchers then systematically reviewed the hospital records and, when necessary, interviewed mothers and pediatricians for both groups of babies. They compared prenatal factors, labor and delivery characteristics, postnatal complications, and patterns of neonatal care between the two groups. In so doing, they investigated no fewer than 47 potential risk factors as part of the same basic research design: studying each factor required just gathering another piece of information about each subject. Moreover, the information needed on the 53 RLF cases and 298 no-RLF controls concerned events that had already occurred by the time data collection began, so the study could be completed quickly.

For three factors, the observed differences between groups were larger than chance alone could easily explain. Compared to controls, the RLF cases were less likely to be a first-born child, spent an average of ten more days in the newborn nursery after birth, and received supplemental oxygen for an average of nine more days. The authors noted that longer time in the nursery and on oxygen might have reflected worse general health among the cases. Many other factors proved to be similar between RLF cases and controls, making it less likely that they were important causes of RLF.

The second study by Kinsey and Zacharias built on the observation that the number of RLF cases each year had risen sharply at their hospital during the mid-1940's, an era when several changes had occurred in treatment patterns for premature babies. They sought to determine whether changes over time in use of any particular treatment coincided with changes in the frequency of RLF. As shown in Figure 1–4, they identified three factors that looked suspicious: use of iron supplements ($FeSO_4$), use of water-miscible vitamins (thought to be better absorbed than the previously used lipid-soluble vitamins), and amount of supplemental oxygen used. Of these, they considered the temporal correlations with iron and vitamins to be the most striking.

The third study reported by Kinsey and Zacharias was motivated by two other observations: first, the incidence of RLF seemed to differ considerably among hospitals; and second, hospitals had different policies and practices about how they treated premature babies, which led to wide variation in treatment patterns. Kinsey and Zacharias reasoned that the hospital-to-hospital variation in RLF

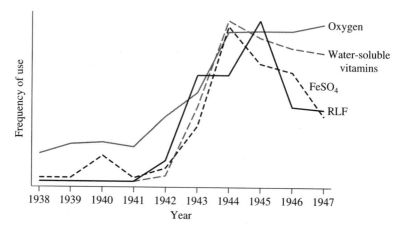

Figure 1–4. Trends Over Time in Use of Water-Miscible Vitamins, Use of Iron Supplements, Days of Oxygen Supplementation, and Incidence of Retrolental Fibroplasia among Babies Who Weighed 3–4 lbs. at Birth, Born at Boston Lying-In Hospital, 1938–1947 (from Kinsey and Zacharias, 1949).

frequency and in treatment might be linked. Accordingly, they gathered data from eight urban hospitals, focusing especially on the use of water-miscible vitamins and on iron supplementation in relation to RLF incidence.

As shown in Table 1–2, the Boston hospital (their own) with the highest incidence of RLF had used water-soluble vitamins and iron supplements frequently. At a hospital in New York that reported using no water-miscible vitamins and no iron, RLF had affected fewer than 1% of babies. Yet the overall pattern of

Table 1–2. Treatment of Babies Weighing 3–4 lbs. at Birth and Incidence of Retrolental Fibroplasia at Eight Urban Hospitals

LOCATION	USE OF WATER-MISCIBLE VITAMINS	USE OF IRON	INCIDENCE OF RLF (%)
Boston	None	Low	0.9
Boston	High	High	20.2
Baltimore	Low	Low	1.0
New York	None	None	0.7
Cincinnati	None	High	6.8
Birmingham, England	None	Low	0.0
Providence	High	Low	5.2
Providence	None	Low	4.0

[*Source:* Kinsey and Zacharias (1949).]

variation failed to implicate one treatment over the other. Nonetheless, after reviewing these results, the investigators arranged to have use of water-soluble vitamins and iron supplements curtailed at their hospital. Unfortunately, the number of new RLF cases remained high and apparently unaffected by the change (Kinsey and Chisholm, 1951).

Half a world away, an Australian pediatrician, Dr. Kate Campbell (1951), began to suspect that the oxygen–RLF association might not be an artifact of worse general health or of treatment for RLF. She had learned that clinicians in England had noted a striking increase in RLF after new, tightly-sealed incubators had been installed, permitting delivery of oxygen at higher concentrations than before. Campbell conducted a small study of her own, comparing three groups of premature babies treated in the Melbourne area who had been subject to different treatment practices with regard to supplemental oxygen. Most babies treated at Institution I had been placed in a cot (incubator) that delivered oxygen at high concentration. Babies treated at Institution II wore a catheter or face mask that delivered lower inhaled oxygen concentrations. A third group of babies under private care had been treated with various oxygen delivery methods that also provided relatively low concentrations of oxygen. She found that RLF had occurred in 19% of premature babies at Institution I, compared with only 7% of the babies treated in other two settings. While acknowledging the small size of her study, she questioned in print whether oxygen supplementation might actually be causing RLF.

Other reports from around the world painted a confusing picture, however. At Charity Hospital in New Orleans (Exline and Harrington, 1951), no cases of RLF were found, despite what was regarded as liberal use of oxygen supplementation. (It was noted later that incubators in the large newborn unit there were frequently opened, however, allowing oxygen to escape, and that oxygen levels were seldom directly measured.) Other hospitals in Oxford, England, and Paris, France, had seen no reduction in RLF after oxygen use was restricted (Houlton, 1951; Lelong et al., 1952), but it was not clear whether babies receiving high vs. low oxygen were otherwise similar.

IMPLICATING OXYGEN: EXPERIMENTAL EVIDENCE

One of many clinicians following these developments was Dr. Arnall Patz, then an ophthalmology resident at Gallinger Municipal Hospital in Washington, D.C. He, too, had become suspicious about the possible role of oxygen when he was called to see more and more babies with RLF after closed incubators were introduced. Although he began some animal studies, he reasoned that more direct and convincing evidence about whether oxygen supplementation was a cause of

RLF or simply an artifact would have to come from a study of human babies. Such a study would have to manipulate the level of oxygen delivery for premature babies, comparing the outcome in those on high oxygen with others on low oxygen. Patz and colleagues applied for, and eventually received, a $4,000 grant from the then-fledgling National Institutes of Health to set up such a study.

Babies weighing under 3.5 pounds were assigned alternately to one of two groups. Group I was to receive 65–70% oxygen for four to seven weeks. Group II was to receive oxygen only at 40% concentration or less, only in response to a clinical need, and only for one to fourteen days. To help allay fears raised during review of their grant proposal about the possible risks of hypoxia, Patz and colleagues stipulated that all babies in both groups would be given enough oxygen to maintain a healthy pink color.

Nonetheless, it proved to be a difficult study to carry out: some nurses questioned the wisdom of curtailing oxygen for premature babies and turned up the oxygen concentration at night for some of them. Ultimately, 11 of 76 babies were excluded due to insufficiently constant oxygen levels or lack of follow-up data. Yet findings for the other 65 babies were striking: 17 of 28 (61%) in the high-oxygen group developed RLF, versus only 6 of 37 (16%) of babies in the restricted-oxygen group. The researchers concluded that "in view of the bizarre manner in which the incidence of the disease fluctuates, additional rigidly controlled observations are necessary. . . ." (Patz et al., 1952).

That recommendation did not go unheeded. The National Institutes of Health soon convened a working group to plan a larger randomized experiment on oxygen supplementation. Ultimately this study, one of the earliest randomized trials supported by NIH, was conducted in 18 hospitals that agreed to follow a common protocol. The study compared high vs. restricted oxygen regimens among babies with birth weights of 1500 grams or less who had survived at least 48 hours after birth. Because of the emerging concern about the safety of administering oxygen at high concentrations, for the first three months of the study, two babies were to be assigned to the restricted-oxygen regimen for every one assigned to the high-oxygen regimen. Thereafter, if no adverse effect of restricted oxygen on mortality appeared, all babies would receive the low-oxygen regimen. Babies in both groups were followed closely with standardized eye examinations to determine the incidence of RLF.

On September 19, 1954, results of the cooperative study were publicly announced, and they were published the following year (Kinsey, 1955). As shown in Table 1–3, the incidence of RLF was nearly three-fold higher among babies in the high-oxygen group. Total mortality in both groups was similar. A smaller randomized trial of oxygen supplementation in Colorado was reported in the same year by Lanman and colleagues (1954), reaching similar conclusions.

Table 1–3. All-Causes Mortality and Incidence of Retrolental Fibroplasia (RLF) in
Relation to Oxygen Treatment among Babies Enrolled During the First
Three Months of the National Cooperative Study

	Mortality		Incidence of RLF	
TREATMENT GROUP	DEATHS/N	PERCENT	CASES/N	PERCENT
Routine high oxygen	15/68	22.0	12/53	22.6
Curtailed oxygen	36/144	25.0	8/104	7.7

[*Source:* Greenhouse (1990).]

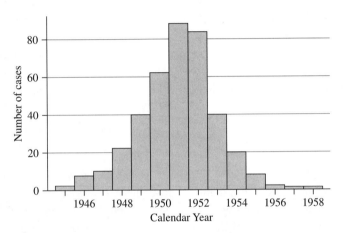

Figure 1–5. Number of Retrolental Fibroplasia (RLF) Cases by Calendar Year in Southern
California, Pre-1946 to 1958 (from Silverman, 1980).

DECLINING INCIDENCE

Early evidence about possible adverse effects of oxygen had already begun to
influence treatment in the early 1950s, but release of the National Cooperative
Study findings hastened the trend toward restricting use of supplemental oxygen.
The American Academy of Pediatrics and other influential professional organizations soon revised their recommendations to clinicians on care of premature
babies, advocating more sparing use of oxygen and use of oxygen supplementation only when clinical circumstances required it. The number of cases of RLF in
the United States fell rapidly—Figure 1–5 shows the trend in Southern California.
The epidemic was over.

MECHANISM

A perplexing aspect of RLF was that implicating oxygen as a culprit seemed contrary to so much other biological knowledge. Oxygen was obviously essential for human life, and it was well known that premature babies often suffered from respiratory problems that led to low blood oxygen levels. Why was more of a good thing not better? Laboratory research on RLF was stymied for some time by lack of a good animal model for the disease. But in 1953 Ashton and colleagues reported research findings from work on kittens. They found that the retina of a newborn kitten, like that of a prematurely born human baby, was incompletely vascularized. Development of retinal vessels was normally completed after birth, probably stimulated by mild hypoxia in areas of the retina that were not yet fully vascularized. Prolonged exposure to high oxygen levels after birth was found to produce constriction and ultimately obliteration of immature retinal vessels. When supplemental oxygen was then withdrawn, areas of the retina that had never become fully vascularized now became severely oxygen-deprived. This led to inflammation and disordered vessel growth, followed in severe cases by scarring and destruction of the retina.

EPILOGUE

The rapid shift to more conservative use of oxygen supplementation in the 1950s is now generally credited as being the main cause of the rapid decline in RLF. But later evidence suggests that the change may not have occurred without cost. In 1960, Avery and Oppenheimer reported that deaths from hyaline membrane disease (now called respiratory distress syndrome) at Johns Hopkins Hospital had increased over the period from 1954 to 1958 after oxygen use was restricted. In the United States and in England and Wales, the rate of infant deaths on the first day of life, which had been declining steadily for more than 15 years, began to rise again in the early 1950s and did not start falling again for another decade (James and Lanman, 1976). While many other changes in care were occurring during those years, it is thought that some clinicians may have been overzealous in their efforts to prevent RLF through sparing use of oxygen. None of the three experimental studies of oxygen described above had involved the number of participants that would be needed to detect small to moderate adverse effects of oxygen curtailment on mortality. In addition, the National Cooperative Study had only enrolled babies who had survived for at least 48 hours after birth. Its results thus did not directly address the possible consequences of oxygen restriction during the first two days of life, when many infant deaths occurred.

Retrolental fibroplasia has not disappeared. Its modern name is *retinopathy of prematurity,* a term that encompasses a wider spectrum of pathological features and that recasts prematurity from being a strong risk factor to being a required precondition. With further advances in technology, survival of ever-smaller premature babies has improved. Many such babies *must* have supplemental oxygen to survive. But clinicians are now far better able to monitor and regulate oxygen levels received by the tissues of premature infants undergoing treatment, so they can better steer a path between benefit and retinal toxicity.

CONCLUSIONS

This chapter is not intended just to recount the history of retrolental fibroplasia. Rather, it is an attempt to illustrate the value of information gained from studying variations in disease frequency in human populations. Epidemiologic research turned out to occupy center stage in this episode of medical history, enabling relatively rapid recognition of an important cause of disease that stemmed directly from the actions of well-meaning physicians.

Among other lessons, the history of RLF suggests that some kinds of research should have greater impact than others on our beliefs and actions. One goal of this book is to explore what features of a research design make one study better than another, and how this should affect our confidence in the validity of the results. For example, early enthusiasm for ACTH as treatment for RLF came from experience with a series of treated cases, but there was no comparable group of cases treated without ACTH. When a control group was added in a subsequent study, conclusions about the effectiveness and safety of ACTH were completely reversed. Later, the sequence of research on oxygen and RLF evolved from observational studies, to a small non-randomized intervention trial, then to a multi-center randomized controlled trial. The broad conclusions of these studies proved to be similar, and the quality and consistency of evidence from better and better studies overcame skepticism and guided practice even before a mature biological theory of the pathogenesis of RLF had emerged.

From that viewpoint, some leading "characters" in the story of RLF are the study designs themselves. Several of these designs will be explored in depth in chapters to come. To unmask some of them now:

- Owens and Owens conducted a *prospective cohort* study to confirm the role of prematurity. They first formed two groups of babies on the basis of birth weight, then monitored babies in both groups over time to measure and compare the incidence of RLF between groups.
- Kinsey and Zacharias carried out a *case-control* study to investigate various perinatal risk factors. They first identified one group of babies with RLF and

another group without RLF, then measured and compared the frequency of past exposure to various possible risk factors in those groups.

- In another part of the Kinsey and Zacharias study, and in the study by Campbell, *ecological* research designs were used to investigate possible hospital-level associations between treatment patterns and RLF incidence.
- Patz's study of oxygen supplementation was a *non-randomized intervention trial*. Whether a study baby received high- or low-dose supplemental oxygen was under the investigators' control. However, allocation of babies alternately between treatment regimens made the sequence of treatment-group assignments entirely predictable, not truly random.
- The National Cooperative Study was a true *randomized controlled trial*. As in the Patz study, the investigators controlled which oxygen regimen each study baby received, but in this instance they used formal random assignment to do so.

The story of RLF also introduces several other key concepts in epidemiology that we shall return to in depth, including using counts and rates as measures of disease frequency (Chapter 3), quantifying excess risk (Chapter 9), detecting and controlling confounding factors (Chapter 11), and determining whether associations are truly causal (Chapter 8).

Finally, we should note that few of the investigators who conducted these studies regarded themselves as epidemiologists, even though they were using epidemiologic methods. Most epidemiologists at that time worked on infectious diseases, although the attention given to other types of epidemiologic studies had begun to grow. But epidemiologic concepts and methods are broadly applicable, and they are available to everyone. This book seeks to introduce many of the tools of epidemiology, and to provide guidance about how to use them well.

FURTHER READING

Several more-complete accounts of the history of RLF and its control have been published. Silverman's 1980 book includes personal anecdotes and reflections of several clinicians and researchers whose work is mentioned here. James and Lanman (1976) edited a monograph about the history of RLF published as a supplement to *Pediatrics* by the American Academy of Pediatrics Committee on the Fetus and Newborn. More recently, Jacobson and colleagues (1992) reviewed a decade of clinical research on RLF and offered a detailed methodological critique. Duc (1999) reflected on lessons of the RLF story for practitioners seeking to apply evidence-based medicine.

REFERENCES

Ashton N, Ward B, Serpell G. Role of oxygen in the genesis of retrolental fibroplasia. A preliminary report. Br J Ophthalmol 1953; 37:513–20.

Avery ME, Oppenheimer EH. Recent increase in mortality from hyaline membrane disease. J Pediatr 1960; 57:553–9.

Blodi FC, Silverman WA, Day R, Reese AB. Experiences with corticotrophin (ACTH) in the acute stage of retrolental fibroplasia. Am J Dis Child 1951; 1951:242–3.

Campbell K. Intensive oxygen therapy as a possible cause of retrolental fibroplasia: a clinical approach. Med J Aust 1951; 2:48–50.

Duc G. From observation to experimentation at the cotside: Lessons from the past. Pediatr Res 1999; 46:644–9.

Exline AL, Harrington MR. Retrolental fibroplasia: clinical statistics from the premature center of Charity Hospital of Louisiana at New Orleans. J Pediatr 1951; 38:1–7.

Greenhouse SW. Some historical and methodological developments in early clinical trials at the National Institutes of Health. Stat Med 1990; 9:893–901.

Houlton ACL. A study of cases of retrolental fibroplasia seen in Oxford. Tr Ophth Soc U Kingdom 1951; 71:583–90.

Ingalls TH. Congenital encephalo-ophthalmic dysplasia. Pediatrics 1948; 1:315–25.

Jacobson RM, Feinstein AR. Oxygen as a cause of blindness in premature infants: "autopsy" of a decade of errors in clinical epidemiologic research. J Clin Epidemiol 1992; 45:1265–87.

James LS, Lanman JT. History of oxygen therapy and retrolental fibroplasia. Pediatrics 1976; 52(Suppl.):591–642.

Jefferson E. Retrolental fibroplasia. Arch Dis Child 1952; 27:329–36.

Kinsey VE. Etiology of retrolental fibroplasia and preliminary report of the Cooperative Study of Retrolental Fibroplasia. Tr Am Acad Ophth Otol 1955; 59:15–24.

Kinsey VE, Chisholm JF. Retrolental fibroplasia: evaluation of several changes in dietary supplements of premature infants with respect to the incidence of the disease. Am J Ophthalmol 1951; 34:1259–68.

Kinsey VE, Zacharias L. Retrolental fibroplasia. Incidence in different localities in recent years and a correlation of the incidence with treatment given the infants. JAMA 1949; 139:572–78.

Lanman JT, Guy LP, Dancis J. Retrolental fibroplasia and oxygen therapy. JAMA 1954; 155:223–6.

Laupus WE. Comment on experiences with corticotrophin (ACTH) in the acute stage of retrolental fibroplasia. Am J Dis Child 1951; 82:243.

Lelong M, Rossier A, Fontaine M, LeMasson C, Michelin et Audibert J. Sur la retinopathie des prematures (fibroplasie retrolentale). Arch Fr Pediatr 1952; 9:897–914.

Owens WC, Owens EU. Retrolental fibroplasia in premature infants. Am J Ophthalmol 1949; 32:1–21.

Patz A, Hoeck LE, De La Cruz E. Studies on the effect of high oxygen administration in retrolental fibroplasia. Am J Ophthalmol 1952; 35:1248–53.

Pratt EL. Comment on experiences with corticotrophin (ACTH) in the acute stage of retrolental fibroplasia. Am J Dis Child 1951; 82:243–4.

Reese AB, Blodi FC, Locke JC, Silverman WA, Day RL. Results of use of corticotropin (ACTH) in treatment of retrolental fibroplasia. Arch Ophthalmol 1952; 47:551–5.

Silverman WA. The lesson of retrolental fibroplasia. Sci Am 1977; 236:100–7.
Silverman WA. Retrolental fibroplasia: a modern parable. New York: Grune and Stratton, 1980.
Terry TL. Extreme prematurity and fibroblastic overgrowth of persistent vascular sheath behind each crystalline lens. Am J Ophthalmol 1942; 25:203–4.
Terry TL. Retrolental fibroplasia in premature infants. V. Further studies on fibroplastic overgrowth of persistent tunica vasculosa lentis. Arch Ophthalmol 1945; 33:203–8.

2

DISEASES AND POPULATIONS

If public health is a branch of knowledge distinct from medicine, and the separation is believed well made, then public health must rest on some fundamental discipline which is characteristic of its activities and individual to it. Public health deals with groups of people, and epidemiology is the study of disease behavior as manifested by groups. For this reason epidemiology is stated to be the basic science of public health.

John Gordon

If you wish to converse with me, define your terms.

François Voltaire

The story of retrolental fibroplasia in Chapter 1 showed epidemiologic research in action. It illustrated what these studies seek to achieve, how they are conducted, and how the information they produce can fit together. Now it is time to try to formalize some key ideas that underlie almost all epidemiologic studies.

In broad terms, epidemiologic research involves describing and interpreting patterns of disease occurrence in populations, in order to generate knowledge that can be used to prevent disease and avoid human suffering. To this end, nearly all epidemiologic studies are based on the concept of trying to identify *all cases of a disease in a defined population at risk*. Disease cases are studied in relation to the base population from which they arose.

As will be described in Chapter 3, the number of disease cases and the size of the population at risk often become the numerator and denominator, respectively, of a numerical measure of disease frequency, such as a rate, which quantifies the burden of disease in a population. This measure is used to compare different populations or subpopulations in the search for patterns of variation. Specifically how this strategy is implemented depends on features of the disease and on the kind of population being studied. This chapter focuses on characteristics of diseases and of populations that are of special importance in epidemiologic research.

DISEASES

The term *disease* is used very broadly in this book to mean almost any departure from perfect health. Diseases can be acute or chronic illnesses, congenital or acquired conditions, medical diagnoses, psychiatric disorders, symptoms, syndromes, or injuries. About the only firm requirement is that there be some way to decide whether someone does or does not qualify as a case. In a specific study, this requirement is met by developing a *case definition*.

Case Definition

A case definition is the operational definition of a disease for study purposes. Several factors come into play in developing a case definition, and much can depend on how much is already known about the disease.

According to Aristotle, any good definition has two parts: it specifies characteristics shared by all members of the class being defined, and it specifies what distinguishes them from others outside the class (Aristotle, 1994). Because many epidemiologic studies are motivated by a search for causes of disease, some elements of the case definition can be intended to identify ill people whose disease is thought to have shared causes. These elements follow from a theory, perhaps tentative and limited in scope, about disease causation. As theory about disease etiology evolves over time, the case definition may be revised.

Example: Early in the AIDS epidemic, several cases of rare opportunistic infections and of Kaposi's sarcoma were noted by clinicians among gay men in California and New York (Centers for Disease Control and Prevention, 1981a,b). The cases occurred near each other in space and time, and their various illnesses had all previously been seen mainly in patients who had a compromised immune system. Accordingly, although their clinical features were quite different, all of these illnesses were suspected of representing instances of a single underlying disease. Over time, additional forms of opportunistic infection were added to the AIDS case definition, based on the belief that they reflected the same acquired defect in the immune system and thus had a common etiology. Subsequent discovery of the human immunodeficiency virus in persons with those conditions confirmed this suspicion.

Especially when little is known about a disease, a case definition may have to be developed inductively, based on shared, readily observable clinical characteristics. At the extreme, the disease may never have been recognized or described before, as with retrolental fibroplasia (Terry, 1942). Because the occurrence of clinically similar illnesses close to each other in space and time can suggest shared causes, place and time of occurrence are themselves sometimes included in the case definition, especially in an acute outbreak, as discussed further in Chapter 19 (Grimm et al., 1994).

For some diseases, specific pathological changes have been identified that are thought to be responsible for the more readily observable clinical manifestations. For example, hallmarks of Alzheimer's disease include presence of neuritic plaques, amyloid deposits, and neurofibrillary tangles in the brain (National Institute on Aging and Reagan Institute Working Group, 1997). Unfortunately, a case definition of Alzheimer's disease based on the presence or absence of these pathological changes would require examining a sample of brain tissue, which clearly limits the applicability of such a case definition on a population scale! Instead, operational case definitions in epidemiologic studies must normally rely on readily available or obtainable data, such as the type and degree of cognitive impairment. It is sometimes possible, however, to evaluate an epidemiologic case definition against a more definitive "gold standard," at least for a sample. For example, autopsy findings have been used to assess the validity of alternative case definitions for Alzheimer's disease (Breitner and Welsh, 1995).

At times there is no generally accepted criterion against which an operational case definition can be validated. Examples include chronic fatigue syndrome, Gulf War syndrome, and fibromyalgia (Hyams, 1998). Nonetheless, precedents for case definition may be available from previous studies of the same disease. Consistent case definitions at least allow a more valid comparison of results across studies and settings. For example, Table 2–1 shows a case definition for Kawasaki syndrome, an acute systemic illness in early childhood. Case definitions for this

Table 2–1. Example of a Case Definition: Kawasaki Syndrome

A febrile illness of at least five days' duration, with at least four of the five following physical findings and no other more reasonable explanation for the observed clinical findings:

- Bilateral conjunctival injection
- Oral changes (erythema of lips or oropharynx, "strawberry tongue," or fissuring of the lips)
- Peripheral extremity changes (edema, erythema, or generalized or periungual desquamation)
- Rash
- Cervical lymphadenopathy (at least one lymph node 1.5 cm. or greater in diameter)

If fever disappears after intravenous gamma globulin therapy is started, fever may be of <5 days' duration, and the clinical case definition may still be met.

[*Source:* Centers for Disease Control and Prevention (1990).]

and other reportable diseases were developed by the Council of State and Territorial Epidemiologists and the Centers for Disease Control and Prevention in order to standardize reporting among states for surveillance purposes (Centers for Disease Control and Prevention, 1990).

Should a case definition be broad or narrow? Brenner and Savitz (1990) showed that low specificity in the case definition (resulting in the inclusion of some bogus cases) can lead to bias and reduced statistical power in case-control studies (see Chapter 10), even though the total number of cases may increase. On the other hand, when uncertainty is great and when resources permit, there can be an advantage in erring on the side of inclusiveness during case surveillance. This strategy leaves open the option of focusing on more narrowly defined subsets of cases in the analysis stage. Otherwise, if a restrictive case definition is later suspected to be too narrow, it may be difficult and time-consuming to go back and find the missed cases.

Epidemiologic Case Definition vs. Clinical Diagnosis

Epidemiologic studies sometimes use a case definition that depends heavily on diagnoses made by clinicians. But it should be kept in mind that epidemiology and clinical practice have different goals. Clinicians need an accurate diagnosis to choose proper treatment and to predict prognosis, while epidemiologists studying the same disease focus more on how the disease was caused and how it might be prevented. A disease definition developed for one purpose may not be optimal for the other.

For example, an emergency-room physician who provides care for someone with a head injury may be most concerned with determining the precise anatomical location and extent of the injury, such as whether there is brain damage, internal bleeding, breaching of the skin barrier, and so on, so that prompt and proper treatment can be given. But for the epidemiologist, a key concern is likely to be the mechanism of injury, such as whether it occurred during a motor-vehicle collision, during an assault, or after a fall from a height. The preventable contributing causes leading to anatomically similar head injuries may be very different depending on the mechanism. For epidemiologic purposes, it may even be appropriate to combine clinically diverse injuries across many different body locations like, say, cases of motor-vehicle crash injury, even though their clinical management and prognosis may be very different.

In other situations, a disease feature that is important for epidemiologic case definition may be of little relevance to clinicians:

Example: In investigating an outbreak of gastroenteritis due to *E. coli* O157:H7, Grimm and colleagues (1994) used molecular "fingerprinting" to identify the particular strain of *E. coli* that had infected each patient. Which particular strain was involved in each case had little bearing on treatment, but it allowed epidemiologists to distinguish between sporadic cases due to diverse bacterial strains and a subgroup of cases who had been infected by one particular strain. Nearly all cases in that subgroup could be linked to having eaten insufficiently cooked ground beef purchased through a certain restaurant chain. The same strain of *E. coli* was later found in uncooked samples of contaminated beef, further substantiating an inference of cause and effect.

Disease Models

Thinking about disease occurrence in a population is often helped by considering first how different diseases evolve over time in affected individuals. The disease models described below are somewhat idealized (as all models are) in order to emphasize certain key features. Most of the models are illustrated using simple time-line diagrams, which show an individual's disease experience over time as a horizontal line of varying thickness or shading. In later chapters, these individual time-lines will be stacked vertically to portray disease occurrence in a population.

Disease states

Some diseases are naturally thought of as *states* of ill health that characterize a person over a period of time. For example, Alzheimer's disease is a chronic form of dementia for which no cure is currently known. The disease state lasts from the time of onset to death. Various other diseases that persist from onset until death include atherosclerotic cardiovascular disease, osteoarthritis, and sickle cell anemia.

The time line for a hypothetical case of such a disease is shown in Figure 2–1 as thin during the early non-diseased period, thick during the period with disease, and ending with death.

Another type of disease is characterized by periods of illness that may not necessarily last until death, but that can recur. Urinary tract infection is an example: an affected person can recover spontaneously or with treatment. But infection may later recur, possibly many times, during a person's lifetime (see Figure 2–2).

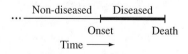

Figure 2–1. Diagram of Disease State.

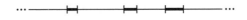

Figure 2–2. Diagram of a Recurrent Disease State.

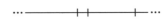

Figure 2–3. Diagram of Recurrent Disease Events.

Urinary tract infection is thus a (potentially) *recurrent* disease, while Alzheimer's disease is *non-recurrent*. Other recurrent-state diseases include depression, skull fracture, and the common cold. The distinction between recurrent and non-recurrent diseases matters in deciding which individuals should be included as part of the population at risk for developing a particular disease.

Disease events

Yet another class of diseases can be naturally regarded as adverse health *events* that occur at a point in time but that have negligible duration. Examples include spontaneous abortions, falls, and premature ventricular contractions. The time line for an affected individual can be portrayed as in Figure 2–3.

Just as some disease states are potentially recurrent while others are non-recurrent, the same can be said of diseases that are intrinsically events. Falls and premature ventricular contractions are examples of potentially recurrent disease events. Spontaneous abortion is a non-recurrent event from the fetus's perspective, although it could be recurrent from the mother's perspective. Sudden infant death syndrome and homicide are other examples of non-recurrent events.

Returning to disease states, note that *onset* of the diseased state can be considered an event that occurs at a particular point in time. It marks a transition from one health state to another. Death, or recovery from disease, can also be viewed as an event, in that it occurs (at least in theory) at a certain point in time.

Whether a disease is regarded as a state or as an instantaneous event, and whether it is regarded as potentially recurrent or non-recurrent, can depend heavily on the case definition, not just on biological considerations. In other words, the investigator may have some latitude in choosing a disease model, depending on how he or she formulates the case definition. For example:

- Epilepsy is traditionally considered to be a chronic condition characterized by recurrent seizure episodes. Epilepsy could thus be defined as a disease state that characterizes a person over a long period of time, even when he or she is not actually having a seizure. Individual seizure episodes, however, which are often very brief, could be defined as recurrent events.

- A study of sociodemographic risk factors for falls might stipulate that only the first fall for a person qualifies as a case. Without this restriction, other falls after the first could be viewed as recurrent disease events; with the restriction, a *first* fall must, by definition, be non-recurrent.

Susceptibility

So far, by focusing on disease states and events, we have allowed absence of disease to remain in the background. But often an important distinction must be made between people who are capable of developing the disease and those who are not. For example, men clearly cannot develop cancer of the uterus, and women cannot develop prostate cancer.

In epidemiologic usage, someone who is capable of becoming a case of the disease is said to be *susceptible* or *at risk* for the disease. Someone who cannot become a case is *non-susceptible* or *not at risk*. A few finer points about this terminology should be noted, however:

- Being classified as *susceptible* does not imply that a person will develop the disease with certainty in the future, or even that the risk of developing the disease is high. It just means that the risk is not zero. Much epidemiologic research can be regarded as an attempt to discern *degrees* of risk among susceptibles. By contrast, being classified as *non-susceptible* or *not at risk* implies zero risk of becoming a case.
- Whether a person is or is not considered susceptible could, in principle, depend on how far into their future we look. For example, a woman who has just had a spontaneous abortion is not at risk for having another one the next day (assuming there is only one fetus). But over the longer term, she may become pregnant again and may have another spontaneous abortion. Hence at the same moment, right after a spontaneous abortion, she could be considered both susceptible (over the long term) and non-susceptible (over the short term). The *short-term* perspective is the one usually implied unless stated otherwise. That is, a person is normally considered to be at risk at a certain time if, in the next instant, there is a non-zero probability that he or she could become a case.
- Whether a person is considered susceptible can also depend heavily on features of the case definition. For example, the case definition in a study of falls may specify that only the first fall for a given person qualifies as a case for study purposes. If a study subject has fallen once, he or she is no longer at risk for becoming a case, since any subsequent falls would not meet the case definition.

Note that *susceptibility* and *non-susceptibility* are both states, as they can characterize an individual over a period of time. Especially for infectious diseases, persons who are non-susceptible are sometimes said to be *immune*.

To illustrate how susceptibility can be incorporated into our time-line diagrams, consider a typical person's experience with measles. A newborn baby normally receives enough protective antibody across the placenta from its mother, if she is immune, to render the baby non-susceptible to measles for a few weeks after birth. After the maternally derived antibody dissipates, the child is at risk for measles. If illness occurs, he or she is sick for a few days, then develops antibodies that normally protect permanently against recurrence. This experience can be diagrammed as in Figure 2–4.

For many diseases, individuals who currently have the disease are not at risk for *developing* that disease. (You cannot enter a room if you are already inside it!) For example, someone who already has Alzheimer's disease cannot then become a new case of Alzheimer's disease a second time. But there are exceptions to this rule—bone fractures, for example—as described below.

Generic Disease Model

These and other common patterns of disease evolution in individuals can be viewed as special cases of a more general model, as shown in Figure 2–5. Each of the three boxes corresponds to a *state*, while the transitions between them correspond to *events*. The model can also be adapted to apply for diseases that are intrinsically

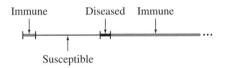

Figure 2–4. Time-Line Diagram for Measles.

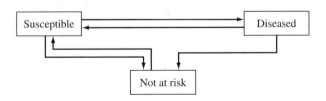

Figure 2–5. Generic Model of Disease Evolution in an Individual over Time.

events if we stipulate that anyone who enters the diseased box immediately exits from it to one of the other boxes, so that the time spent as diseased is only an instant.

Anticipating Chapter 3, the generic disease model in Figure 2–5 relates closely to the two main kinds of disease frequency measures, prevalence and incidence. *Prevalence* refers to how members of a population are distributed among the boxes at a given moment in time—in particular, the number or the proportion who are in the diseased state at that time. *Incidence* refers to the rate of flow from susceptible to diseased over time. More generally, these epidemiologic tools provide useful ways to quantify the distribution of health states and the transitions between them in populations.

Each of the arrows in Figure 2–5 corresponds to a rate of flow between states that can be relevant to disease control. Prevention efforts attempt to minimize the flow from susceptible to diseased. One strategy for doing so is to try to shift people from the susceptible box to the not-at-risk box through strategies such as immunization. Therapeutic care tries to increase rates of flow out of the diseased box. A permanent cure moves the patient from the diseased box to the not-at-risk box; a temporary cure for a disease that may recur moves the patient from the diseased box back to the susceptible box. For some diseases, being not at risk is only a temporary state, as when maternally derived antibodies against measles dissipate after the first few weeks of an infant's life, or when a woman becomes pregnant and thus becomes susceptible to medical complications of pregnancy. The only transition between states that is not possible, by definition, is from not at risk to diseased.

Parts of the generic model may not apply to some diseases, which can thus be described by a simpler model, usually a subset of the generic one. For Alzheimer's disease, no non-susceptible state is known, and recovery does not occur. Hence the model is reduced to just two boxes, a susceptible box with a one-way arrow to a diseased box. For urinary tract infection, there is again no non-susceptible state, but the possibility of recovery calls for arrows in both directions between the susceptible and diseased boxes. People can oscillate between them over time. For appendicitis, surgical removal of the appendix, either preventively or during an attack of acute appendicitis, moves a person permanently to the not-at-risk box, so that no arrow need be drawn from not at risk to susceptible. For still other diseases, a non-susceptible state may be logically possible but so rare as to be of little concern when estimating the size of the population at risk for the disease in question. For example, people in whom a mechanical artificial heart has been implanted are technically not at risk for coronary heart disease, but so far the number of such people in the population is so small that there is no need to account for their presence when seeking to gauge the magnitude of the at-risk population.

Beyond the Generic Model

The generic disease model presented above offers a useful way to organize one's thinking about diseases from an epidemiologic perspective. But while quite broadly applicable, it cannot capture all of the complexities of the real world. Still, such a model and the concepts behind it may be useful as a starting point that, with a little improvisation, can be used to create an extended model that fits a particular situation better. Two examples follow.

Disease onset as an abrupt event

Alzheimer's disease was described earlier as a chronic disease state with onset at a certain point in time. Representing disease onset as an abrupt transition, however, may be questionable. Clinically, memory loss worsens gradually over months or years, and the underlying brain lesions may have begun forming long before symptoms are recognized or diagnosed. What, then, should be regarded as the time of onset?

One option is to re-frame the situation to fit the standard model. Any formal study of Alzheimer's disease needs an operational case definition, and at any given time, a person either meets that definition or does not. *For study purposes,* then, a person could be considered a case when disease manifestations first cross the threshold needed to meet study criteria for Alzheimer's disease. This approach recognizes that an epidemiologic case definition and a clinical diagnosis need not always be tightly coupled.

Another approach involves defining additional event milestones in the course of illness for someone who is destined to develop Alzheimer's disease: for example, when symptoms first began, when medical care was first sought, when the medical diagnosis was made, and so on. Each such milestone would be a possible choice as a disease-onset time. (The time at which the first brain lesions occurred might be attractive in theory, but in practice that time is probably unknowable.)

It may then be useful to employ different milestones for different purposes, even within the same study. For example, Time A might be when symptoms began and Time B when the study criteria for Alzheimer's disease were first met (see Figure 2–6).

For surveillance of Alzheimer's disease in a population, it may not be possible or practical to use Time A as the onset date for each case, even though Time A may be closer to when the disease had its biological onset. One problem is that

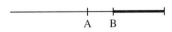

Figure 2–6. Two Possible Times of Disease Onset for Alzheimer's Disease.

surveillance is usually carried out over certain periods of calendar time, counting all cases that occurred in each period. But if the disease progresses slowly—so that the time between A and B is long—then cases who reach Time A in a certain period may not actually seek care or be recognized until long after that period has ended. This delay may at a minimum necessitate postponing compilation of the occurrence data, so that the results become available only after the time period they refer to is long past. Even if special surveys were mounted to identify promptly anyone who had experienced mild memory loss that could represent the first symptoms of Alzheimer's disease, such a strategy could instead yield a meaninglessly mixed set of cases. Many of those with mild memory loss could later prove not to have Alzheimer's disease at all. For these reasons, it may be preferable to use Time B as the disease-onset time for surveillance purposes.

For epidemiologic research into antecedent causes, however, a different choice of onset time may be preferable. For example, a study might involve interviewing family members about experiences in the case's past that may have contributed to development of Alzheimer's disease. It would almost certainly be better to ask about experiences before Time A than before Time B because, in retrospect, early disease was probably present during the A–B time interval. Hence, experiences during that interval would be hard to implicate as causes of the disease. Some exposures during that period, such as X-rays to the head or head trauma, might even have resulted from early manifestations of disease.

Concurrent disease and susceptibility

As noted earlier, someone who already has a disease is usually not considered to be at risk for developing that disease anew. But what about dental caries? Someone with decay in one tooth would seem to be still at risk for developing decay in other teeth.

Dental caries could be forced into the generic model by stipulating that decay in any number of teeth qualifies as a case. But this clearly ignores a major part of the problem by failing to distinguish between mild decay in only one tooth and rampant decay in all teeth. Instead, the extent of dental caries has often been measured on a continuum, rather than simply as present or absent (Hujoel et al., 1991; Klein et al., 1938). For example, the 1988–1994 U.S. National Health and Nutrition Examination Survey III recorded the *number* of teeth decayed, missing, or filled for each participant (Vargas et al., 1998). Under such a model, a study of risk factors for future dental decay might investigate whether characteristics found at an initial examination were associated with movement along the dental-decay continuum between baseline and follow-up examinations. Disease would thus be modeled as a series of ordered states, while still incorporating some features of the generic model.

POPULATIONS

Defined vs. Undefined Populations

Relating cases of disease to the base population they arose from is central to epidemiologic thinking. At a minimum, the size of the population at risk is needed to calculate common and useful measures of disease frequency, such as incidence and prevalence, and a population must be defined before its size can be known. In addition, generalizability of results from one population to another depends in part on how similar those populations are, which can best be judged if the populations are well defined. Finally, as will be described in Chapter 15, in a population-based case-control study, the defined population that generates cases becomes the natural sampling frame for controls.

As with case definition, perhaps the most useful way to define a population is to specify the characteristics that its members have in common and that set them apart from non-members. Characteristics typically used for this purpose include *personal attributes,* such as age, gender, or membership in a predefined group, such as a factory work force or a health insurance plan; *geographic scope,* such as residence in a certain state or city; and the *time* or *time period* in which the cases are identified. Table 2–2 lists a range of examples of defined populations.

Yet not every group of people necessarily qualifies as a defined population for epidemiologic purposes. Characteristics that might describe a population informally may be too vague to determine in practice who is and who is not included. For example, what constitutes "a typical primary-care patient population" can vary across settings and by the experience of the care provider. "The population of people who would have sought care at hospital X had they been injured in a motor-vehicle collision" may be appealing in theory but is almost impossible to identify in practice.

Table 2–2. Examples of Defined Populations

- The civilian, non-institutionalized population of the U.S. during 1999–2000
- Passengers and crew on Alaska Airlines Flight #261 on February 10, 2000
- All persons covered under the New York State Medicaid program as of April 1, 2000
- All babies born alive in Ghana during 1999
- Patients hospitalized in the surgical intensive care unit at San Francisco General Hospital during August, 1993
- Residents of Dublin, Ireland, on June 16, 1904

Link Between Cases and the Population at Risk

As noted earlier, epidemiologic research commonly involves seeking to identify *all cases of a disease in a defined population at risk*. Besides being well defined, the population must truly correspond to the disease cases under study. Two questions can be used to check this linkage:

1. If each of the cases had *not* developed the disease, would he or she still have been included in the population?
2. If each of the non-cases in the population had developed the disease, would he or she have been included as a case?

The answer to both questions should be *yes*.

Sometimes the stimulus for doing an epidemiologic study arises after a set of cases of some disease has already been identified. There may be interest in knowing whether the observed number of cases is greater or less than would be expected, or in knowing how the cases differ from non-cases selected from the same setting. Addressing these questions epidemiologically begins with trying to identify the defined population from which the cases arose. This task may not be easy, as shown by the following example:

Example: Suppose that a group of cardiologists has identified all cases of myocardial infarction (heart attack) who were admitted to a certain hospital during a certain year. You have been asked to help them use these cases as the starting point for an epidemiologic study of myocardial infarction. Your first task is to identify the corresponding population at risk.

First you might consider all patients who are admitted to the study hospital during the same year with any diagnosis. This group qualifies as a defined population—you could actually construct a list of them and specify exactly who is and who is not a member—and the group includes the heart attack cases. Unfortunately, however, you realize that this population fails our first check: we cannot assume that each of the heart attack cases would necessarily have been admitted to the hospital with some other diagnosis during the year if he or she had *not* suffered a heart attack. Noting this leads you to realize that there are undoubtedly other people "out there" who would have become cases at the study hospital if they had suffered a heart attack during the year. This part of the population at risk has not been captured by considering only hospitalized patients.

In addition, the population of all hospitalized patients may also fail the second test if some patients hospitalized with other diagnoses would have gone elsewhere if they had had a heart attack instead. For example, if the hospital specializes in bone-marrow transplants, it may draw referrals from a wide region, even though many of those patients would have been hospitalized elsewhere closer to home if they had had a heart attack.

So you now realize that you need to look outside the hospital for the real population at risk. Accordingly, you might next consider trying to define a geographic "catchment area" from which the hospital is thought to draw its heart-attack patients, then figure out the population of that catchment area. To pass the first check, you could exclude any heart-attack cases who resided outside the catchment area. In most settings, however, the catchment area population would still fail the second check. The study hospital may be only one of several local hospitals that treat heart attack patients, and there would be no guarantee that someone who resides in the catchment area would necessarily go to the study hospital if he or she suffered a heart attack. Thus, case ascertainment within the catchment area may be incomplete, and there is no way to know from the study of hospital cases alone how many other cases were missed.

Unfortunately, it is often not possible to identify the true population at risk that generated the cases drawn from a particular clinical site, which limits the kinds of epidemiologic research that can be done with them. They are a clinical case series, not necessarily representing all cases in any defined population.

Yet there are situations in which a set of clinical cases *does* correspond to an identifiable population at risk. These situations are thus very favorable for epidemiologic research, and epidemiologists are often on the lookout for them:

- There may be essentially only one source of care for a relatively isolated community. For example, the Mayo Clinic provides nearly all health care for residents of Rochester, Minnesota (Melton, 1996), and the Marshfield Clinic does so for residents of Marshfield, Wisconsin (Nordstrom et al., 1994).
- There are several sources of care, but all contribute to a single population-wide case registry. For example, the National Cancer Institute's Surveillance, Epidemiology, and End Results program supports population-based cancer registries in several regions of the U.S. (Hankey et al., 1999).
- All health care for members of a single health insurance plan is provided by, or billed to, that plan. In the U.S., most health maintenance organizations (HMOs) fit this description and have become important settings for epidemiologic research (Nordstrom et al., 1994). Note that HMO enrollees constitute an administratively (not geographically) defined population.

- The research focuses only on the *outcome* of illness among patients at one or more clinical sites. These patients then become a defined population in their own right, and the research issue is complete ascertainment of disease outcomes among them. This kind of research has been called *clinical epidemiology* (Weiss, 1996).

Defined Populations Observed over Time

Once the characteristics that define a population have been specified, it is easy in theory (if not necessarily in practice) to determine its size and composition at a single point in time. Everyone who meets the defining criteria at that time is a member, and counting them yields the population size.

But once we "start the clock" and monitor a population over a certain period of time, its size and composition may change.

- If membership in the population remains constant, except possibly for loss of members in whom the disease of interest has already occurred before they depart, the population is termed *closed*. Such a population is also sometimes called a *fixed cohort.*
- If membership in the population changes in any other way—for example, if new members are added, and/or if people who have not developed the disease are lost—the population is termed *open*. Such a population is also sometimes called a *dynamic population.*

The distinction between closed and open populations will soon become important when we consider approaches to measuring disease incidence in Chapter 3.

Closed populations

Some examples of closed populations are listed in Table 2–3. One situation that favors stable population membership is when the period of observation is short,

Table 2–3. Examples of Closed Populations

- Passengers on an airplane over the duration of the flight
- Participants in a clinical trial in which all study procedures and observations are completed in a single encounter
- Motor-vehicle occupants involved in a police-investigated collision, considered from the moment of impact until police arrive
- Soldiers who fought in the Persian Gulf War, monitored for death from any cause for 25 years after the end of the war (and assuming that ascertainment of deaths is complete)

---

as the first three examples illustrate. In the last example, however, the observation is long—25 years. Deaths would be sure to occur in such a large population over such a long time, and members who die are not normally retained as population members after they die. Thus the population membership would change. It would, however, still qualify as a closed population because: *(1)* no new members could be added after the war ends, since they would have no opportunity to satisfy the population's eligibility criteria; and *(2)* losses would occur only due to death, which is itself the disease end-point under study.

Open populations

Examples of open populations are shown in Table 2–4. In practice, open populations are more common than closed populations in epidemiologic research, chiefly because of the fairly stringent conditions for what can qualify as a closed population.

Many open populations of interest to epidemiologists are defined by residence in a certain geopolitical area, such as a city, county, state, region, or nation, because population counts and health statistics are often routinely collected and aggregated for such areas. New members may be gained over time in these populations through birth or in-migration, and members may be lost through death or out-migration.

Other open populations are defined administratively. For example, having a certain tie to an organization, such as employment at a factory, enrollment in a health insurance plan, or registration with a school system, may be one of the population's main defining characteristics. Often that relationship may change over time, so that people gain or lose eligibility for membership.

Changes over time in eligibility for membership can occur for other reasons as well. If being in a certain age range is required, new members may be gained as persons who were too young to qualify at the start of the study period become old enough to join. Members who originally met the age requirements may no longer qualify for membership once they pass the upper age limit.

Table 2–4. Examples of Open Populations

- Factory workers employed at a certain automobile assembly plant at any time during a two-year study period
- Residents of Chicago, Illinois, during 2001
- High-school students in Miami public schools during the 1999–2000 school year
- Washington State Medicaid program beneficiaries during 2001

EXERCISES

1. For each of the following diseases, would you consider the disease to be recurrent or non-recurrent? Who is susceptible? Who, if anyone, is not at risk?

    (a) Coronary heart disease   *N*
    (b) Myocardial infarction (heart attack)   *R*
    (c) First myocardial infarction   *N*
    (d) Asthma   *R*
    (e) Spontaneous abortion   *N*
    (f) Cancer of the uterine cervix   *R*
    (g) Post-traumatic epilepsy (repeated seizures after head trauma)   *R*

2. *Febrile seizures* occur at some time in about 2% to 4% of all children. While ill with a fever, the child loses consciousness and develops jerking movements, usually in all four limbs, often lasting several minutes.

    At least 26 studies have followed up a group of such children to determine what proportion develop epilepsy, a chronic seizure disorder. On reviewing these studies, Ellenberg and Nelson (1980) noticed a pattern:

    bigger Lge pop. N Defined area Defined pop

    • Seven studies followed up all children who had experienced a febrile seizure in some defined population, such as a prepaid health plan or a geographic area. Estimates of the percentage of children who later developed epilepsy ranged across studies from 1.6% to 4.6%, with a median of 3.0%.

    • Nineteen studies followed up all children with a febrile seizure who had been treated in a certain hospital clinic or by a particular specialist in seizure disorders. The conclusions of these studies were much more variable but generally described a worse prognosis: the percentage of children who later developed epilepsy ranged across studies from 2.6% to 76.9%, with a median of 18.8%.

    specific hospital specific

    The definition of epilepsy and the duration and completeness of follow-up appeared to be generally similar between groups of studies. Why do you think the results differed so markedly between the groups of studies?

3. Epidemiologic study of a condition often begins by trying to identify all cases of the condition that occur in a defined population. For each of the following sets of cases, identify, if possible, the corresponding defined population at risk.

    (a) All cases of hospital-acquired (nosocomial) infection among inpatients at Metropolitan General Hospital during 1999.   *All pts Admitted to the hospital without admission diagnosis of infection*
    (b) All cases of sudden cardiac death occurring in Cook County, Illinois, during 1999.   *Death Certificates w cause of death listed as Cardiac.*
    (c) All cases of influenza who were treated by one of several hundred volunteer "sentinel physicians" throughout the U.S. during December, 1999, through March, 2000.   *Pt Reports. Every patient who was See during D'99 M 2000*

ANSWERS

1. *(a)* Coronary heart disease is treatable but not completely curable, and it does not go away spontaneously. Thus it is non-recurrent. Anyone who does not already have coronary heart disease is at risk.

   (b) A person who has had one myocardial infarction can have another, so it is a recurrent disease. Everyone is at risk.

   (c) Although a person can have more than one myocardial infarction, nobody can have more than one *first* myocardial infarction. Thus anyone who has never had a myocardial infarction is at risk. Anyone who has had at least one myocardial infarction is no longer at risk of having another *first* one.

   (d) Acute asthma attacks are usually regarded as events, but asthma can also be regarded as a chronic condition or state characterized by repeated acute attacks. Either viewpoint is legitimate and useful; which definition is chosen depends on the purpose of the study. Both the acute attacks and the chronic condition may be recurrent. The population at risk includes anyone who does not already have asthma.

   (e) Although a spontaneous abortion can happen at most once during a pregnancy, it can happen to the same woman two or more times and is thus potentially recurrent. The population currently at risk consists solely of pregnant women. Men and non-pregnant women are clearly not at risk.

   There is an interesting additional feature of this example, however. A fetal loss occurring after the twentieth week of gestation is classified as a fetal death by most state vital statistics offices, while a fetal loss occurring earlier in pregnancy is classified as a spontaneous abortion. Under this definition, the population at risk for spontaneous abortion would consist only of pregnant women whose pregnancy has not yet lasted 20 weeks. Women who have been pregnant for more than 20 weeks are no longer at risk: by definition, any fetal loss they experience would be classified as a fetal death, not as a spontaneous abortion. Note how the operational definitions of spontaneous abortion and fetal death in turn influence definition of the population at risk.

   (f) Very early cancer of the cervix can sometimes be treated with local excision and then recur. The population at risk is any woman who still has a uterine cervix. Men are clearly not at risk, and women who have had a hysterectomy are not at risk.

   (g) Like asthma, epilepsy is a state characterized by recurrent acute attacks (in this case, seizures). Depending on the case definition, post-traumatic epilepsy could be deemed to have been resolved or cured, then recur. The population at risk is anyone who has experienced an episode of head trauma and who does not already have post-traumatic epilepsy. People who

have not had an episode of head trauma are not at risk for post-traumatic epilepsy.

2. A likely explanation is that the cases seen at hospital clinics or in the practices of seizure specialists may not be typical of all cases occurring in any defined population. Often these clinical centers receive referrals of patients with a relatively severe or difficult-to-manage form of the disease. Less complicated and less severe cases remain under the care of primary-care physicians and are seldom referred.

In fact, the risk of epilepsy has been found to be greater in children who have had "atypical" febrile seizures—for example, "focal" seizures starting in one part of the body, or lasting an unusually long time, or occurring repeatedly within 24 hours. These are just the kinds of cases that a primary-care physician might be uncomfortable managing alone. Hence they tend to be over-represented in a clinic-based case series.

3. (a) The defined population at risk would be all people admitted to Metropolitan General Hospital during 1999.

(b) We can get fairly close by using all residents of Cook County during 1999 as the defined population at risk. It is, however, possible for a visitor to the area who resides elsewhere to die of sudden cardiac death in Cook County. This is a problem, because these cases did not arise from the population at risk as we have defined it and should therefore not be counted. On the other hand, some cases of sudden cardiac death affecting people who reside in Cook County may occur while they are outside the county, and these may be quite difficult to identify and enumerate. Often we depend on the number of such cases' being small enough to ignore and hope that the two kinds of errors cancel out. The smaller the geographic area, however, the bigger this problem of border-crossing becomes.

(c) Unfortunately, there is no defined population corresponding to these cases. There is no good way of identifying and counting everyone who would choose go to one of these sentinel physicians if they developed influenza. About the best we can do is to assume that whatever that hypothetical population is, it remains relatively stable over time, allowing us to track the raw count of cases over time to detect influenza outbreaks.

REFERENCES

Aristotle. Posterior analytics. (Translated by Jonathan Barnes). Book II, Chapter 13. New York: Oxford University Press, 1994.

Breitner JCS, Welsh KA. Genes and recent developments in the epidemiology of Alzheimer's disease and related dementia. Epidemiol Rev 1995; 17:39–47.

Brenner H, Savitz DA. The effects of sensitivity and specificity of case selection on validity, sample size, precision, and power in hospital-based case-control studies. Am J Epidemiol 1990; 132:181–92.

Centers for Disease Control and Prevention. *Pneumocystis* pneumonia—Los Angeles. MMWR Morb Mortal Wkly Rep 1981a; 30:250–52.

Centers for Disease Control and Prevention. Kaposi's sarcoma and *Pneumocystis* pneumonia among homosexual men—New York City and California. MMWR Morb Mortal Wkly Rep 1981b; 30:305–8.

Centers for Disease Control and Prevention. Case definitions for public health surveillance. MMWR Morb Mortal Wkly Rep 1990; 39 (RR-13):1–42.

Ellenberg JH, Nelson KB. Sample selection and the natural history of disease. Studies of febrile seizures. JAMA 1980; 243:1337–40.

Gordon JE. "Epidemiology—old and new." In: Buck C, Llopis A, Najera E, Terris M (eds.). The challenge of epidemiology. Issues and selected readings. Washington, D.C.: Pan American Health Organization, 1988.

Grimm LM, Goldoft M, Kobayashi J, Lewis JH, Alfi D, Perdichizzi AM, et al. Molecular epidemiology of a fast-food-restaurant–associated outbreak of *Escherichia coli* 0157:H7 in Washington State. J Clin Microbiol 1994; 84:2155–58.

Hankey BF, Ries LA, Edward BK. The Surveillance, Epidemiology, and End Results program: a national resource. Cancer Epidemiol Biomarkers Prev 1999; 8:1117–21.

Hujoel PP, Weyant RJ, DeRouen TA. Measures of dental disease occurrence. Community Dent Oral Epidemiol 1991; 19:252–56.

Hyams KC. Developing case definitions for symptom-based conditions: the problem of specificity. Epidemiol Rev 1998; 20:148–56.

Klein H, Palmer CE, Knutson JW. Studies on dental caries. I. Dental status and dental needs of elementary school children. Public Health Rep 1938; 53:751–65.

Melton LJ. History of the Rochester Epidemiology Project. Mayo Clin Proc 1996; 71:266–74.

National Institute on Aging and Reagan Institute Working Group. Consensus recommendations for the postmortem diagnosis of Alzheimer's disease. Neurobiol Aging 1997; 18 Suppl:S67–70.

Nordstrom DL, Remington PL, Layde PM. The utility of HMO data for the surveillance of chronic diseases. Am J Public Health 1994; 84:995–97.

Terry TL. Extreme prematurity and fibroblastic overgrowth of persistent vascular sheath behind each crystalline lens. Am J Ophthalmol 1942; 25:203–4.

Vargas CM, Crall JJ, Schneider DA. Sociodemographic distribution of pediatric dental caries: NHANES III, 1988–1994. J Am Dent Assoc 1998; 129:1229–38.

Voltaire FMA. Quoted in: Durant W. The story of philosopy. New York: Washington Square Press, 1961.

Weiss NS. Clinical epidemiology. The study of the outcome of illness (2nd ed.). New York: Oxford University Press, 1996.

3

DISEASE FREQUENCY: BASICS

In your otherwise beautiful poem, there is a verse which reads:

Every moment dies a man
Every moment one is born

It must be manifest that, were this true, the population of the world would be at a standstill. In truth the rate of birth is slightly in excess of that of death. I would suggest that in the next edition of your poem, you have it read:

Every moment dies a man
Every moment 1–1/16 is born

Strictly speaking this is not correct. The actual figure is a decimal so long that I cannot get it on the line, but I believe 1–1/16 will be sufficiently accurate for poetry. I am, etc.

Charles Babbage
(Inventor of the first programmable computer,
in a letter to poet Alfred Lord Tennyson)

The basic tools of epidemiology are quantitative measures of disease frequency in populations, and any epidemiologist needs to be skilled in their use. Fortunately, our toolbox is well stocked.

One aspect of skill is knowing the right tool for the job. This chapter seeks to provide an overview of several commonly used measures of disease frequency, including when each applies and examples of its use. Our main purpose is to lay out the "big picture," so many details are deferred.

Another aspect of skill is knowing your tools well. Chapter 4 returns to discuss in more depth several of the measures introduced in this chapter, including some of their statistical properties. It also describes useful relationships among different measures.

OVERVIEW

Choosing an approach to measuring disease frequency for a certain purpose involves considering two main factors: what kind of information is needed, and

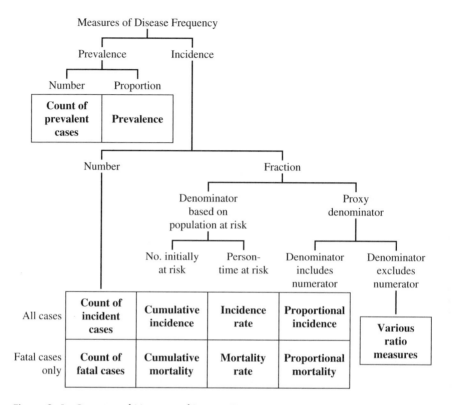

Figure 3–1. Overview of Measures of Disease Frequency.

what kind of information is obtainable. Figure 3–1, a classification scheme for measures of disease frequency, incorporates both factors. It will serve roughly as our itinerary for this chapter.

In broad terms, needs for disease frequency information can be grouped into two main types. First, in some situations we need to know how common a disease is *as of a certain time.* For example:

- Suppose that a new study has just been published, showing that surgical bypass of atherosclerotic lesions in the carotid arteries is effective for preventing stroke. The medical director of a health insurance plan asks: How many of our enrollees currently have carotid atherosclerosis that would make them candidates for this surgery?
- Suppose that an international medical aid organization seeks to reduce parasite infection among children in villages in a less developed country. They ask: What proportion of children are infected? In which villages is the proportion especially high?

• Suppose that, having mounted a treatment-and-prevention program in certain villages, the same organization wants to evaluate the success of its intervention approach. They ask: What proportion of children in these villages have parasitic infection now, two years after the program was implemented?

These kinds of questions are best answered by data on disease *prevalence,* which captures the frequency of disease *as of a certain time.* It is a static measure, closely tied to the notion of disease states. The time point of interest may be on any of several time scales, such as a calendar date, a specified age, or a milestone after some event. Prevalence is static because time is "frozen"—anyone who is in the diseased state at the specified time is counted as a case.

Second, in other situations we need to know how often new cases of disease develop in a population *as time passes.* For example:

• Suppose that a health insurance plan has decided to cover the cost of a self-care program, which is designed to train people with newly diagnosed diabetes about how to monitor their glucose level and adjust their diet and insulin dosage. The plan's medical director asks: How many new cases of diabetes should be expected over the next year?
• Concern about possible side effects of silicone breast implants has raised the question: Is rheumatoid arthritis any more likely to develop over time among women with such implants than among women without them?
• Suppose that state legislators are considering enactment of a mandatory helmet-use law for motorcycle drivers in their state. They ask: Are motorcycle-crash deaths any less common in states with a helmet-use law than in states without one?

These kinds of questions are best answered by data on disease *incidence,* which captures the frequency at which disease develops *over a period of time.* It is a dynamic measure, closely tied to the notion of disease events. The disease event may be an instantaneous occurrence, such as death in a motorcycle crash, or it may be the onset of a more persistent disease state, such as onset of rheumatoid arthritis.

Regardless of whether the need calls for prevalence or incidence, sometimes just knowing the *number* of disease cases is sufficient. For example, the health plan medical director simply needed to know the number of existing cases of carotid atherosclerosis, or the number of new cases of diabetes to expect.

But in many other situations, comparisons of disease frequency are to be made between populations of different sizes or observed over different periods of time. Case counts alone do not account for these differences. Instead, more valid comparisons can be based on measures that take the form of a fraction: the numerator is the number of cases, and the denominator captures the base of population experience that generated those cases.

For incidence, the denominator should ideally reflect the size of the population at risk. Some incidence measures also incorporate the amount of time at risk into the denominator. But sometimes information on the size of the true population at risk is unobtainable. Instead, a proxy denominator may be better than none at all. It is hoped that the proxy denominator will be approximately proportional to the true population at risk.

Finally, the need for data may concern only fatal cases, or data on fatal cases may be the only information available. If so, measures of *mortality*—really a form of incidence that considers only fatal cases—can be used.

PREVALENCE

The *count of prevalent cases* of a disease is the number of persons in the population who are in the diseased state at a specified time. *Prevalence* is a proportion obtained by dividing the count of prevalent cases by the population size at that time:

$$\text{Prevalence} = \frac{\text{Number of prevalent cases}}{\text{Size of population}}$$

Example: In 1944, the cities of Newburgh and Kingston, New York, agreed to participate in a study of the effects of water fluoridation for prevention of tooth decay in children (Ast and Schlesinger, 1956). Initially, the water in both cities had low fluoride concentration. In 1945, Newburgh began adding fluoride to its water to increase the fluoride concentration tenfold, while Kingston left its water supply unchanged. At baseline, the frequency of dental caries among children in both cities was similar. To assess the effect of water fluoridation, a dental health survey was conducted among all schoolchildren in certain grades in both cities during the 1954–1955 school year. One measure of dental decay in children aged 6–9 years was whether at least one of a child's 12 deciduous cuspids or first or second deciduous molars was missing or had clinical or X-ray evidence of caries. Of the 216 first-graders examined in Kingston, 192 had decay by this definition, compared with 116 of the 184 first-graders examined in Newburgh.

Assuming complete survey coverage, there were 192 *prevalent cases* of dental decay among first-graders in Kingston at the time of the study and 116 in Newburgh. These counts themselves could be useful to local health officials for estimating the number of dental personnel and other resources needed to provide restorative dental care for children in each city. A fair comparison, however, of the frequency of dental decay in the two cities would need to account for differences in the number of children examined. Prevalence serves this purpose. The *prevalence* of dental decay was 192/216 = 89% in Kingston and 116/184 = 63% in Newburgh.

The style in which prevalence is expressed can be chosen for convenience to avoid an awkward number of leading or trailing zeros, or for ease of comparison with other published estimates. For example, the prevalence of dental decay among Newburgh first-graders could be expressed as 63%, as 0.63, as 630 per 1000, as 6300 per 10,000, etc.

Prevalence involves "stopping the clock" and assessing disease frequency at a point in time. Confusion may arise, however, when trying to define just what is meant by "a point in time." Figure 3–2 diagrams the data collection process in, say, Newburgh for the dental-decay example. A total of 184 first-graders were examined, each corresponding to a row in the figure, here arranged in chronological order by examination date. The dental-decay status of each child was known only at his or her survey examination, shown as a small "porthole" through which we glimpse a tiny portion of the child's dental-disease time line. As in Chapter 2, that line is thick if the child was a case at the time and thin if not. Given the brevity of the examination in relation to the pace at which dental decay develops, in effect each child's disease status was assessed at a point in time. The rest of her or his time line was unobserved, as implied by dots before and after the porthole.

The figure shows that these examinations were not all done simultaneously, which would have required 184 examination teams on the same day. Instead, they were distributed over several months during the school year as the examiners worked their way through different schools and grades. The point in time to which the prevalence refers is thus not a point in calendar time. Nor is it a point on the age time scale: the first-graders were examined at various ages, albeit within a

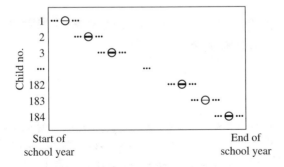

Figure 3–2. Diagram of Data Collection for Dental Survey of Newburgh, N.Y., First-Graders.

fairly narrow range. Rather, the point in time is the *time of observation* for each child. The fact that each child's disease status was observed only as of one point in time, not monitored over a period of time, is the key feature. The calendar time period and age range over which the examinations were done are relevant as descriptors, along with place and other population-defining characteristics, to put the prevalence estimate in its proper context. Prevalence can be compared across time periods or age groups, just as other disease frequency measures can.

In some studies, the observation times on individuals may indeed be synchronized in calendar time, by age, or on another time scale. Then prevalence also pertains to a specific time point on that time scale.

Example: A study of Crohn's disease and ulcerative colitis in Manitoba, Canada, used administrative data from the province's only health insurer to identify persons who had received care for one of these chronic gastrointestinal diseases (Bernstein et al., 1999). Prevalent cases as of December 31, 1994, were those who had made the requisite number of medical visits for the condition during the preceding two years and who had not died or emigrated from Manitoba before the end of 1994. The resulting prevalence estimate pertained to what can be considered a point in calendar time—December 31, 1994.

Example: The prevalence of HIV infection among inmates entering U.S. correctional facilities was estimated from HIV-1 antibody tests on routine blood samples obtained upon entry to jail or prison (Vlahov et al., 1991). These intake examinations occurred on various calendar dates, but they pertained to the same point on the time scale that chronicled each inmate's incarceration.

INCIDENCE

Incidence measures how frequently susceptible individuals become disease cases as they are observed over time. It is based on disease events, each of which represents a transition from being at risk to being diseased.

Counts

An *incident case* occurs when an individual changes from being susceptible to being diseased, by the study's case definition. The *count of incident cases* is the number of such events that occur in a defined population during a specified time period. Recurrences of disease in the same person may or may not qualify as incident cases, depending on the study's operational definition of disease, as discussed in Chapter 2.

Simple counts of incident cases can sometimes be sufficient to guide health planning. For example, knowing the number of lower-extremity amputations per year in a certain health plan could be used to project the number of limb prostheses likely to be needed.

Counts may also be adequate for comparing incidence across populations that can safely be assumed to be of similar size.

Example: Phillips and colleagues (1999) found that, over a 16-year period, 113.8 deaths due to substance abuse occurred in the U.S. during the first week of the month for every 100 such deaths in the last week of the month. They hypothesized that the excess may be related to receipt of government benefit payments from Social Security, welfare, or military benefits at the beginning of each month. Because the population at risk would be nearly the same size across different weeks of the month, the study could be based simply on the number of deaths in each one-week period.

Example: In 2000, 702,093 new cases of genital *Chlamydia trachomatis* infection were reported to the U.S. Centers for Disease Control and Prevention (CDC), compared with 358,995 new cases of gonorrhea (Centers for Disease Control and Prevention, 2001b). Assuming similar completeness of reporting for both diseases, these counts by themselves should accurately reflect differences in incidence between these two sexually transmitted diseases. This is because the sizes of the populations at risk for each disease should be about the same (or nearly so, after subtracting prevalent cases).

Cumulative Incidence

Cumulative incidence is the proportion of initially susceptible individuals in a closed population who become incident cases during a specified time period.

$$\text{Cumulative incidence} = \frac{\text{Number of incident cases}}{\text{Number of persons initially at risk}}$$

Cumulative incidence is also sometimes called the *incidence proportion* or *attack rate*. It is the simplest measure of incidence to account explicitly for the size of the population at risk.

Example: A jumbo jet full of tourists bound from Tokyo to Copenhagen stopped at Anchorage, Alaska, for refueling and reprovisioning. Upon reaching cruising altitude again, passengers were served breakfast. Somewhere over the polar ice cap, an illness characterized by cramps, vomiting, and diarrhea swept through the plane, and by the time they reached Copenhagen, $196/344 = 57\%$ of passengers had become ill. Epidemiologists who investigated the outbreak used interview data and food service records to calculate the cumulative incidence of illness among those who did and those who did not eat various food items. Eating ham proved to be strongly associated with becoming ill. Among those who ate ham that had been prepared by a particular cook, 86% got sick, compared with none of those who ate ham prepared by a different cook. Microbiological tests found heavy staphylococcal contamination of the suspected ham, which was eventually found to have resulted from improper food handling (Eisenberg et al., 1975).

The time period cumulative incidence refers to is usually fixed, specified, and the same for all members of the study population. For example, the proportion of patients undergoing a surgical procedure who develop deep venous thrombosis during the two weeks after surgery could be termed the "two-week cumulative incidence" of that complication.

In some situations, the time period that cumulative incidence refers to may not be stated and may, in fact, vary among individuals. For example, the cumulative incidence of death before discharge among hospitalized patients is sometimes used as a measure of disease severity or outcome. Because of differences in length of hospital stay, however, the amount of time at risk for death varies among patients.

Cumulative incidence is easy to calculate and to interpret, but unfortunately it can only be measured directly in closed populations (as defined in Chapter 2). In particular, the population cannot gain or lose members during the period of follow-up, except for losses that occur after disease occurs. The reason is that cumulative incidence is designed to estimate the proportion of persons initially at risk who develop disease during follow-up. If gains or losses in the study population took place, the essential correspondence between the case count in the numerator, and the defined population at risk in the denominator, would be broken. For example, if a new member were to join the population partway through follow-up and then become a case, he or she would be added to the numerator, even though she or he had not been counted as a member of the denominator population at risk. If an original member of the denominator population were lost to follow-up, he or she might actually go on to become a case during the study period who would go undetected.

Chapter 4 describes how cumulative incidence can be estimated indirectly under certain assumptions, even when follow-up data on some original population members are incomplete. It also describes methods for obtaining confidence limits.

Incidence Rate

The *incidence rate* is the count of incident cases divided by the amount of at-risk experience from which they arose. Its denominator is usually measured in units of person-time.

$$\text{Incidence rate} = \frac{\text{Number of incident cases}}{\text{Amount of at-risk experience}}$$

Whether disease recurrences are counted in the numerator depends on the study's case definition, as discussed in Chapter 2.

The incidence rate also goes by several other names, including *incidence density* (a term originally suggested by Miettinen, 1976), *person-time incidence rate,* or sometimes simply *incidence.*

Example: Gardner et al. (1999) studied on-the-job back sprains and strains among 31,076 material handlers employed by a large retail merchandise chain. Payroll data for a 21-month period during 1994–1995 were linked with job injury claims, which provided data on the timing of each injury, body part injured, and mechanism of injury. A total of 767 qualifying back injuries occurred during 54,845,247 working hours, yielding an *incidence rate* of 1.40 back injuries per 100,000 worker-hours. Higher incidence was found among males and among employees whose work was more physically demanding.

The work force in this example comprised an open, defined population. Thousands of workers joined or left the company during the study period. Only on-the-job back injuries were of interest, so each worker's at-risk experience consisted of many discontinuous time periods at work, separated by periods away from work. These features of the research situation made an incidence-rate approach to measuring disease frequency attractive and a good match to the available data.

The basic rationale behind the incidence rate is straightforward. Other things being equal, the number of new cases of disease should be proportional to *(1)* the size of the population at risk and *(2)* the amount of time over which susceptible individuals are observed. The denominator simply combines these two elements.

The number of cases and the number of persons at risk are unitless counts, while the time component of the denominator has units, so an incidence rate has units of $time^{-1}$.

Incidence rates can be used across a wide range of epidemiologic research situations. They can be applied to both closed and open populations, with or without detailed information on the time at risk for each individual, and for both recurrent and non-recurrent disease events—circumstances in which cumulative incidence may be impossible to apply.

Estimating incidence rate with detailed data on individual times at risk

In many epidemiologic studies, detailed information is available on the amount of time at risk for each individual and the timing of each disease event. In the Gardner back-injury study, for example, payroll records furnished each worker's time on the job right down to the hour, and injury claims contained data on the timing of each back injury.

To see how a person-time denominator is calculated from detailed individual data, consider the small population shown in Figure 3–3. It deliberately involves several features that would make cumulative incidence impossible to apply but that can be accommodated easily under an incidence-rate approach. Four cases occur among six individuals during a 30-day period. Some people enter late in the study period, some are observed only intermittently, some drop out early, one (person no. 4) is not at risk for part of the time, and one (person no. 5) has two separate disease events.

Depending on the study purpose, recurrent disease events in the same person might or might not be relevant and qualify for inclusion. In this instance, that decision affects the contributions of several individuals to both the numerator and

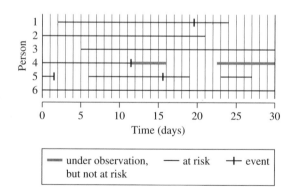

Figure 3–3. Hypothetical Population to Illustrate Incidence Rate Estimation with Detailed Data on Individual Times at Risk.

Table 3–1. Example of Incidence Rate Calculation, Keyed to Figure 3–3

PERSON	If All Cases Qualify		If Only First Cases Qualify	
	CONTRIBUTION TO NO. OF CASES	DAYS AT RISK	CONTRIBUTION TO NO. OF CASES	DAYS AT RISK
1	1	22	1	17.5
2	0	21	0	21
3	0	25	0	25
4	1	11.5	1	11.5
5	2	18.5	1	1.5
6	0	30	0	30
Total cases	4		3	
Total person-days		128		106.5
Incidence rate—per 100 person-days	3.13		2.82	

the denominator of the incidence rate estimate. Table 3–1 shows the calculations both ways.

- If recurrent events qualify, then both of the disease events in person no. 5 are added to the numerator. In addition, anyone who becomes a case may continue thereafter to contribute person-time at risk to the denominator, because he or she remains at risk for recurrence.
- If recurrent events do *not* qualify, then person no. 5 contributes only one event to the numerator. In addition, anyone who becomes a case contributes no further person-time to the denominator thereafter, because he or she is no longer at risk for a first event.

Estimating incidence rate without detailed data on individual times at risk

Often detailed information about each population member's time at risk is unknown and not feasibly obtainable. This problem often arises, for example, when the defined population of interest consists of residents of a geographic area over some time period. The number of incident cases may be readily available, but the challenge is to estimate the total amount of person-time at risk from which those cases arose.

Figure 3–4 provides a graphical example. It shows gradual growth in the size of a true population at risk over an observation period that extends from Time A to Time E. Total person-time at risk corresponds to the area of the shaded region, which could be calculated exactly if moment-by-moment details about the size

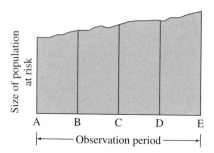

Figure 3–4. Estimating Average Size of the Population at Risk.

of the population at risk were known. Otherwise, the area must be estimated by sampling the size of the population at risk at one or more time points, averaging these population-size estimates, and multiplying by the duration of the observation period. Variations of this approach include:

1. Using estimated population size at mid-period (here, Time C) as an estimate of the average. This method might be suitable when a single population count is made at or near the middle of the observation period. This could apply, for example, to a county or state observed over the four-year period from 1998 to 2001, because 2000 was a census year.
2. Averaging the estimated population size at the start and at the end of the observation period (here, Times A and E). This method might be suitable if, for example, the observation period spans a 10-year period between two decennial censuses.
3. Averaging several population size estimates made periodically during the observation period. For example, government planning agencies in many areas publish year-by-year estimates of population size and composition for geopolitical areas. Average population size over a four-year observation period could then be estimated by averaging four annual estimates.

Example: Some 702,093 new cases of genital *Chlamydia trachomatis* infection were reported in the U.S. in 2000 (Centers for Disease Control and Prevention, 2001b). The U.S. Census Bureau estimates that the population of the U.S. on July 1, 2000 was about 282.1 million. Under method no. 1 above, 282,100,000 can be treated as an estimate of the average size of the population at risk during the one-year period from January 1, 2000, through December 31, 2000, yielding an estimated 282,100,000 *person-years at risk*. The estimated incidence rate of genital *Chlamydia trachomatis* infection would therefore be $702,093/282,100,000 = .00249 = 2.49$ cases per 1000 person-years at risk.

By similar logic, it is sometimes possible to calculate an incidence rate from a published paper even if the results are not reported as such. If a cohort of N persons is described as having been followed for an average of $\overline{T}$ years, then they experienced $N\overline{T}$ person-years in all. If all of this person-time can be considered at-risk time, and if c incident cases occur, then $c/N\overline{T}$ is an estimate of the incidence rate.

For some diseases, the prevalence of disease may be high enough, or a not-at-risk state common enough, that the discrepancy between total population size and size of the true population at risk is too large to be ignored. Corrections may then need to be based on the estimated prevalence of disease or the estimated proportion of the population that is not at risk. For example, the estimated incidence of dementia in the elderly has been found to increase considerably after prevalent cases of dementia were subtracted from the denominator (Rocca et al., 1998). For uterine cancer, higher and almost certainly more accurate incidence estimates have been obtained when the estimated number of women with a prior hysterectomy were subtracted from the denominator (Marrett, 1980).

Denominators other than person-time

In some areas of epidemiologic research, such as the study of injuries, metrics other than person-time are often used to quantify the amount of at-risk experience from which a set of incident cases arose. For example, the incidence of motor-vehicle collision injuries can be expressed as injuries per 100,000 person-years, as injuries per 100,000 licensed-driver-years, or as injuries per million vehicle-miles traveled. The extent to which older adults are a high-risk group for motor-vehicle collision injuries has been shown to depend strongly on which measure of incidence is used (Massie et al., 1995). Relative to younger adults, a smaller percentage of older adults have a valid driver's license, and even those who do have a driver's license drive fewer miles per year than younger drivers. Hence the increase in incidence by age is more marked when the denominator is vehicle-miles traveled.

Comparison of Cumulative Incidence and Incidence Rate

The distinction between cumulative incidence and incidence rate was appreciated by early epidemiologists and health statisticians (Vandenbroucke, 1985). The differences are both conceptual and statistical (Morgenstern et al., 1980; Elandt-Johnson, 1975). Table 3–2 summarizes and contrasts several properties of these two measures of incidence.

Despite the differences, the generic term *incidence* is widely applied to both cumulative incidence and incidence rate throughout the epidemiologic literature. The specific kind of incidence being discussed must often be inferred from the context. To accustom readers to this widespread practice, and for brevity,

Table 3–2. Comparison of Cumulative Incidence and Incidence Rate

CHARACTERISTIC	CUMULATIVE INCIDENCE	INCIDENCE RATE
Units	None	Time^{-1}
Range	0–1	0–infinity
Directly calculable by:	Observing a closed population over time	Observing a closed or open population over time with detailed data on individual times at risk
Indirectly calculable by:	Survival-analysis methods in presence of censoring[a]	Estimating total person-time as (average size of population at risk) × (duration of observation period)
Individual-level counterpart	Risk (probability)	Hazard rate[a]

[a] Discussed in Chapter 4.

this book often simply uses the generic term *incidence* when its meaning seems unambiguous.

Chapter 4 describes how confidence limits for incidence rates can be obtained; how cumulative incidence and the incidence rate are related mathematically and, under certain assumptions, computable from each other; and how incidence rates in a population relate to individual-level hazard rates.

Variants of Incidence

Incidence can actually be thought of as a family of disease-frequency measures. Some members of this family traditionally go by names of their own, but in reality they are just special types of incidence.

Mortality

Mortality is the incidence of fatal cases of a disease in the population at risk for dying of the disease. The denominator includes both prevalent cases of the disease as well as persons who are at risk for developing the disease. Subtypes are *cumulative mortality* and *mortality rate*. *Mortality density* and *death rate* are essentially synonyms for the mortality rate.

Example: Some 8,911 deaths due to AIDS were recorded in the U.S. in 2000 (Centers for Disease Control and Prevention, 2001a). Essentially the entire U.S.

population is considered to be at non-zero risk for dying of AIDS, although the level of risk clearly varies greatly from person to person. Hence the denominator for the mortality rate is (estimated average size of the U.S. population during 2000) × (length of observation period) = 282,100,000 × 1 year. The mortality rate for AIDS in 2000 was thus 8,911/282,100,000 = 3.16 deaths per 100,000 person-years.

Fatality

Fatality refers to the incidence of death from a disease *among persons who develop the disease.* The difference between fatality and mortality is in their denominators. Fatality reflects the prognosis of the disease among cases, while mortality reflects the burden of deaths from the disease in the population as a whole.

In principle, *cumulative fatality* and *fatality rate* can be defined as special types of cumulative incidence and incidence rate, respectively, with appropriate restrictions on who counts toward the numerator and denominator. In practice, these terms are rarely used, although the underlying theory still applies.

Instead, *case fatality* is a commonly used measure of fatality. It is:

$$\text{Case fatality} = \frac{\text{Number of fatal cases}}{\text{Total number of cases}} \tag{3.1}$$

Case fatality can be viewed as the cumulative incidence of death due to the disease among those who develop it. As with *attack rate,* a fixed time period after disease onset may or may not be explicitly specified and must often be inferred from the context. As a variant of cumulative incidence, case fatality is most readily applied for diseases of relatively short duration, in which there are few losses to follow-up or deaths from other causes.

Example: The National Highway Traffic Safety Administration (2001) reported that 4,739 deaths occurred in the U.S. during 2000 when a pedestrian was struck and killed by a motor vehicle. They estimate that 78,000 pedestrians were injured in pedestrian/motor-vehicle collisions during that year. Based on these data, the case fatality of pedestrian/motor-vehicle collision injury in 2000 was 4,739/78,000 = 6.1%.

Proxy Measures of Incidence

Sometimes good denominator data for the desired measure of incidence cannot feasibly be obtained. Yet case counts alone are likely to be inadequate for comparing incidence between populations that differ in size or other key characteristics. Under those circumstances, a proxy denominator may be better than none at all.

Proportional mortality

The *proportional mortality* for a disease is:

$$\text{Proportional mortality} = \frac{\text{Deaths from the disease}}{\text{Deaths from all causes}}$$

As its name indicates, it is simply the proportion of all deaths that are due to a particular cause for a specified population and time period of interest. This proportion can provide useful descriptive information in its own right: for example, the statement that heart disease accounted for 30% of all deaths among Americans in 1999 refers to proportional mortality (National Center for Health Statistics, 2001).

For comparing disease frequency between populations, the main advantage of proportional mortality is that its denominator—total number of deaths—can usually be ascertained from the same source that furnishes its numerator. The count of all deaths serves as a proxy for person-time at risk under the assumption that, other things being equal, one would expect total deaths to vary in proportion to population size and in proportion to the duration of the monitoring period.

A potential limitation of comparing proportional mortality between populations or subpopulations can be illustrated by an example:

Example: Berkel and de Waard (1983) studied mortality among Seventh-day Adventists (SDA) in the Netherlands over a ten-year period. The church proscribes its members from using tobacco or alcoholic beverages and recommends a vegetarian diet. These policies led the investigators to expect a reduced death rate among SDA from cancer (particularly lung cancer, which is strongly related to smoking) and heart disease.

The second column of Table 3–3 shows the observed number of deaths among SDA, and the third column shows the percentage of those deaths due to each cause. For comparison, the fourth column shows the percentage of deaths by cause in a similarly aged sample of the full population of the Netherlands during the same ten years. Based on a comparison of proportional mortality (columns 3 and 4), there seems to be no evidence of a reduced occurrence of death due to lung cancer and only a slight reduction in mortality due to cardiovascular disease.

But in this instance, the investigators also had detailed year-by-year data on the size of the SDA population, from which they could determine the number

Table 3–3. Proportional Mortality and Mortality Rate Analyses of Deaths among Dutch Seventh-Day Adventists (SDA)

CAUSE OF DEATH	OBSERVED DEATHS IN SDA	Proportional Mortality		Expected Deaths in SDA, Based on:	
		SDA	NETHERLANDS	NETHERLANDS PROPORTIONAL MORTALITY	NETHERLANDS MORTALITY RATES
Lung cancer	12	2.5%	2.5%	12	27
Other cancer	103	21.3%	18.9%	91	204
Cardiovascular	227	47.1%	50.8%	245	547
Other causes	130	27.0%	27.7%	134	299
All causes	482	100.0%	100.0%	482	1077

[*Source:* Based on Berkel and de Waard (1983).]

of person-years at risk contributed by SDA during the study period, by age and gender. They obtained the age- and sex-specific mortality rates for the Netherlands as a whole from published sources. By applying these published Dutch mortality rates to the SDA denominator data, they were able to estimate how many deaths would have been expected among the SDA if they had experienced the mortality rates in effect for all Dutch people of similar age and gender.

The rightmost column of Table 3–3 shows these results, and they lead to quite a different conclusion. The observed numbers of lung cancer and cardiovascular disease deaths in SDA were in fact sharply lower than the number of such deaths expected based on rates for all Dutch people of similar age and gender. But deaths from *other* causes were also substantially lower than expected among SDA. Hence the *proportions* of SDA deaths from lung cancer and heart disease differed very little from those in the Netherlands in general. In this example, we would have been led astray if only a proportional mortality analysis had been possible. The total number of deaths was actually a poor proxy for population size because of a major difference in all-causes mortality between populations.

Other proxies for incidence are based on the same basic idea, applied to non-fatal events. For example, hospital admissions for diabetes can be expressed as a proportion of all hospital admissions if no good data are available on the size of the true population at risk for hospitalization. Similarly, incident cases of colon cancer can be expressed as a proportion of all incident cancer cases. The same potential pitfall applies, however: comparisons could be misleading if the overall hospitalization rate or the overall cancer incidence rate were to differ between populations being compared. Contrasts based on proxy measures must therefore be cautiously interpreted.

Fetal death ratio

In perinatal epidemiology, the frequency of fetal death in a certain population over a specified time period is quantified as:

$$\text{Fetal death ratio} = \frac{\text{Number of fetal deaths}}{\text{Number of live births}}$$

The denominator for a cumulative-incidence measure of fetal death would be the total number of pregnancies. But some pregnant women may undergo spontaneous or elective abortions that can be difficult to ascertain and count. Hence the number of live births is used as a proxy for the total number of pregnancies.

In contrast to proportional mortality, the fetal death ratio and other analogues that do not include the numerator as part of the denominator are not proportions.

OTHER MEASURES OF DISEASE FREQUENCY

Period Prevalence

Earlier, *prevalence* was described as reflecting the frequency of the diseased state at a specified point in time. Especially when *prevalence* refers to a point in calendar time, the term *point prevalence* is often used (Last, 2000). In contrast, *period prevalence* is a hybrid of prevalence and cumulative incidence. Like cumulative incidence, it refers to a period of time, rather than a point in time. Cases counted in its numerator, however, include both *(1)* cases that are extant when the observation period begins, and *(2)* new cases that occur during the period. Referring to Figure 3–5, persons no. 1, no. 3, no. 4, and no. 5 would all count as cases. The denominator includes both *(1)* extant cases when the period starts and *(2)* persons

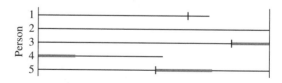

Figure 3–5. Illustration of Period Prevalence.

at risk when the period starts. For Figure 3–5, the period prevalence would thus be $4/5 = 0.8$.

Period prevalence is essentially uninterpretable except in a closed population, for the same reasons that apply to cumulative incidence. For a closed population, if P = point prevalence when the observation period starts, and CI = cumulative incidence among individuals at risk at that time, then period prevalence can be seen to be:

$$\text{Period prevalence} = P + (1 - P) \cdot CI$$

For Figure 3–5, this would be $1/5 + (1 - 1/5) \times 3/4 = 0.8$.

The main limitation of period prevalence is that point prevalence and cumulative incidence convey very different kinds of information about disease frequency. Those distinctions are lost when they are combined in this way, which limits the usefulness of period prevalence as a summary measure. When possible, point prevalence and cumulative incidence are generally better kept separate as two more interpretable components.

Yet sometimes this separation cannot be made from the data available. For example, the U.S. Centers for Disease Control (1998) reported that 25.3 per 1000 U.S. women who delivered a live-born infant during 1993–1995 had diabetes during the pregnancy, according to data on the baby's birth certificate. Some of these mothers had diabetes before becoming pregnant, while others developed diabetes during pregnancy. In any event, all reportedly had diabetes sometime during the period of pregnancy, so 25.3/1000 is probably best regarded as a period prevalence.

Years of Potential Life Lost

As noted earlier, case counts alone can be used to compare the frequency of two or more diseases within the same population. For example, the purpose may be to help guide allocation of resources among different programs aimed at specific diseases. Because of the special importance often attached to fatal cases, and because mortality data are often readily available, such comparisons are often based on the number of deaths from each disease.

Implicitly, these comparisons weight all deaths equally. It has been argued, however, that "premature" deaths—those occurring at younger ages—have greater social and economic impact than do deaths in old age, and that age at death should be considered when comparing diseases (Centers for Disease Control and Prevention, 1986). One measure designed to do this is *years of potential life lost (YPLL)* (Gardner and Sanborn, 1990). One version, used in reporting of national health

Table 3–4. Top Ten Causes of Death by Years of Potential Life Lost Before Age 75 Years
and by Total Deaths: United States, 1998

	By Years of Potential Life Lost		By Number of Deaths	
RANK	DISEASE CATEGORY	YPLL$_{75}$ [a]	DISEASE CATEGORY	NUMBER OF DEATHS
1	Cancer	1716	Heart disease	724,915
2	Heart disease	1343	Cancer	549,787
3	Unintentional injuries	1052	Stroke	167,340
4	Suicide	365	COPD[b]	124,153
5	Homicide	301	Unintentional injuries	97,298
6	Stroke	233	Diabetes mellitus	68,379
7	COPD[b]	186	Pneumonia and influenza	63,686
8	HIV infection	177	Alzheimer's disease	44,507
9	Diabetes mellitus	174	Chronic renal disease	35,524
10	Chronic liver disease	159	Septicemia	30,670

[a] Years of potential life lost to age 75 years, per 100,000 persons age <75 years
[b] COPD = Chronic obstructive pulmonary disease
[*Source:* National Center for Health Statistics (2001).]

statistics for the U.S., is:

$$\text{YPLL} = \sum_{a=1}^{X} d_a (X - a)$$

where a denotes age at death (in years), d_a denotes number of deaths at age a, and X denotes a particular cutoff age, often 65 or 75 years. Essentially, YPLL weights each death by the number of years before age X at which the death occurs. Deaths in infancy get the most weight; deaths at or after age X years get zero weight. YPLL can also be expressed per 1000 population (say), but this is not really necessary if all comparisons are made within the same population.

The impact of this weighting by age at death is shown in Table 3–4. For the U.S. in 1998, it shows the top ten disease categories as ranked by YPLL with $X = 75$ and the top ten as ranked by number of deaths. Disease categories such as injuries, which tend to kill people at younger ages, rise higher in the ranking by YPLL.

Criticisms of YPLL include the fact that the choice of a cutoff age X is somewhat arbitrary; rankings by YPLL depend on the age distribution of the population at risk, which also affects comparability of YPLL between populations or over time; and the implicit assumption that persons who died of a certain disease before age X years would otherwise have lived to age X or beyond (Gardner and Sanborn, 1990; Lai and Hardy, 1999). Nonetheless, YPLL is increasingly reported as a measure of disease impact on a population and conveys information that other such measures may not readily capture.

EXERCISES

1. Atrial fibrillation (AF) is a heart rhythm abnormality that can be either chronic or "paroxysmal" (occurring in repeated episodes). AF increases the risk of stroke, but the excess risk can be reduced by taking anticoagulants.

    To estimate the prevalence of AF among older adults in a certain region of England, 4843 persons were sampled at random from a list of all persons aged 65 years or older who were registered with a National Health Service primary care physician. Of the 3678 who participated and had an electrocardiogram, 207 were found to have AF.

    To check for participation bias, medical records were also reviewed for a sample of participants and for a sample of nonparticipants. A diagnosis of AF was found somewhere in the medical record for 139/1413 in the participant sample and for 40/382 in nonparticipants.

    (a) Based on these results, what is your best estimate of the prevalence of AF among older adults in the region? $207/3678 = 5.6\%$ 10% (9.8)

    (b) Do the results from medical record review for a subsample of participants and nonparticipants suggest that persons with AF were any more or less likely to be surveyed?

    (c) Why do you think the percentage of patients with AF in the medical record substudy was so much higher than the percentage found to have AF in the survey?

2. The so-called "sex ratio" is usually calculated as the number of male cases of a condition divided by the number of female cases.

    (a) You are studying patterns of disease occurrence in your community using data on hospital discharges. The sex ratio in 80 cases of pyloric stenosis, which is almost always diagnosed during the first year of life, is found to be 3:1. (Duplicate hospitalizations by the same patients have been eliminated.) Does this finding suggest that male babies are at higher risk for pyloric stenosis than are female babies in your community? Why or why not?

    (b) Below age 75, the sex ratio for myocardial infarction is found to be 2:1. Above age 75, it is about 1:2. Does this imply that men in the area are more prone to heart attacks below age 75, but that women are more prone after that age? Why or why not?

3. Lenaway et al. (1992) described epidemiologic characteristics of school-related injuries among 5,518 students in nine schools in the Boulder, Colorado, area during a particular school year. During this period, 509 injuries were reported, which occurred at the following times:

TIME	PERCENT
Before school	2%
Morning	41%
Lunch	27%
Afternoon	16%
After school	14%
Total	100%

From this information, can you conclude that the risk of injuries was highest during the morning hours? Why or why not?

4. If a hen and a half lay an egg and a half in a day and a half, how many eggs would one hen lay in three days?

5. Vancouver, British Columbia, and Seattle, Washington, are geographically near each other and are quite similar with regard to population size and several measures of socioeconomic status. Over a seven-year period, the following data were obtained from the respective police departments concerning homicides, according to the weapon used.

Percentage of Homicides Committed Using Each Weapon Type

TYPE OF WEAPON	SEATTLE	VANCOUVER
Firearm	42.5%	14.3%
Knife	27.4%	50.0%
Other	30.1%	35.7%

A newspaper reporter is sitting beside you when these data are shown at a press conference. He voices his conclusion that a Seattle resident may be more likely than a Vancouver resident to be shot to death by someone else, but that Seattleites can at least take comfort in knowing that they are less likely to be stabbed to death or killed by other weapons than are Vancouver residents. Do you agree? Why or why not?

ANSWERS

1. *(a)* Prevalence $= 207/3678 = .056$.
   (b) AF was found for $139/1413 = 9.8\%$ of participants and $40/382 = 10.5\%$ of nonparticipants, suggesting little participation bias.
   (c) The kind of prevalence measured in the community survey was *point prevalence* as of the time the electrocardiogram was taken for each participant. The kind of prevalence measured in the medical record review is better considered *period prevalence*. It referred not to the proportion of patients who had AF at a particular *point* in time, but over the *period* of time during which patients had received care from the clinic whose medical record was reviewed.

2. *(a)* In this instance, yes. At least in most societies, it would be safe to assume that there are about equal numbers of male and female babies at risk during the first year of life, even though the exact numbers at risk may be unknown.
   (b) Not necessarily. The shift in the sex ratio with advancing age might be largely due to differences in the gender composition of the population at risk, with women outnumbering men at the older ages because they generally live longer.

3. No. We can convert the percentages back to the number of cases that occurred during each time period to get a set of numerators for some kind of incidence measure. We could also probably assume that the number of students at risk during each of the time periods shown was about the same. But the *duration* of each time period, while not specified, undoubtedly differed among the time periods. The lunch period, for example, probably lasted only an hour or less, while morning could have spanned three or four hours. Clearly, the longer the time period, the more injuries we would expect to see in the period, even if the intrinsic risk to students per unit of time were the same.

   A good incidence measure here would be the incidence rate, computed using a person-time denominator. We cannot calculate it from the data given for lack of the time component of the denominator.

4. This familiar riddle is actually an incidence-rate problem. The number of eggs laid should be proportional to the number of hens and to the amount of time spent waiting for eggs. The "incidence rate" of egg-laying is 1.5 eggs/(1.5 hens × 1.5 days) $= 2/3$ eggs/hen-day. One hen on the job for three days amounts to 3 hen-days, so we would expect $3 \times 2/3 = 2$ eggs.

5. The table concerns only "numerator data" on the distribution of homicides by weapon type. It does not show whether the incidence of homicides, overall or of any type, is higher in one city than in the other.

Here are the actual homicide incidence rates from the two cities during 1980–1986 (Sloan et al., 1988):

Incidence of Homicide per 100,000 Person-Years by Weapon Type

TYPE OF WEAPON	SEATTLE	VANCOUVER
Firearm	4.8	1.0
Knife	3.1	3.5
Other	3.4	2.5
All types	11.3	7.0

The overall incidence of homicide was higher in Seattle, and the difference in rates for firearms accounted for most of the excess. The incidence of homicide carried out with knives was slightly higher in Vancouver, but the incidence of murder involving other weapons was actually higher in Seattle than in Vancouver.

REFERENCES

Ast DB, Schlesinger ER. The conclusion of a ten-year study of water fluoridation. Am J Public Health 1956; 46:265–71.

Babbage C. Letter to Alfred Lord Tennyson. Quoted in: Newman JR (ed.). The world of mathematics. Volume 3, p. 1487. New York: Simon and Schuster, 1956.

Berkel J, de Waard F. Mortality pattern and life expectancy of Seventh-day Adventists in the Netherlands. Int J Epidemiol 1983; 12:455–59.

Bernstein CN, Blanchard JF, Rawsthorne P, Wajda A. Epidemiology of Crohn's disease and ulcerative colitis in a central Canadian province: a population-based study. Am J Epidemiol 1999; 149:916–24.

Centers for Disease Control and Prevention. Premature mortality in the United States: public health issues in the use of years of potential life lost. MMWR 1986; 35:1S–11S.

Centers for Disease Control and Prevention. Diabetes during pregnancy—United States, 1993–1995. MMWR 1998; 47:408–14.

Centers for Disease Control and Prevention. HIV/AIDS Surveillance Report 12 (No. 2). Atlanta, Ga.: Centers for Disease Control and Prevention, 2001a.

Centers for Disease Control and Prevention. Sexually transmitted disease surveillance, 2000. Atlanta, Ga.: U.S. Department of Health and Human Services, Centers for Disease Control and Prevention, 2001b.

Eisenberg MS, Gaarslev K, Brown W, Horwitz M, Hill D. Staphylococcal food poisoning aboard a commercial aircraft. Lancet 1975; 2:595–99.

Elandt-Johnson RC. Definition of rates: some remarks on their use and misuse. Am J Epidemiol 1975; 102:267–71.

Gardner JW, Sanborn JS. Years of potential life lost (YPLL)–what does it measure? Epidemiology 1990; 1:322–29.

Gardner LI, Landsittel DP, Nelson NA. Risk factors for back injury in 31,076 retail merchandise store workers. Am J Epidemiol 1999; 150:825–33.

Lai D, Hardy RJ. Potential gains in life expectancy or years of potential life lost: impact of competing risks of death. Int J Epidemiol 1999; 28:894–98.

Last JM (ed.) A dictionary of epidemiology (4th edition). New York: Oxford, 2000.

Lenaway DD, Ambler AG, Beaudoin DE. The epidemiology of school-related injuries: new perspectives. Am J Prev Med 1992; 8:193–98.

Marrett LD. Estimates of the true population at risk of uterine disease and an application to incidence data for cancer of the uterine corpus in Connecticut. Am J Epidemiol 1980; 111:373–78.

Massie DL, Campbell KL, Williams AF. Traffic accident involvement rates by driver age and gender. Accid Anal Prev 1995; 27:73–87.

Miettinen O. Estimability and estimation in case-referent studies. Am J Epidemiol 1976; 103:226–35.

Morgenstern H, Kleinbaum DG, Kupper LL. Measures of disease incidence used in epidemiologic research. Int J Epidemiol 1980; 9:97–104.

National Center for Health Statistics. Health, United States, 2001, with urban and rural health chartbook. Hyattsville, Md.: National Center for Health Statistics, 2001.

National Highway Traffic Safety Administration. 2000 Motor vehicle traffic crashes, injury and fatality estimates, early assessment. Washington, D.C.: U.S. Department of Transportation, 2001.

Phillips DP, Christenfeld N, Ryan NM. An increase in the number of deaths in the United States in the first week of the month. An association with substance abuse and other causes of death. N Engl J Med 1999; 341:93–98.

Rocca WA, Cha RH, Waring SC, Kokmen E. Incidence of dementia and Alzheimer's disease. A reanalysis of data from Rochester, Minnesota, 1975–1984. Am J Epidemiol 1998; 148:51–62.

Sloan JH, Kellermann AL, Reay DT, Ferris JA, Koepsell T, Rivara FP, et al. Handgun regulations, crime, assaults, and homicide. A tale of two cities. N Engl J Med 1988; 319:1256–62.

Vandenbroucke JP. On the rediscovery of a distinction. Am J Epidemiol 1985; 121:627–28.

Vlahov D, Brewer TF, Castro KG, Narkunas JP, Salive ME, Ullrich J, et al. Prevalence of antibody to HIV-1 among entrants to U.S. correctional facilities. JAMA 1991; 265:1129–32.

4

DISEASE FREQUENCY: ADVANCED

Chapter 3 offered an overview of ways to measure disease frequency in populations. In this chapter we return to take a closer look at several of the main techniques, highlighting properties and relationships among them that may not be apparent on a first encounter.

People embark on the study of epidemiology from varying backgrounds and with varying amounts of statistical training. Readers without much prior statistical training may find parts of this chapter challenging but are encouraged to try to follow the basic reasoning and conclusions without getting too bogged down in mathematical details. Those with more statistical experience should find a few helpful connections between new terminology and familiar concepts.

PREVALENCE

Prevalence and Length-Biased Sampling

Not all cases of a disease necessarily have an equal chance of being included in a set of prevalent cases, which are counted in the numerator of a prevalence estimate. The reason is that the time course of many diseases is quite variable from person to person, and an individual's chance of being a case at the time of a prevalence survey depends on how much time he or she spends in the diseased state.

Coronary heart disease, for example, can take several forms, including chronic cardiac chest pain (angina pectoris), acute myocardial infarction, or sudden cardiac death. Figure 4–1 shows the time course of coronary heart disease for three hypothetical cases in a workforce population of middle-aged men during a one-year period. At mid-year, case no. 1 develops chronic angina pectoris, which lasts through the end of the year and beyond. Case no. 2 experiences a myocardial infarction early in the year and dies a week later. Case no. 3 remains disease-free until late in the year, when he suddenly collapses with ventricular fibrillation and soon dies of sudden cardiac death.

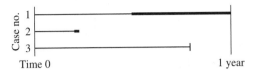

Figure 4–1. Three Hypothetical Cases of Coronary Heart Disease.

Now suppose that an employee health survey seeks to measure the prevalence of coronary heart disease by enumerating all prevalent cases in the workforce. For simplicity, say that a questionnaire is sent to all employees simultaneously and that all eligible cases are identified. This protocol is tantamount to drawing a vertical line somewhere in Figure 4–1, at a horizontal position reflecting the date of the survey, and counting all active cases crossed by that line. If a survey date is chosen at random, case no. 1 has about a 50% chance of being included as a prevalent case. Case no. 2 has about a 1/52 chance of being included, because only a few potential survey dates would fall within the week when he is an active case. Case no. 3 has an infinitesimal chance of being included—the survey would have to reach him between the onset of ventricular fibrillation and when he dies a few minutes later.

Other things being equal, a person's probability of being captured as a prevalent case is proportional to the duration of his or her disease. A set of prevalent cases thus tends to be skewed toward cases with more chronic forms of the disease. This principle has important implications for the design of some kinds of epidemiologic research—particularly case-control studies, to be discussed in Chapter 15. For example, a set of prevalent cases may not be ideal for use in a case-control study of etiologic risk factors, because the frequency of any risk factor that is also associated with chronicity of the disease may be distorted among such cases (Wang et al., 1999). The same principle arises in evaluating the effects of disease screening programs: screening is like a prevalence survey, and cases detected by screening tend to be skewed toward more slowly progressive forms of pre-symptomatic disease (Morrison, 1992).

Confidence Limits

Prevalence is a proportion. Methods of obtaining confidence limits for an estimate of a proportion based on a simple random sample are described in Appendix 4A.

Example: In the Newburgh, New York, dental-decay survey described in Chapter 3, 116 first-graders were found to meet the case definition for dental decay, out of 184 first-graders examined. The estimated prevalence was $116/184 = .63$. The 95% confidence limits for this estimate may be calculated as follows.

$$c = \text{number of cases} = 116$$

$$n = \text{number of examinees} = 184$$

$$\hat{p} = \text{point estimate of prevalence}$$

$$= c/n = .63$$

$$se(\hat{p}) = \text{standard error of } \hat{p}$$

$$= \sqrt{\frac{\hat{p}(1 - \hat{p})}{n}}$$

$$= \sqrt{\frac{.63(1 - .63)}{184}}$$

$$= .0356$$

$$Z_\alpha = \text{standard normal deviate for desired confidence level}$$

$$= 1.96 \text{ (for 95% confidence limits)}$$

The desired 95% confidence limits for prevalence are:

$$\hat{p} \pm Z_\alpha \times se(\hat{p}) = .63 \pm 1.96 \times .0356$$

$$= (.56 \text{ to } .70)$$

When an observed prevalence is based on a complete enumeration of all cases in the population, an argument can be made that no sampling error is involved and that confidence limits are unnecessary. Even in this situation, however, an observed prevalence is ordinarily treated as an estimate of the true prevalence in a larger source population from which the study population has been sampled at random. The study sample may also be regarded as a random sample in time.

CUMULATIVE INCIDENCE

Estimating Cumulative Incidence in the Presence of Censoring

Sometimes we would like to estimate cumulative incidence but cannot do so directly because some persons drop out during the observation period, even though they had not become a case before dropping out. Disease occurrence information on such subjects is termed *censored*. Censoring can occur for many reasons, including voluntary withdrawal, departure from the disease-surveillance system's coverage area, death from some unrelated disease, or the scheduled end of study data collection. *Survival analysis* encompasses a family of biostatistical methods that can allow the epidemiologist to estimate cumulative incidence in the presence of censoring, under certain assumptions (Kalbfleisch and Prentice, 1980; Hosmer and Lemeshow, 1999; Kleinbaum, 1996). A simple and widely used method that requires relatively few assumptions is described here: the *Kaplan-Meier* or *product-limit* method (Kaplan and Meier, 1958).

To see how the method works, a specific context will be helpful. An abdominal aortic aneurysm is a balloon-like expansion of the abdominal aorta caused by weakening of the aortic wall. Theory predicts that the larger the aneurysm grows, the weaker the vessel wall becomes and the greater the chance of still further expansion and potentially catastrophic rupture. But surgical repair of an unruptured aneurysm involves significant risk, pain, and cost in its own right. To help decide between early surgery and watchful waiting, doctors and patients need to know the risk of rupture and how it varies over time.

As a "thought experiment," we could imagine monitoring a group of newly diagnosed aneurysm patients over time, without censoring. The cumulative incidence of rupture would rise over time. How high and how quickly the risk rises would help determine the urgency of elective surgery.

In practice, however, aneurysm patients would be diagnosed on widely varying calendar dates, and it would be almost impossible to follow them all until rupture occurred. Censoring could happen due to death from other causes, elective surgical repair, or the scheduled end of data collection.

Example: A study by Nevitt and colleagues (1989) involved tracking the experience of 176 residents of Rochester, Minnesota, who were first diagnosed with an unruptured abdominal aortic aneurysm between 1951 and 1984. Among them, 11 ruptures were identified within eight years after diagnosis. However, even by five years after diagnosis, only 76 of the original patients were actually still at risk for rupture and being followed. Had all 176 patients been tracked for a full eight years without censoring, the cumulative incidence of rupture no doubt would have exceeded 11/176, possibly by a large amount.

Figure 4–2 portrays five hypothetical patients who are diagnosed with an aneurysm at different times during a five-year study period. In the top panel, each patient's experience is shown as a horizontal line that begins at diagnosis and terminates either with rupture (a bold vertical bar) or with censoring (a vanishing line).

In the second panel, the time scale is changed to "time since diagnosis," which bears more directly on the research question at hand. To make this conversion, the

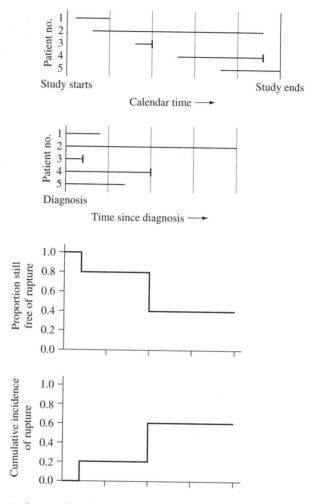

Figure 4–2. Application of Kaplan-Meier Method to Estimate Cumulative Incidence for Five Hypothetical Subjects.

line for each person is moved leftward to align its start with the vertical axis, keeping its length and manner of termination unchanged.

The third panel is the Kaplan-Meier survival curve derived from these data. (Such "curves" normally have a stair-step shape like this one.) Although we are mainly interested in cumulative incidence, it is mathematically more convenient to focus first on "survival"—here, the probability of *not* having had a rupture. To construct the curve, we proceed from left to right. By definition, all patients with a newly discovered unruptured aneurysm are free of rupture at diagnosis (Time 0), so the survival curve begins at height 1.0. Here, no ruptures occurred until halfway through the first year. Of the five patients then under surveillance, four remained rupture-free immediately after patient no. 3's rupture. Hence the curve drops at that point to $1.0 \times (4/5) = 0.8$. The next rupture (patient no. 4) occurred two years after diagnosis. At that time, one of the two patients still at risk and under surveillance remained rupture-free after patient no. 4's rupture. Hence the curve drops to $0.8 \times (1/2) = 0.4$ at that time. Between the two ruptures, patients no. 1 and no. 5 dropped out due to censoring. Those losses have no effect on the height of the survival curve at the times they occurred, but they increase the size of the drop at the time of patient no. 4's later rupture. After patient no. 4's rupture, no further ruptures occurred through year 4, when the last person under surveillance dropped out.

The bottom panel of Figure 4–2 shows the desired plot of cumulative incidence over time, obtained by calculating cumulative incidence = $1 -$ (proportion still free of rupture) at each follow-up time. In effect, it is the third panel turned upside-down. Note that the estimated cumulative incidence of rupture at four years is 0.6, not $2/5 = 0.4$, as might have been guessed naïvely without accounting for censoring. A more generic description of the Kaplan-Meier method and related methods can be found in references on survival analysis (Kaplan and Meier, 1958; Kalbfleisch and Prentice, 1980; Kleinbaum, 1996).

When there is no censoring, the Kaplan-Meier method yields the same cumulative incidence estimate as the simpler direct method described earlier. When censoring is present, the method uses the experience of those remaining at risk and under follow-up to estimate the shape of the curve. The validity of the resulting curve and cumulative incidence estimates depends on an assumption that censoring is unrelated to risk. In other words, it is assumed that, had they been observed to completion, the survival curve for persons with censored data would look the same as the curve for everyone else, aside from sampling variability. This assumption is usually not empirically testable, but a judgment about its plausibility can often be made by considering the reasons for censoring. In our aneurysm example, censoring due to the arbitrary end of the study period might well be unrelated to risk and create no bias. But censoring due to surgical repair might be triggered by the onset of symptoms or by evidence of rapid aneurysm growth, so that the surgeon's hand may have been forced by an impending rupture. To the extent that censoring for that reason is common, we might suspect that the cumulative incidence of rupture without surgical intervention could be underestimated by the Kaplan-Meier method.

Survival analysis includes several other conceptually similar but computationally more complex methods for estimating cumulative incidence when adjustment must be made for subject characteristics (covariates) that may differ across comparison groups (Kalbfleisch and Prentice, 1980; Hosmer and Lemeshow, 1999; Kleinbaum, 1996).

Confidence Limits

Cumulative incidence, like prevalence, is a proportion. When it is estimated directly from data on a closed population, methods described in Appendix 4A can be used to obtain confidence limits. When the estimate is obtained by the Kaplan-Meier method, confidence limits must be obtained by more complex techniques, as described in several statistical texts (Kalbfleisch and Prentice, 1980; Hosmer and Lemeshow, 1999; Kleinbaum, 1996; Rosner, 1995).

INCIDENCE RATE

Population-Level and Individual-Level Perspectives

Measures of disease frequency in populations have a dual interpretation. First, they estimate the burden of disease on a population as a whole. This perspective bears directly on such public health activities as detection and tracking of epidemics, health planning and resource allocation, and evaluation of policies and programs, which focus on the population as a unit.

Second, disease frequency in a population is also used to estimate disease *risk* in individuals. From this perspective, the population is viewed as a collection of individuals who have certain characteristics in common. The population is a set of replicate observations. Viewed this way, data on disease frequency in the population provide input for inductive reasoning: predictions about the likely fate of one individual can be based on the observed experience of others.

For example, the percentage of newborn babies weighing less than 2500 grams at birth has been found to be higher among babies of mothers who smoked cigarettes during pregnancy than among babies of non-smoking mothers. For any particular mother, there is no way to know for sure whether she will or will not have a low-birth-weight baby. Yet based on the experience of other mothers, we infer that the *risk* or *probability* that she will have a low-birth-weight baby is greater if she smokes than if she does not. This view of a population as a set of replicate observations also underlies statistical theory for obtaining confidence limits for measures of disease frequency.

Duality of perspectives applies to many disease-frequency measures, not just incidence rates, and epidemiologists are used to moving freely between them. But there are situations in which population-level disease frequency does not necessarily translate directly into individual-level risk estimates, and then it becomes important to distinguish between the perspectives. This issue has special relevance to incidence rates.

Incidence Rate and Hazard Rate

A key feature of the person-time incidence rate is that its denominator is a "lump sum." Person-time is regarded as a freely interchangeable commodity, and all that matters in the final calculation is the total amount. Observing one susceptible person for 12 years, 12 people for one year, or 144 people for a month all result in adding 12 person-years to the denominator. This property was assumed in the calculations shown in Table 3–1.

This feature of the incidence rate can be both a strength and a limitation. The examples in Figure 3–3 and Table 3–1 illustrated that the ability to combine person-time across people and over time makes the incidence rate a much more broadly applicable measure of incidence than cumulative incidence. But to appreciate the implications of this pooling, it is helpful to consider a model that breaks down the population's disease experience into smaller building blocks.

Looking again at Figure 3–3, the vertical lines divide the total observation period into 30 one-day periods. Taken one day at a time, many of the original complicating factors that interfered with direct calculation of cumulative incidence—censoring, recurrent cases, periods not at risk, multiple observation periods per person—become less problematic. On any given day, recurrent events in the same person and gains and losses to the population at risk are rare or non-existent.

Furthermore, we can imagine that if we had detailed data on the timing of events, we could extend this divide-and-conquer strategy still further, splitting days into hours, hours into minutes, and so on, rather like viewing a movie one frame at a time. No two disease events occur in the same person at exactly the same time on a sufficiently fine time scale, so in principle it is always possible to choose a time increment short enough that the chance of multiple cases occurring within the same increment is negligible.

In addition, there is a fixed number of instances when some population member joined or left the population, or moved into or out of the susceptible state. But again, there is no limit on how short a time increment we could select. Hence the *proportion* of intervals involving censoring of this sort can be made as small as we wish, and ultimately rare enough to be negligible.

So suppose that we specify a certain short time increment, such as a minute or a second—short enough to eliminate recurrent cases within a single interval and short enough to allow censoring and susceptibility changes to be ignored. Call this increment Δt. The entire study period of interest is then split into a series of intervals, each of duration Δt. The population's disease experience over time could now be represented as a very large matrix, as illustrated in Figure 4–3. Each row refers to a different individual who belongs to the population for at least part of the study period. Consecutive columns refer to consecutive short time intervals throughout the observation period. Each cell corresponds to a tiny piece

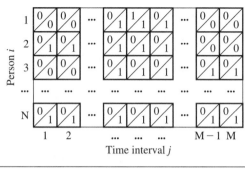

Figure 4–3. Matrix Representation of Population Disease Experience.

of person-time. Rows (individuals) are numbered 1 through N, while columns (time intervals) are numbered 1 through M. Any particular cell can be referred to by its row number (i) and column number (denoted j).

This matrix can be thought of as a "digitized" version of the kind of population line diagram shown in Figure 3–3. Each row of the line diagram in Figure 3–3 maps to a row of the matrix in Figure 4–3. The horizontal resolution is adjustable by the choice of Δt, with smaller values of Δt yielding finer resolution.

Each cell in Figure 4–3 contains two numbers. The upper left number in cell ij is 1 if the person in row i became a case during time interval j; otherwise it is 0. In other words, this number is the value of a *disease* indicator, d_{ij}. The lower right number in that cell is 1 if person i was at risk and under observation at the start of time interval j; otherwise it is 0. It is the value of a *susceptibility* indicator, s_{ij}.

Cells for which $s = 0$ are of little interest, corresponding to persons who were non-susceptible, not under observation, or already ill at the time. We know in advance that $d = 0$ for those cells—there is no uncertainty, and the observed value of d provides no real information. But every cell for which $s = 1$ corresponds to a brief "experiment of nature," or binomial trial, as considered earlier for cumulative incidence. "Chance" (as a euphemism for our incomplete knowledge about disease causes) determines whether d is 1 or 0. Each of these *trial-cells* captures the experience of a single at-risk individual over a short, fixed time period: person i either develops disease during time interval j or does not.

Associated with each trial is an underlying probability p_{ij} that person i would become a case during interval j. Because Δt was already made short enough to let us ignore the possibility of recurrent disease events within one interval, p_{ij} can also be interpreted as the *expected number* of disease events in that trial-cell. The true values of these p's are not observable. A trial-cell, however, contains either 0/1 or

1/1, either of which can be read as the observed cumulative incidence in a certain one-person population over a certain brief time interval. It is a crude estimate—the crudest possible estimate, in fact—of the corresponding p. Symbolically, $\widehat{p_{ij}} = d_{ij}/s_{ij} = d_{ij}$, because the denominator is always 1 for all trial-cells.

The total number of trial-cells, and the probability that a case occurs in one of them, clearly depend on the choice of Δt. The binomial-trial model fits better and better as Δt gets shorter, so it is worth considering what happens as Δt approaches 0. The smaller Δt is, the more trial-cells there are, and the less likely it is that any given one of them contains a case. Moreover, as Δt gets near enough to 0, p_{ij} becomes *proportional* to Δt. This is because a fixed number of cases is being spread over an increasingly large number of cells. Over a short enough period, p remains essentially constant for the same person from one instant to the next. Dividing p expected cases among, say, k still shorter sub-intervals puts p/k expected cases into each sub-interval of duration $\Delta t/k$. The k's cancel out, and the *ratio* of expected events to interval duration remains unchanged.

This ratio is variously termed the *hazard* or *hazard rate* (our preferred terms), *event rate, probability rate, force of morbidity,* or *instantaneous probability*. It is usually denoted with the Greek lambda (λ):

$$\lambda_{ij} = \frac{p_{ij}}{\Delta t}$$

For a given individual, a value of λ can be associated with each *point* in time by taking the limiting value of λ as $\Delta t \to 0$ for the interval that includes that time point.

The hazard rate merits some contemplation. It is the expected number of disease events per unit of time for a certain person at a certain moment (which explains why *event rate* is one of its aliases). Computed as the ratio of a unitless probability to an amount of time, the hazard rate has units of time^{-1}, just as does the incidence rate. But we must remember that incidence is an observable population measure of disease occurrence over a period of time, while the hazard rate is an unobservable individual measure of disease risk per time unit, evaluated at a moment in time.

We can now re-aggregate the data in the many trial-cells back toward what we as epidemiologists observe at the population level. The observed number of cases, c, is the total number of trial-cells for which $d = 1$, summed over all rows and columns:

$$c = \sum_i \sum_j d_{ij}$$

The total time at risk (call it T with no subscript), summed for all population members, is the number of trials for which $s = 1$, times the duration of each trial:

$$T = \sum_i \sum_j s_{ij} \cdot \Delta t$$

The total number of trials is:

$$N = T/\Delta t$$

Finally, the *mean hazard rate* across all persons and time intervals at risk is:

$$\bar{\lambda} = \frac{\sum_i \sum_j \frac{p_{ij}}{\Delta t}}{N}$$

$$= \frac{\sum_i \sum_j \frac{p_{ij}}{\Delta t}}{T/\Delta t}$$

$$= \frac{\sum_i \sum_j p_{ij}}{T}$$

We noted earlier that p_{ij} is interpretable as the expected number of cases in cell ij, so the numerator of the last expression is the total expected number of cases for the population. The *expected* total number of cases is not directly observable, but in a particular set of data, the *observed* number of cases c, is an estimate of it. Hence:

$$\text{Incidence rate (IR)} = \frac{c}{T} \text{ estimates } \bar{\lambda}$$

In words, the incidence rate is an estimate of the mean hazard rate over all person-time at risk contributed by population members during the study period. This interpretation holds true regardless of how variable the hazard rate may be within individuals and over time. It also does not require that the p_{ij} be independent of one another.

Incidence rate as a weighted average

As noted earlier, one of the main uses of incidence data in a population is to infer disease risk in individual population members. Later in this chapter, we will examine a "weighted-average rule," showing that the rate for a population is always a weighted average of rates for the population's component parts, which are usually subgroups of the population. The weight for each subgroup is its size—here, how much person-time it contributes. In the present context, the weighted-average rule says that the overall incidence rate will be most heavily influenced by hazard rates that apply over the largest amounts of person-time.

- Suppose the hazard rate is constant for all individuals and over time. Then the incidence rate estimates a weighted average of this constant, which is just the constant itself.
- Suppose each individual has his or her own possibly unique hazard rate, λ_i, which remains constant over time. Then the incidence rate estimates a weighted average of the λ_i. The weight for each λ_i is the proportion of the total person-time at risk contributed by person i. Hazard rates that apply to persons who are at risk and under observation longer are thus weighted more heavily. This can be important if censoring is more or less common among individuals with relatively high hazard rates. The incidence rate will tend to be skewed toward hazard rates among those persons who are least subject to censoring.
- Suppose the hazard rate changes over time but is similar for all at-risk individuals who are under observation at a given time. This situation might apply, for example, in a cohort of similar individuals who are tracked for occurrence of new cases over a long time. As cohort members age, their hazard rates may change. Concurrently, members of the cohort may be lost to attrition, so that more person-time comes from earlier in the study period than from later. The incidence rate will be skewed toward hazard rates in effect during early parts of the observation period, when more people were being observed.

Confidence Limits

As noted earlier, few assumptions are needed in order to interpret the incidence rate as an estimate of the mean hazard rate. To obtain confidence limits for an incidence rate estimate, however, additional assumptions must be made. Three models are discussed here and some research situations to which each might correspond.

Constant hazard

The simplest and probably most widely used assumption is that the hazard rate is constant across individuals and over time. Under this assumption, all person-time within the observation period is freely interchangeable. An analogy from physics is decay of a radioactive element: the hazard rate of fissioning in a certain atom at a certain moment is thought to be constant across all atoms of the same isotope and over time (Armitage and Berry, 1994).

In the human health arena, there are probably not many exact counterparts—perhaps the hazard of being struck by a giant meteor from outer space—but some situations come closer than others. The constant-hazard assumption is most plausible for a relatively homogeneous population observed over a relatively short time period. "Relatively homogeneous" and "relatively short" need to be interpreted in the context of the disease in question. In occupational epidemiology, for example, cases and person-time at risk are routinely partitioned into categories defined by job title, age range, gender, and calendar year, with incidence being estimated separately for each of the resulting categories (Checkoway et al., 1989).

When this constant-hazard assumption is met, methods based on the Poisson distribution can be used to obtain confidence limits for an incidence rate estimate (Mendenhall et al., 1986; Armitage and Berry, 1994; Breslow and Day, 1987). Specifically, say that c cases are observed in T person-time. T is considered a fixed quantity, not subject to sampling error, and confidence limits for the rate are based on confidence limits for c alone. If $c > 100$, the following expression (based on the normal approximation to the Poisson distribution) is reasonably accurate (Armitage and Berry, 1994, p. 142):

$$\text{Confidence limits} = \frac{c \pm Z_\alpha \cdot \sqrt{c}}{T}$$

where Z_α is the standard normal deviate for the desired confidence level ($Z_\alpha = 1.96$ for two-sided 95% confidence limits). The second term in the numerator is subtracted to get the lower confidence limit and added to get the upper limit.

If $c \leq 100$, more accurate confidence limits can be obtained by basing them directly on the Poisson distribution. Table 4–3 in Appendix 4B can be used to obtain a lower and an upper multiplier for c, the observed case count. Multiplying each of these by the observed point estimate of incidence yields the desired lower and upper confidence limits.

Example: In the study of back injuries by Gardner et al. (1999) described in Chapter 3, nine back injuries were reported in 322,193 working hours by female department managers who had been employed for less than eight months, for a rate of 2.79 cases per 100,000 worker-hours. Using the table in Appendix 4B, the upper and lower multipliers needed to obtain Poisson 95% confidence limits for an incidence rate that is based on nine cases are 0.457 and 1.898. The desired confidence limits therefore extend from 2.79 × 0.457 = 1.28 to 2.79 × 1.898 = 5.30 cases per 100,000 worker-hours.

Hazard varying randomly among individuals

In some situations, theory or available data suggest that the hazard rate varies among individuals, even after accounting for measured differences in exposure to risk factors and other personal characteristics. This variation could arise, for example, from differences in genetic susceptibility, differences in exposure to unmeasured risk factors, or just biological variation. In the biostatistical literature, random inter-individual differences in hazard rates are called differences in *frailty* (Aalen, 1994; Clayton, 1994).

This model seems particularly applicable to studies of recurrent illness (Glynn et al., 1993; Glynn and Buring, 1996; Cumming et al., 1990). Under the constant-hazard assumption considered earlier, someone who has had one disease event is no more or less likely than anyone else to have another event in the future. But for many diseases, evidence suggests that future risk is often elevated among persons who have already experienced an initial event. For example, victims of assault have been found to be at greatly increased risk of being assaulted again (Dowd et al., 1996). Children treated for an unintentional injury are more likely than are other children to experience a future unintentional injury (Johnston et al., 2000). Postmenopausal women who experience a vertebral fracture are at high risk of having an additional fracture within the next year (Lindsay et al., 2001). Possible mechanisms include continued exposure to a hazardous environment, existence of a chronic underlying health condition that predisposes to recurrent complications, or effects of the initial illness event itself, as might occur if an assault victim confronted his or her attacker. Whatever the reason, an initial event may serve as a marker for a subpopulation with a systematically higher hazard rate. Statistically, the problem is known as *extra-Poisson variation*. When it is present, confidence limits based on the Poisson distribution, which assumes constant hazard, are too narrow (Glynn and Buring, 1996; Clayton, 1994).

Several statistical approaches have been proposed to deal with this problem (Glynn and Buring, 1996; Clayton, 1994; Sturmer et al., 2000). One involves computing an individual event rate for each population member based on his or her observed number of events and person-time at risk, and basing confidence limits for the overall incidence rate on the observed variance in those event rates across persons (Glynn and Buring, 1996). When follow-up times are unequal among individuals, the individual rates can be weighted by amount of time at risk (Stukel et al., 1994). More complex multivariate methods include logistic regression using generalized estimating equations, Poisson regression with correction for overdispersion, or adaptations of proportional-hazards survival analysis (Sturmer et al., 2000).

Variation in hazard rates among individuals can have another effect in the context of non-recurrent disease in closed populations. It can affect the degree to which changes in incidence rates in the population over time reflect corresponding changes in individual risk (Aalen, 1994, 1988). For example, suppose that a population under surveillance initially consists of a 50:50 mixture of a high-risk subgroup and a low-risk subgroup. The earliest cases arise mainly from the high-risk subgroup. But as those early cases occur, they also preferentially deplete the high-risk subgroup. Over time, the original 50:50 mixture thus shifts toward an increasing predominance of low-risk individuals, which in turn yields a decline over time in incidence for the population as a whole. The observed decline in incidence could be misinterpreted as implying a decline in risk to individual population members, either as they age or as calendar time passes, when in fact the decline would be due at least in part to changes in the composition of the population at risk.

Hazard varying over time

As noted earlier, the simple and common model of constant hazard rates can be expected to hold best over relatively short observation periods. As time passes, changes in such factors as exposure to environmental causes, diagnostic methods, and disease classification commonly occur and can affect disease frequency. Closed populations also age. To reduce variation in hazard over time in the face of these factors, a long period of observation is often subdivided into shorter sub-periods or "time bands" for analysis. Other analytic strategies include modeling the effects of time itself on incidence—for example, by including time as a predictor in the kinds of multivariate models to be described later (Chapter 11).

Often, however, changes in hazard rates over time are not of main interest and are instead just a potential source of bias when making comparisons among subgroups or populations. This viewpoint has helped make the proportional-hazards model popular in epidemiology (Cox, 1972; Kalbfleisch and Prentice, 1980; Kleinbaum, 1996). Briefly, under this model, the "baseline" hazard may change over time in an arbitrary way, and these changes are assumed to apply to all individuals. But at any given moment, an individual's hazard relative to that of other individuals then at risk is assumed to depend on his or her measured personal characteristics, at least one of which is exposure to a potential risk factor of main interest.

Incidence Rate and Mean Time to Disease Onset

The incidence rate has units of $time^{-1}$. Under somewhat idealized circumstances, the *reciprocal* of incidence, which is in units of time, can be interpreted as the mean time to disease onset. Although this odd fact is perhaps of more theoretical than practical importance in epidemiology, its basis is explained here. It will soon play a role in linking prevalence, incidence, and disease duration.

Consider a hypothetical population of N susceptible individuals who are followed indefinitely for development of a non-recurrent disease. Say that incidence rate remains constant at some value IR throughout the follow-up period. If there are no competing risks, and if the population is followed long enough, then everyone in it must eventually develop the disease. Before becoming a case, person i

contributes a certain amount of person-time at risk, T_i. Total person-time, $T = \sum_i T_i$, stops increasing when the last case occurs. At that time, N cases would have occurred in T person-time. By definition, the incidence rate was constant throughout follow-up, so $IR = N/T$.

Now suppose we are interested in how much time goes by, on average, until a susceptible person becomes a case. This would be $\sum_i T_i/N = T/N = 1/IR$. In other words, the reciprocal of the incidence rate estimates the mean time to disease onset under the circumstances described. Although a proof is beyond the scope of this text, this property also holds for recurrent diseases.

Example: Say that upper respiratory infections occur at the (very high) incidence of three per person-year in a population. The average time to the next upper respiratory infection for a person at risk would be $1/(3 \text{ year}^{-1})$, or 4 months.

For lower-incidence diseases, the required assumption of no competing risks will rarely be satisfied, in which case the resulting numerical estimate of mean time to disease onset may not be very meaningful. But the algebraic rule itself will prove useful below.

RELATIONSHIPS AMONG MEASURES OF DISEASE FREQUENCY

Populations and Their Subpopulations

Many commonly used measures of disease frequency take the form of fractions. The numerator is usually a case count, and the denominator is a measure of population size or of the amount of person-time in which those cases occurred. Prevalence, cumulative incidence, person-time incidence rate, mortality rate, case fatality, and various other measures all fit this description. It will be convenient to call all such measures "rates" for now, recognizing that "rate" has a narrower meaning in other contexts.

A simple and very useful algebraic relationship connects the value of any such rate in the whole population to its value in subpopulations formed from the whole.

Suppose that, for a certain study population, an overall rate of disease, r, is calculated by dividing the total number of cases, c, by an appropriate denominator, n, so that $r = c/n$. The population can be divided in various ways into a set of *mutually exclusive and collectively exhaustive* subgroups—for example, by gender, by age category, or by exposure to some environmental factor. A separate "local" rate can then be calculated for each subgroup, simply by restricting both the numerator and the denominator to members of that subgroup.

Imagine that the population is separated into males and females, and that the gender-specific rates are $r_m = c_m/n_m$ for males and $r_f = c_f/n_f$ for females. The rate in the full population is:

$$r = \frac{c_m + c_f}{n_m + n_f}$$

Some algebra shows that:

$$r = \frac{c_m}{n_m + n_f} + \frac{c_f}{n_m + n_f}$$

$$= \frac{c_m}{n_m} \cdot \frac{n_m}{n_m + n_f} + \frac{c_f}{n_f} \cdot \frac{n_f}{n_m + n_f}$$

$$= r_m \cdot w_m + r_f \cdot w_f$$

where $w_m = n_m/(n_m + n_f)$ is the proportion of the overall denominator contributed by males, and w_f is the proportion contributed by females. Note also that $w_m + w_f = 1$. The w's can be interpreted as *weights* for the corresponding gender-specific rates.

Example: In a population of 700 women and 300 men, there are 35 prevalent cases of diabetes among the women and 30 cases among the men. The overall prevalence of diabetes is thus $(35 + 30)/(700 + 300) = 65/1000 = 6.5\%$, while the gender-specific prevalences are $35/700 = 5.0\%$ in women and $30/300 = 10\%$ in men. The overall prevalence is a 700:300 weighted average of 5% and 10%: $6.5\% = (5\%)(0.7) + (10\%)(0.3)$.

The algebra above can be extended to cover any number of mutually exclusive and collectively exhaustive subgroups. The general rule is:

> The overall disease rate in a population is a weighted average of the rates in its subpopulations. The weight for each subpopulation rate is the proportion of the overall rate's denominator contributed by that subpopulation.

This property applies to all disease-frequency measures that are fractions. Among other uses, the rule underlies direct and indirect standardization of rates (discussed in Chapter 11)—techniques that enable valid comparison of rates across populations that differ with regard to sociodemographic or other characteristics.

Cumulative Incidence and Incidence Rate

A useful relationship between the two main measures of incidence can be developed for non-recurrent diseases. Consider again what would happen over time in a closed, susceptible population in which the incidence rate of a certain

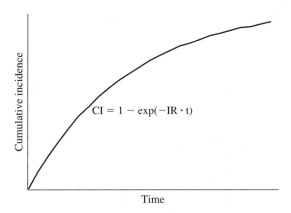

Figure 4-4. Cumulative Incidence over Time When Incidence Rate Is Constant.

non-recurrent disease remains constant. As new cases occur, they are subtracted from the population at risk. It can be shown with calculus that the population at risk declines *exponentially* over time—a process analogous to the exponential decay of a radioactive element.

Say that N_0 is the number of persons originally at risk, N_t is the number remaining at risk at time t, IR is the incidence rate (assumed to be constant), and e is the base of natural logarithms, approximately 2.71828. Then:

$$N_t = N_0 \cdot e^{(-IR \cdot t)} = N_0 \cdot \exp(-IR \cdot t) \qquad (4.1)$$

Because of the steadily declining population at risk, a smaller and smaller *number* of new cases occurs per unit of time. Cumulative incidence (CI) continues to rise, but with decreasing slope. Specifically:

$$CI = 1 - \exp(-IR \cdot t) \qquad (4.2)$$

Figure 4-4 illustrates this relationship.

Relation (4.2) can be handy, for example, when comparing results from two or more studies that used different incidence measures. As we have seen, the incidence rate applies to a broader range of populations and disease types, while cumulative incidence is more easily interpretable in terms of disease probability or risk. Relation (4.2) provides one way to use incidence rate data to address "What if . . . ?" questions involving cumulative incidence.

Example: Table 4-1 is based on results from a study by Morris and colleagues (1953) of coronary heart disease incidence among London bus drivers and conductors. It was among the first studies to suggest a link between regular physical

Table 4–1. Using Incidence Rate to Project Cumulative Incidence of Coronary Heart Disease in London Bus Drivers and Conductors

JOB/AGE	Results from Morris Study			Projected Experience of 1000 Hypothetical Workers		
	CASES	PERSON-YEARS	INCIDENCE RATE[a]	AGE	STILL AT RISK	CUMULATIVE INCIDENCE SINCE AGE 35[b]
Drivers						
35–44	8	12,360	0.6	35	1000	—
45–54	29	11,698	2.5	45	994	0.6%
55–64	43	6668	6.4	55	969	3.1%
				65	909	9.1%
Conductors						
35–44	0	9622	0.0	35	1000	—
45–54	11	5522	2.0	45	1000	0.0%
55–64	20	4022	5.0	55	980	2.0%
				65	933	6.7%

[a] Per 1000 person-years   0.05. pu
[b] In the absence of competing risks
[*Source:* based on Morris et al. (1953).]

activity and lower heart disease risk. The conductors moved around the bus all day collecting fares, climbing up and down stairs. Meanwhile, drivers remained relatively sedentary while seated driving the bus. Because the work force was an open population, the results were reported as coronary heart disease cases per 1000 worker-years for each job type and for each of three 10-year age categories.

In each age group, the incidence rate of heart disease was higher in drivers than in conductors, consistent with the hypothesis that physical activity lowers the risk of heart disease. The implications of these results in terms of individual risk can be clarified by using the incidence rate data to estimate the cumulative incidence of coronary heart disease in two hypothetical cohorts of 1000 drivers and 1000 conductors from age 35 to 65 years.

On the right side of Table 4–1, relation (4.1) was applied to each age decade in turn. The number of cohort members still at risk for incident coronary heart disease was estimated for the end of each decade, based on how many were at risk at the start of the decade and on the incidence rate for that decade from the Morris study. Cumulative incidence follows directly from the projected number still at risk. For example, among 1000 bus drivers at risk starting at age 35, the number expected *not* to develop coronary heart disease in the next decade would be:

$$1000 \times \exp(-.0006 \cdot 10) = 994$$

Thus, the projected cumulative incidence of coronary heart disease over the 35–44 age decade would be $(1000 - 994)/1000 = .006 = 0.6\%$. For the 45–54 age decade, the same formula is applied again, substituting 994 for 1000 and .0025 for .0006, and so on down the table. We estimate that, in the absence of competing risks, a man who began working as a London bus driver at age 35 would stand a 9.1% chance of developing coronary heart disease within the next 30 years. The corresponding 30-year risk in a conductor would be 6.7%.

In many situations, the disease is rare enough and the observation period short enough that very little reduction in the size of the population at risk takes place during observation. Expressed with like denominators, incidence rate and cumulative incidence may thus appear to be numerically very close. For example, the incidence rate of coronary heart disease among London bus drivers aged 35–44 years was 0.6 cases per 1000 person-years. Based on (4.2), the projected one-year cumulative incidence among 1,000 such drivers would be $1 - \exp(-0.6/1000 \cdot 1) = 0.0005998 = 0.5998$ per 1000 drivers.

Prevalence, Incidence, and Duration

Under certain circumstances, prevalence and incidence can be easily related to each other. Consider a closed population in which a recurrent disease state occurs, such as urinary tract infection, the common cold, or depression. Assume that all individuals who do not have the disease are susceptible (that is, there is no third not-at-risk state), and that the incidence rate is constant at some value *IR* among all susceptibles and over time. Under this simple two-state model, people move back and forth between the states over time (Fig. 4–5).

The flow along the disease-onset path, measured in the number of events per unit of time, depends on *(1)* the size of the susceptible pool and *(2)* the incidence rate. Because the disease is recurrent, there is also a counter-flow of individuals from diseased back to susceptible, which we may call *recovery*. The number of recovery events per unit of time depends on *(1)* the size of the diseased pool, and *(2)* what we may call a *recovery rate,* which is just like the incidence rate but operates in the opposite direction. We shall further assume that this recovery rate is constant over time and is the same for all diseased individuals at some value *RR*.

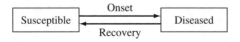

Figure 4–5. Two-State Model to Illustrate the Relationship Among Prevalence, Incidence, and Duration.

As demonstrated earlier, $1/IR$ can be interpreted as the mean time to disease onset among susceptibles. By similar logic, $1/RR$ can be interpreted as mean time to recovery among diseased individuals. In other words, $1/RR$ is the *mean duration* of disease, which it will be convenient to call $\overline{d}$.

Now suppose we begin with all individuals in the susceptible state and imagine what happens over time. People start to develop the disease at a rate determined by IR. In the process, they start emptying the susceptible compartment and start filling the diseased compartment. As the diseased compartment accumulates prevalent cases, recoveries begin to occur. The more prevalent cases accumulate, the more recoveries occur, which tends to empty the diseased compartment and to refill the susceptible compartment. As long as the two opposing flows are unequal, one compartment will grow and the other shrink, which in turn will act to equalize the two flows. Eventually an equilibrium is reached, in which the flow of incident cases is exactly balanced by the flow of recoveries. Because the flows into and out of each compartment are equal at that point, both compartments maintain a stable size.

More formally, suppose that the flows and compartment sizes at equilibrium are labelled as follows:

$$S = \text{number of susceptible persons}$$

$$D = \text{number of diseased persons (prevalent cases)}$$

$$i = \text{number of incident cases per time unit } \Delta t$$

$$r = \text{number of recoveries per time unit } \Delta t$$

At equilibrium,

$$i = r$$

$$IR \cdot S = RR \cdot D$$

$$\frac{D}{S} = IR \cdot \frac{1}{RR}$$

$$= IR \cdot \overline{d} \qquad (4.3)$$

Relation (4.3) says that, under the specified assumptions and at equilibrium, D/S is the product of incidence rate and mean duration of disease. D/S is not quite the prevalence, which would be $D/(S + D)$. Rather, D/S is the *prevalence odds,* which expresses the relative frequency of the diseased state as an odds rather than as a proportion. For many realistic situations, however, the prevalence of disease is low, so that $S \gg D$, and therefore $D/S \approx D/(S + D)$. The final result is then:

$$\text{Prevalence} \approx (\text{Incidence rate}) \times (\text{Mean disease duration}) \qquad (4.4)$$

Relation (4.4) links two key measures of disease frequency. It is a time-honored rule of thumb in epidemiology. Nonetheless, it is probably best regarded as a conceptual aid rather than as a relation that can be expected to hold true consistently in real data. The main reason is that the assumptions behind the hypothetical model are often poorly or only approximately met under real-world conditions. For example, the incidence rate and recovery rate may not remain constant long enough for an equilibrium to be achieved, because of changes in environmental or behavioral exposures, disease-control activities, diagnostic technologies, disease treatments, and so on. Also, the population of interest may not be closed, so that in- and out-migration of prevalent cases is possible. Nonetheless, relation (4.4) is quite useful for understanding the two main determinants of disease prevalence and for predicting how prevalence may change as a result of changes in incidence or disease duration.

Example: To illustrate how relation (4.4) works, imagine a population of married women aged 15–45 years in whom the incidence and prevalence of pregnancy are studied. Table 4–2 shows three scenarios. In the "base case," the incidence rate of pregnancy is 8 per 100 woman-years. Full-term pregnancies last 9 months, or 0.75 years. If all pregnancies go to term, and if incidence has been stable long enough for equilibrium to be reached, then a prevalence survey would be expected to find about $8/100 \times 0.75 = 6/100$ of women pregnant on a random survey date.

Now suppose that highly effective oral contraceptives become available for the first time, and a random 50% of women choose to use them. No other changes in reproductive practices occur. Use of the "pill" should reduce the incidence of pregnancy by half to 4 per 100 woman-years, but it should not affect the duration of pregnancies that do occur. Once a new equilibrium is achieved, we would expect another prevalence survey to find about $3/100$ women pregnant on a random date.

Table 4–2. Incidence, Duration, and Prevalence of Pregnancy in a
Hypothetical Population of Women of Reproductive Age

	Pregnancy		
BIRTH CONTROL USE	INCIDENCE RATE[a]	DURATION (YEARS)	PREDICTED PREVALENCE (APPROX.)
None	8	0.75	6%
50% use "pill"	4	0.75	3%
50% have abortion at 3 months	8	0.50	4%

[a] Pregnancies per 100 woman-years

Starting over from the "base case" without oral contraceptives, suppose instead that elective abortions become available. A random 50% of women who become pregnant decide to terminate the pregnancy at three months, while the rest carry the child to term. Abortion would have no effect on the rate at which women become pregnant, so incidence would remain at 8 per 100 woman-years. But abortions would reduce the average duration of a pregnancy from 9 months to $(0.5)(3) + (0.5)(9) = 6$ months. Hence we would expect fewer women—about $4/100$—to be in the pregnant state on a random survey date.

Mortality, Incidence, and Case Fatality

The following relations follow directly from the definitions of mortality, incidence, and case fatality:

$$\text{Mortality rate} \approx \text{incidence rate} \times \text{case fatality}$$

$$\text{Cumulative mortality} \approx \text{cumulative incidence} \times \text{case fatality}$$

Intuitively, we can think of the risk of dying of a disease as (the risk of getting the disease) × (the risk of dying of it if you get it). These relations are shown as approximations because *(1)* the denominators of mortality and incidence differ slightly with regard to inclusion of prevalent cases; and *(2)* some time must pass between disease onset and death from the disease. The incidence rate when disease-related deaths occur may differ from the rate in effect when those cases arose.

For the pedestrian/motor-vehicle collision injury example described in Chapter 3, neither of these caveats would be of serious concern. The United States' population in 2000 was about 282,100,000, so:

$$\text{Mortality rate} \approx \frac{4739 \text{ deaths}}{282,100,000 \text{ person-years}}$$

$$\approx \frac{78,000 \text{ cases}}{282,100,000 \text{ person-years}} \times \frac{4739 \text{ deaths}}{78,000 \text{ cases}}$$

$$\approx (\text{incidence rate}) \times (\text{case fatality})$$

APPENDIX 4A

Confidence Limits for a Proportion

Several measures of disease frequency are *proportions,* including prevalence, cumulative incidence, and proportional mortality. Let c be the number of cases in the numerator and n the number of persons in the denominator. If $c \geq 10$ and $n - c \geq 10$, the normal approximation to the binomial distribution gives reasonably accurate confidence limits (Armitage and Berry, 1994, p. 122) based on the estimated standard error (s.e.) of $\hat{p}$:

$$s.e.(\hat{p}) = \sqrt{\frac{\hat{p}(1 - \hat{p})}{n}}$$

Confidence limits for $p = \hat{p} \pm Z_\alpha \times s.e.(\hat{p})$

where Z_α is the standard normal deviate for the desired confidence level: $Z_\alpha = 1.96$ for two-sided 95% confidence limits.

If $c < 10$ or $n - c < 10$, confidence limits for p are more accurate if based directly on the binomial distribution and can be obtained by any of the following methods:

1. Using standard statistical software that calculates exact binomial confidence limits.
2. Calculating and summing tail probabilities for the binomial distribution, according to the algorithm described in Rosner, 1995, pp. 176–7.
3. Consulting published statistical tables or figures, as in Rosner, 1995, or Ciba-Geigy, 1982.
4. Using tables of the F-distribution as follows (Armitage and Berry, 1994, p. 121):
   - Set $A = F_{\alpha/2, [2(n-c+1), 2c]}$
   - Set $B = 1/F_{\alpha/2, [2(c+1), 2(n-c)]}$
   - Calculate $p_{lower} = \frac{c}{c + (n-c+1) \times A}$
   - Calculate $p_{upper} = \frac{c+1}{c+1 + (n-c) \times B}$

Confidence limits for proportions estimated from complex probability samples, such as those used in several national health surveys, require special statistical methods beyond the scope of this text—see Levy and Lemeshow, 1991; Korn and Graubard, 1991, 1999.

APPENDIX 4B

Poisson-Based Confidence Limits for Incidence Rate Estimates Based on 100 or Fewer Cases

Table 4–3 provides multipliers that can be used to estimate confidence limits for an incidence rate, based on the Poisson distribution. Select the row that corresponds

Table 4–3. Rate Multipliers to Obtain 95% Poisson Confidence Limits for an Incidence Rate That Is Based on 100 or Fewer Cases

COUNT	Multipliers LOWER	Multipliers UPPER	COUNT	Multipliers LOWER	Multipliers UPPER	COUNT	Multipliers LOWER	Multipliers UPPER
1	0.025	5.572	35	0.697	1.391	68	0.777	1.268
2	0.121	3.611	36	0.701	1.384	69	0.778	1.266
3	0.206	2.922	37	0.704	1.378	70	0.780	1.263
4	0.273	2.560	38	0.708	1.373	71	0.781	1.261
5	0.325	2.333	39	0.711	1.367	72	0.782	1.259
6	0.367	2.176	40	0.715	1.362	73	0.784	1.257
7	0.402	2.060	41	0.718	1.357	74	0.785	1.255
8	0.432	1.970	42	0.721	1.352	75	0.787	1.254
9	0.457	1.898	43	0.724	1.347	76	0.788	1.252
10	0.480	1.839	44	0.727	1.342	77	0.789	1.250
11	0.499	1.789	45	0.730	1.338	78	0.790	1.248
12	0.517	1.747	46	0.732	1.334	79	0.792	1.246
13	0.533	1.710	47	0.735	1.330	80	0.793	1.245
14	0.547	1.678	48	0.737	1.326	81	0.794	1.243
15	0.560	1.649	49	0.740	1.322	82	0.795	1.241
16	0.572	1.624	50	0.742	1.318	83	0.796	1.240
17	0.583	1.601	51	0.745	1.315	84	0.798	1.238
18	0.593	1.580	52	0.747	1.311	85	0.799	1.237
19	0.602	1.562	53	0.749	1.308	86	0.800	1.235
20	0.611	1.544	54	0.751	1.305	87	0.801	1.233
21	0.619	1.529	55	0.753	1.302	88	0.802	1.232
22	0.627	1.514	56	0.755	1.299	89	0.803	1.231
23	0.634	1.500	57	0.757	1.296	90	0.804	1.229
24	0.641	1.488	58	0.759	1.293	91	0.805	1.228
25	0.647	1.476	59	0.761	1.290	92	0.806	1.226
26	0.653	1.465	60	0.763	1.287	93	0.807	1.225
27	0.659	1.455	61	0.765	1.285	94	0.808	1.224
28	0.665	1.445	62	0.767	1.282	95	0.809	1.222
29	0.670	1.436	63	0.768	1.279	96	0.810	1.221
30	0.675	1.428	64	0.770	1.277	97	0.811	1.220
31	0.680	1.419	65	0.772	1.275	98	0.812	1.219
32	0.684	1.412	66	0.773	1.272	99	0.813	1.217
33	0.689	1.404	67	0.775	1.270	100	0.814	1.216
34	0.693	1.397						

to the number of cases counted in the numerator of the rate. Then multiply the observed rate by the "lower" multiplier to get the lower 95% confidence limit, then by the "upper" multiplier to get the upper 95% confidence limit. Using Poisson-based confidence limits assumes constant hazard in the base of experience from which the cases arose.

Confidence limits for incidence rate estimates derived from multi-stage samples, such as those used in several national health surveys, require special statistical methods (Levy and Lemeshow, 1991; Korn and Graubard, 1999).

EXERCISES

1. Table 4–4 shows some fictitious data describing the frequency of hepatitis among high school students in a particular school district. Which of the following explanations could be compatible with the time trends seen in these data? (There may be more than one.)

   (a) More aggressive treatment, resulting in earlier and more frequent cures.
   (b) Adoption of a new treatment that, though it diminishes the severity of hepatitis symptoms, suppresses the immune response and thereby prolongs the clinical course of the disease.
   (c) Success of efforts to prevent new cases of hepatitis.
   (d) A shift toward the occurrence of more aggressive disease, leading to earlier and more frequent deaths among afflicted students.

Table 4–4. Hypothetical Data Showing Incidence and Prevalence of Hepatitis by Year in a Certain School District

YEAR	INCIDENCE[a]	PREVALENCE[b]
1985	24.5	41.8
1986	24.9	41.2
1987	23.8	40.9
1988	24.6	40.1
1989	24.1	38.4
1990	24.7	37.9
1991	24.2	35.3
1992	23.9	33.2
1993	25.1	29.8
1994	24.5	27.2

[a]Cases per 100,000 person-years
[b]Cases per 100,000 persons

Table 4–5. Prevalence of Low Birth Weight, by Town
and Mother's Race

	% of Babies Weighing <2500 Grams at Birth	
RACE	TOWN 1	TOWN 2
Black	12%	18%
White	6%	9%
All babies	8%	15%

2. In the early years of the AIDS epidemic, it was generally accepted that AIDS was almost always fatal. According to the Centers for Disease Control, the incidence of AIDS in the U.S. in 1990 was 17.2 cases per 100,000 person-years, yet the mortality rate in that year was only 12.4 deaths per 100,000 person-years. Can you reconcile these apparently conflicting data?

3. The local health department where you work has received funding to set up one new prenatal clinic in some needy area of the county. You and your colleagues decide that the birth prevalence of low birth weight will be used as the primary indicator of need. You are helping the department decide whether to put the clinic in Allenville or Bakertown. Allenville is predominantly African American, while Bakertown is predominantly white, and neither community contains any significant number of residents of other races. At your request, a data technician has compiled some statistics from birth certificate data for babies born in each town over the last two years. Unfortunately, in his haste, he forgot to write down which town was which. He shows you the results in Table 4–5.

   He apologizes and is about to set off to re-do his analysis and identify the towns. Instead, you ponder the data carefully, then thank him for giving you all the information you need to determine that the needier community is Allenville. How did you reach that conclusion?

4. You are a hospital epidemiologist working with intensive-care specialists to evaluate a new type of indwelling urinary catheter. The clinical team needs to know how the cumulative incidence of urinary tract infection (UTI) increases in relation to how long the catheter has been in place.

   During the month of September, 10 patients received the new catheter. Daily urine cultures were done on all patients. All patients were monitored until they developed a UTI, no longer needed an indwelling urinary catheter, were discharged from the intensive-care unit, or died, whichever came first. Their experience is summarized in Table 4–6. Based on these early data, what is your best estimate of the one-week cumulative incidence of UTI among patients who receive the new catheter?

Table 4–6. Use of New Urinary Catheter Among Ten Patients on an Intensive Care Unit

PATIENT NO.	CATHETER INSERTED ON	LAST URINE CULTURE ON	REASON FOR ENDING FOLLOW-UP
1	9/1	9/8	Discharged
2	9/2	9/5	Developed UTI
3	9/3	9/9	Died
4	9/5	9/8	Discharged
5	9/5	9/7	Developed UTI
6	9/8	9/13	Catheter no longer needed
7	9/9	9/13	Developed UTI
8	9/11	9/19	Died
9	9/13	9/18	Catheter no longer needed
10	9/14	9/20	Developed UTI

ANSWERS

1. Inspection of the data shows that the prevalence of hepatitis was declining, while its incidence was stable. The approximate relation $P \approx ID \cdot \bar{d}$ tells us that the decline in prevalence could be accounted for by a decline in disease duration, however. Explanations (a) and (d) are compatible with this assertion. Explanation (b) is not, since it implies an increase in duration of disease, not a decrease. Explanation (c) suggests that incidence should have been dropping, which it was not.

2. In order for the approximate relation (mortality) $\approx$ (incidence) $\times$ (case fatality) to hold true numerically, incidence and case-fatality rates must be stable over a period of time so that a steady-state situation can develop. This requirement is clearly not met for AIDS: in 1990, its incidence was still rising sharply. Moreover, although AIDS was usually fatal at that time, death did not occur immediately after diagnosis but occurred months or years later. Deaths occurring in 1990 might thus have consisted primarily of patients diagnosed in, say, 1988. The rise in incidence over that period tells us that there were fewer new AIDS patients in 1988 than in 1990.

3. You knew that the overall rate (here, the overall prevalence of weighing under 2500 grams at birth) in a population is always a weighted average of subgroup-specific rates within that population, and that the weights are the proportion of the population in each subgroup. Because most of Allenville's pregnant mothers were African American, the prevalence for "All babies" in Allenville must lie closer to the prevalence for African American mothers than to the prevalence for white mothers. For Town no. 1, the overall prevalence of 8% is closer to the 6% for whites than it is to the 12% for African Americans, so Town no. 1 cannot

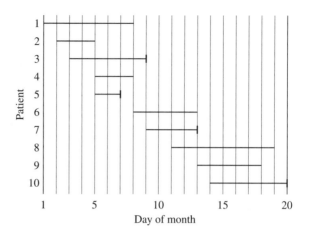

Figure 4-6. Catheter Use by Day of Month in Patients on an Intensive Care Unit.

be Allenville; it must be Bakertown. For Town no. 2, the overall prevalence of 15% is closer to the 18% prevalence for African Americans than to the 9% prevalence in whites, which makes sense if it is, in fact, Allenville.

Having identified which town is which, it is easy to decide which is needier. The race-specific and overall prevalences of low birth weight are all higher in Allenville, so it gets the clinic.

4. Four cases of UTI occurred among 10 patients. But most patients were under observation for less than a full week. Discharge, death, and discontinuation of the catheter were all forms of *censoring*. This is a job for the Kaplan-Meier method. Diagrammatically, the experience of these 10 patients was as shown in Figure 4–6.

The day of the month on which each patient entered and left the study are not really relevant, however. Instead, we are interested in the cumulative incidence of UTI in relation to *time since catheter insertion*. We can change the time scale by aligning the leftmost end of each patient's line along the vertical axis in a new plot. Arithmetically, this is done by just calculating how many days transpired between catheter insertion and the last urine culture for each patient and letting this be the length of that patient's line in the new figure, shown in Figure 4–7.

From these data, we can estimate the proportion "surviving" (*not* having developed a UTI) on each day since catheter insertion, as shown in Table 4–7. The estimated seven-day cumulative incidence is $(1 - .514) = .486$. In other words, our best estimate is that 48.6% of patients with the new catheter develop a UTI within seven days after its insertion.

Table 4–7. Proportion of Patients Remaining Free of Urinary Tract Infection, by Days Since Catheter Insertion

DAYS SINCE INSERTION	NO. STILL UNDER OBSERVATION	NO. OF CASES	PROPORTION "SURVIVING"
0	10	0	1.000
1	10	0	1.000
2	10	1	$1.000 \times 9/10 = .900$
3	9	1	$.900 \times 8/9 = .800$
4	7	1	$.800 \times 6/7 = .686$
5	6	0	.686
6	4	1	$.686 \times 3/4 = .514$
7	2	0	.514

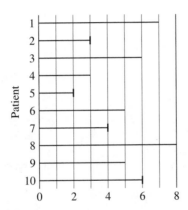

Figure 4–7. Duration of Catheter Use by Time Since Insertion in Patients on an Intensive Care Unit.

REFERENCES

Aalen OO. Heterogeneity in survival analysis. Stat Med 1988; 7:1121–37.

Aalen OO. Effects of frailty in survival analysis. Stat Methods Med Res 1994; 3:227–43.

Armitage P, Berry G. Statistical methods in medical research (3rd edition). London: Blackwell, 1994.

Breslow NE, Day NE. Statistical methods in cancer research. Vol. II—The design and analysis of cohort studies. Lyon, France: International Agency for Research on Cancer, 1987.

Checkoway H, Pearce NE, Crawford-Brown DJ. Research methods in occupational epidemiology. New York: Oxford, 1989.

Ciba-Geigy. Geigy scientific tables. Vol. 2. Introduction to statistics. Statistical tables. Mathematical formulae (8th ed.). Basel, Switzerland: Ciba-Geigy, 1982.

Clayton D. Some approaches to the analysis of recurrent event data. Stat Methods Med Res 1994; 3:244–62.

Cox DR. Regression models and life tables (with discussion). J R Stat Soc B 1972; 34:187–220.

Cumming RG, Kelsey JL, Nevitt MC. Methodologic issues in the study of frequent and recurrent health problems. Falls in the elderly. Ann Epidemiol 1990; 1:49–56.

Dowd MD, Langley J, Koepsell T, Soderberg R, Rivara FP. Hospitalizations for injury in New Zealand: prior injury as a risk factor for assaultive injury. Am J Public Health 1996; 86:929–34.

Gardner LI, Landsittel DP, Nelson NA. Risk factors for back injury in 31,076 retail merchandise store workers. Am J Epidemiol 1999; 150:825–33.

Glynn RJ, Buring JE. Ways of measuring rates of recurrent events. BMJ 1996; 312:364–67.

Glynn RJ, Stukel TA, Sharp SM, Bubolz TA, Freeman JL, Fisher ES. Estimating the variance of standardized rates of recurrent events, with application to hospitalizations among the elderly in New England. Am J Epidemiol 1993; 137:776–86.

Hosmer DW Jr, Lemeshow S. Applied survival analysis: regression modeling of time to event data. New York: Wiley and Sons, 1999.

Johnston BD, Grossman DC, Connell FA, Koepsell TD. High-risk periods for childhood injury among siblings. Pediatrics 2000; 105:562–68.

Kalbfleisch JD, Prentice RL. The statistical analysis of failure time data. New York: Wiley and Sons, 1980.

Kaplan EL, Meier P. Nonparametric estimation from incomplete observations. J Am Stat Assoc 1958; 53:457–81.

Kleinbaum DG. Survival analysis: a self-learning text. New York: Springer, 1996.

Korn EL, Graubard BI. Epidemiologic studies utilizing surveys: accounting for the sampling design. Am J Public Health 1991; 81:1166–73.

Korn EL, Graubard BI. Analysis of health surveys. New York: Wiley, 1999.

Levy PS, Lemeshow S. Sampling of populations: methods and applications. New York: Wiley and Sons, 1991.

Lindsay R, Silverman SL, Cooper C, Hanley DA, Barton I, Broy SB, et al. Risk of new vertebral fracture in the year following a fracture. JAMA 2001; 285:320–23.

Mendenhall W, Scheaffer RL, Wackerly DD. Mathematical statistics with applications (3rd edition). Boston: Duxbury Press, 1986.

Morris JN, Heady JA, Raffle PAB, Roberts CG, Parks JW. Coronary heart-disease and physical activity of work. Lancet 1953; 2:1053–57.

Morrison AS. Screening in chronic disease (2nd edition). New York: Oxford, 1992.

Nevitt MP, Ballard DJ, Hallett JW Jr. Prognosis of abdominal aortic aneurysms: a population-based study. N Engl J Med 1989; 321:1009–14.

Rosner B. Fundamentals of biostatistics (4th edition). New York: Duxbury Press, 1995.

Stukel TA, Glynn RJ, Fisher ES, Sharp SM, Lu-Yao G, Wennberg JE. Standardized rates of recurrent outcomes. Stat Med 1994; 13:1781–91.

Sturmer T, Glynn RJ, Kliebsch U, Brenner H. Analytic strategies for recurrent events in epidemiologic studies: background and application to hospitalization risk in the elderly. J Clin Epidemiol 2000; 53:57–64.

Wang HX, Fratiglioni L, Frisoni GB, Viitanen M, Winblad B. Smoking and the occurrence of Alzheimer's disease: cross-sectional and longitudinal data in a population-based study. Am J Epidemiol 1999; 149:640–44.

5

OVERVIEW OF STUDY DESIGNS

We're all of us guinea pigs in the laboratory of God.

Tennessee Williams

An epidemiologic study generally begins with a question. Once the research question has been specified, the next step in trying to answer it is to choose a study design.

A study design is a plan for selecting study subjects and for obtaining data about them. Study subjects in epidemiology are typically individual people, but at times they can be other kinds of observation units, such as social groups, places, time periods, or even published articles. Information on study subjects can come from pre-existing sources or can be gathered anew by various methods, including direct observation, interviews, examinations, or physiological measurements.

In principle, the number of possible study designs is infinite. But in practice, a few standard designs account for most epidemiologic research. Collectively, these standard designs offer enough flexibility to address a wide range of research questions. Knowledge of their pros and cons can usually guide the investigator to a study design that is well matched to a particular research question. This chapter seeks to provide a broad overview by introducing several standard designs and the terms that are commonly used to describe them and distinguish them from each other. Later chapters cover specific designs in more depth.

DESIGN TREE

Just as there are many possible study designs, there are many possible ways to classify them, depending on which features are highlighted. Figure 5–1 is a tree diagram that organizes designs according to important distinguishing features. Major branches of this tree include:

- *Descriptive* studies are undertaken without a specific hypothesis. They are often among the earliest studies done on a new disease, in order to

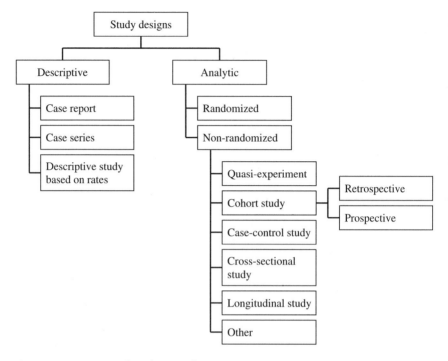

Figure 5–1. Major Epidemiologic Study Designs.

characterize it, quantify its frequency, and determine how it varies in relation to demographic characteristics, place, and time.

- *Analytic* studies are undertaken to test one or more specific hypotheses, usually about whether a certain exposure influences the risk of a disease. Analytic studies, in turn, can be divided into two main kinds:

    — In *randomized* studies, random chance is used to assign subjects to different exposure groups.

    — In *non-randomized* studies, no formal chance mechanism governs which subjects are exposed and which are not. Sometimes the investigator can assign subjects to different exposure conditions and elects to do so non-randomly. But often the investigator is merely an observer, with no control at all over subjects' exposure to the factor of interest.

Another factor that distinguishes study designs is the unit of study itself. In most epidemiologic research, subjects are individual people, each of whom can be determined to have been exposed or not and diseased or not. In *ecological* studies, the units of study are entire groups of people, as when mortality rates by state are examined in relation to per-capita income. As discussed in Chapter 12, ecological studies can themselves be categorized in much the same way as studies of individuals. In short, then, the unit of study can be regarded as a separate dimension, or "layer," on which studies can be classified, beyond those shown in Figure 5–1.

DESCRIPTIVE STUDIES

The hallmark of a descriptive study is that it is undertaken without a specific hypothesis.

Case Reports

A *case report* describes some newsworthy clinical occurrence, such as an unusual combination of signs and symptoms, experience with a novel treatment, or a sequence of events that may suggest previously unsuspected causal relationships. A case report can alert others to be on the lookout for similar occurrences, lead to more formal attempts to quantify the magnitude of the problem, or suggest a possible association for follow-up in other studies. It is generally reported simply as a clinical narrative.

Example: Trivier and colleagues (2001) reported the occurrence of fatal aplastic anemia in an 88-year-old man who had taken clopidogrel, a relatively new drug that inhibits platelet aggregation. Other chemically related drugs had been associated with aplastic anemia, and the victim had no history of exposure to other known causes of the disease. The authors speculated that his fatal illness may have been caused by clopidogrel and wished to alert other clinicians to a possible adverse effect of the drug.

Strictly speaking, a case report may not fully qualify as a "study design." It often results from serendipity rather than a planned strategy for answering a research question that was specified in advance. Nonetheless, a case report can often provide the first empirical evidence of a possible new problem or association.

Case Series

A case report shows that something can happen once; a *case series* shows that it can happen repeatedly. A case series also provides an opportunity to identify common features among multiple cases and to describe patterns of variability among them.

Example: After bovine spongiform encephalopathy (BSE, or "mad cow disease") appeared in British cattle in 1987, there was concern that it might spread to humans. A special surveillance unit was set up to study Creutzfeld-Jakob disease (CJD), a rare and usually fatal progressive dementia in humans that shares some clinical and pathological features with BSE. British neurologists and neuropathologists who encountered cases of CJD were asked to notify the unit about them. In 1996, investigators at the unit described ten cases that met pathological criteria for CJD but had all occurred at unusually young ages, showed distinctive clinical manifestations, and on pathological examination had extensive prion protein plaques throughout the brain, resembling those found in animal brain diseases known to be of infectious origin (Will et al., 1996). The authors expressed concern that this new variant form of CJD could represent human infection by the infectious agent of BSE. They recommended further epidemiologic and laboratory research to evaluate this possibility.

As noted in Chapter 2, case series that include all eligible cases in a defined population can be of special value because they avoid the selection bias that can accompany referral of certain kinds of patients to a particular clinical center. Extrapolating results from one setting to another must always be done with caution, but one can at least be more confident that the cases in a population-based case series are representative of cases in the setting where they arose.

Descriptive Studies Based on Rates

A *descriptive study based on rates* combines data on a population-based set of cases with denominator data. It quantifies the burden of disease on a population, using incidence, prevalence, mortality, or other measures of disease frequency as discussed in Chapter 3. Most such studies use data from existing sources, such as birth and death certificates, ongoing disease registries or surveillance systems, or periodic health surveys. New data collection may be undertaken if the problem is important enough and there are no satisfactory pre-existing data.

This kind of descriptive epidemiologic study often involves exploratory comparisons of disease frequency in relation to personal characteristics, place, and time. Ordinarily these comparisons are made without any advance prediction about what they might show, so the term *descriptive* fits. Descriptive studies can be a rich source of hypotheses that lead to later analytic studies, as illustrated in Chapter 7.

Example: Schwarz and colleagues (1994) conducted a descriptive epidemiologic study of injuries in a predominantly African-American part of Philadelphia. They set up their own injury-surveillance system through hospital emergency departments and vital records in order to capture nearly all fatal or medically treated non-fatal injuries among residents of the study area. Denominator data came from the U.S. census. The findings called attention to the high incidence of intentional interpersonal injury in the inner city and the high risk of recurrent interpersonal injury among persons with an initial injury.

ANALYTIC STUDIES

An analytic study is undertaken to test a hypothesis. In epidemiology, the hypothesis typically concerns whether a certain *exposure* causes a certain *outcome,* such as whether cigarette smoking causes lung cancer. Diagrammatically:

Figure 5–2   Exposure $\xrightarrow{\text{?}}$ Outcome

The term *exposure* is used very generally in epidemiology to refer to any trait, behavior, environmental factor, or other characteristic being investigated as a possible cause. Other essentially synonymous terms include *potential risk factor, putative cause, independent variable,* or *predictor.*

The outcome in epidemiologic studies of disease etiology is occurrence of a disease. But the same research designs that can be used to study disease etiology can also be used to study disease consequences. For example, a randomized trial can be used to determine whether receiving a new vaccine reduces the risk of developing a disease, and a randomized trial can also be used to study whether one treatment is better than another at prolonging survival among patients who develop the disease. The broader term *outcome* thus has the advantage of applying to both etiological and clinical studies. Essentially synonymous terms for *outcome* include *effect, end-point,* or *dependent variable.*

The directional arrow between *exposure* and *outcome* in the preceding diagram is worth noting. It indicates that the hypothesis behind an analytic study usually concerns whether the exposure actually *causes* the outcome, not merely whether the two are associated. Chapter 8 covers various kinds of evidence that support an inference of causality, but one firm requirement is that the exposure must *precede* the outcome in time. As we shall see, some analytic study designs provide stronger evidence than others about whether this condition is met.

Because an analytic study usually focuses from its outset on a particular exposure and a particular outcome, the researcher can choose among alternative study designs based in part on characteristics of that exposure and outcome. Two key factors are *(1)* whether the exposure is potentially modifiable by the investigator, and *(2)* how common the exposure and outcome are expected to be. Special opportunities or barriers, such as availability of a rich pre-existing data set or peculiarities of the study setting, may also greatly influence the choice of a design.

Randomized Trials

Randomized trials occupy a special place among epidemiologic research designs. Other things being equal, results from randomized trials can offer a more solid basis for an inference of cause and effect than results obtained from any other study design. The design's key feature is that a formal chance mechanism is used to assign participants either to receive an intervention of interest or to serve as a control. Subjects are then followed over time to measure one or more outcomes, such as occurrence of a disease. Chapter 13 covers randomized trials in some depth.

A simple two-arm randomized trial is diagrammed in Figure 5–3. From some source of potential study subjects, such as patients receiving care from a certain

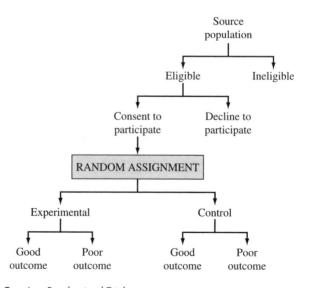

Figure 5–3. Two-Arm Randomized Trial.

clinic, candidates are screened for eligibility. Those found eligible are asked to give their informed consent to participate in the trial. Consenting subjects are then randomized by a formal chance mechanism to one of two groups, here called *experimental* and *control*. Subjects in the experimental arm receive a study intervention to be evaluated; those in the control arm may receive no intervention, a placebo, a specific alternative treatment, or usual care. Both groups are then followed over time, and the incidence of one or more outcomes is compared between groups.

Example: Bacterial vaginosis affects an estimated 800,000 pregnant women each year in the U.S. and has been found to be associated with premature birth and other pregnancy complications. To determine whether treatment with antibiotics could reduce the incidence of adverse pregnancy outcomes, Carey and colleagues (2000) screened 29,625 pregnant women to identify 1953 who had bacterial vaginosis, met certain other eligibility criteria, and consented to participate. These women were randomly assigned to receive either *(1)* two 2-gram doses of the antibiotic metronidazole, or *(2)* two doses of a similar-appearing placebo. Bacterial vaginosis cleared up in 78% of women in the metronidazole group, but in only 37% of women in the placebo group. Nonetheless, pre-term delivery proved to occur with almost equal frequency in both groups: 12.2% in the metronidazole group vs. 12.5% in the placebo group. Pre-term labor, postpartum infections in the mother or infant, and admission to the neonatal intensive care unit were also about equally common in both groups. The results suggested that: *(1)* treatment with metronidazole was ineffective for preventing pregnancy complications among women with bacterial vaginosis, and *(2)* the associations previously found between bacterial vaginosis and pregnancy complications may not have been causal after all.

Randomization generally provides excellent control over confounding (discussed below), even by factors that may be hard to measure or that may be unknown to the investigator. A difference in outcomes between groups formed by randomization that exceeds the limits of chance can be ascribed with high confidence to the difference in exposure that the study was designed to investigate. Randomized trials also provide information on the actual incidence of outcome events, because they involve prospective monitoring of two or more defined groups over time. Finally, as illustrated by the bacterial vaginosis study, they can be used to compare multiple outcomes between treatment arms without having to alter the basic study design.

For all their virtues, randomized trials have not been the source of data underlying most inferences regarding disease causation. For many exposures of concern, such as cigarette smoking or water pollution, it is neither ethical nor feasible to allow chance to dictate which persons are to incur them. Also, randomized trials can be too expensive or impractical if the primary outcome of interest is rare, or if long periods of follow-up would be required before intervention effects appear.

Non-randomized Studies

In non-randomized studies, regardless of what the exposure of concern is—a genetic trait, a lifestyle choice, a feature of the physical or social environment, or whatever—the researcher must assume that it is not distributed at random in the population. Inevitably there are many systematic differences between exposed and non-exposed persons, and some of the characteristics on which they differ may also be risk factors for disease in their own right. Hence a key methodological issue in all non-randomized studies is *confounding*—distortion of the exposure–outcome association due to their mutual association with another factor. This section considers only the basic layout of several standard non-randomized study designs, leaving a fuller discussion of confounding to Chapter 11.

Except for non-randomized intervention studies, non-randomized study designs are sometimes termed *observational* studies, because the investigator plays the more passive role of observer rather than experimenter.

Non-randomized intervention studies

In a *non-randomized intervention trial* or *quasi-experiment,* the investigator actually controls the assignment of study subjects to either an experimental or a control condition, but elects to do so by a process other than randomization. (The term *quasi-experiment* distinguishes these studies from randomized trials, which have been called "true" experiments [Campbell and Stanley, 1966].) This design is most useful when the investigator has some control over which study subjects are exposed to which condition, but when cost, logistics, or political considerations preclude using randomization to make those assignments. A design diagram would look just like Figure 5–3, except that "random assignment" would be replaced by "non-random allocation."

Example: The Minnesota Heart Health Program sought to test whether a community cardiovascular health promotion campaign could reduce the incidence of coronary heart disease and stroke (Luepker et al., 1996). Three Midwestern communities were chosen as intervention sites, based in part on how far they were from study headquarters in Minneapolis. Proximity to the investigators' home institution affected the cost and logistics of mounting the intervention campaign. Three other matched communities were selected as controls. A multi-component prevention program was then implemented over 5–6 years in the intervention sites only. The incidence of coronary heart disease declined about 1.8% per year among men and 3.6% per year among women in intervention communities, but similar declines were observed in the control communities. Stroke incidence remained almost stable in all sites. The investigators concluded that the intervention program had had no appreciable effect on the occurrence of coronary heart disease or stroke.

Note that the primary units of study in this example were entire communities, which were assigned non-randomly to intervention or control conditions.

The main problem with non-randomized trials is that the non-random process of subject allocation can cause the comparison groups to differ systematically on risk factors for study outcomes. This places a greater burden on the researcher to deal with confounding, and it can be a challenge to identify, measure, and control for all relevant confounding factors. Because confounding is also a key methodological issue in observational studies, non-randomized trials are often regarded as more closely akin to cohort studies (see below) than to randomized trials.

Cohort studies

A *cohort study* involves comparing disease incidence over time between groups that are found to differ on their exposure to a factor of interest. The design is discussed in depth in Chapter 14.

Example: During a 14-month period beginning in May, 1968, about 47,000 women of reproductive age were identified from among the patients of 1,400 British physicians who were members of the Royal College of General Practitioners (Beral et al., 1988). By design, half of these women were using oral contraceptives at the time of their recruitment, and the other half were never-users. Over the next two decades, participating physicians provided updated data twice a year on all study women who remained under their care, including month-by-month data on oral contraceptive use and on occurrence of various fatal or non-fatal illnesses. For analysis, each woman contributed person-time as long as she remained under surveillance. Women who were initially in the never-user group but who later began using oral contraceptives were switched to the ever-user group at that time.

Table 5–1 summarizes the incidence of cancers of the reproductive tract in ever-users and never-users. Oral contraceptive use was associated with two to three times higher incidence of cervical cancer and with lower incidence of cancer

Table 5–1. Incidence of Reproductive Malignancies among Women in the Royal College of General Practitioners Oral Contraception Study

| | No. of Cases | | Incidence[a] | | Rate Ratio $(A) \div (B)$ | | Rate Difference[a] $(A) - (B)$ | |
| | EVER- | NEVER- | EVER-USERS | NEVER-USERS | | | | |
CANCER TYPE	USERS	USERS	(A)	(B)	EST.	(95% CI)	EST.	(95% CI)
Uterine cervix								
Invasive	49	16	18	10	1.8	(1.0, 3.3)	8	(0.3, 15.7)
In situ	173	34	62	21	2.9	(2.0, 4.1)	41	(27.3, 54.7)
Uterine body	2	16	1	6	0.2	(0.0, 0.7)	−5	(−8.9, −1.1)
Ovary	12	18	5	9	0.6	(0.3, 1.4)	−4	(−10.6, 2.6)

[a] Cases per 100,000 woman-years, adjusted for age, parity, smoking, social class, number of previously normal cervical smears, and history of sexually transmitted disease.
[*Source:* Beral et al. (1988).]

of the body of the uterus. The incidence of ovarian cancer was slightly lower in ever-users, but this difference was easily compatible with chance given no true difference.

Cohort studies can be distinguished as *prospective* and *retrospective*. Figure 5–4 shows both. The difference concerns when the outcomes of interest occur relative to when the study is begun. As shown at the figure's lower left, in a prospective cohort study, the study is initiated before any of the outcomes that will eventually be tabulated have occurred. The Royal College of General Practitioners Oral Contraception Study was a prospective cohort study: recruitment began in 1968, and all of the cancer cases of interest occurred in subsequent years as the research proceeded.

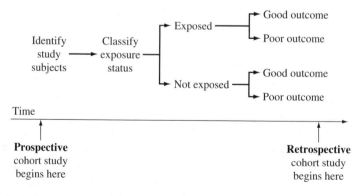

Figure 5–4. Retrospective and Prospective Cohort Studies.

In contrast, here is an example of a retrospective cohort study:

Example: To assess the possible carcinogenic effects of radio-frequency signals emitted by cellular telephones, Johansen and colleagues (2001) conducted a retrospective cohort study in Denmark. The two companies that operate cellular telephone networks in Denmark furnished names and addresses for all 522,914 of their individual clients during the years from 1982 to 1995. The investigators then matched these records to the Danish Central Population Register, which contains a unique 10-digit number for each person and information on vital status and emigration. After removing non-matches, duplicates, persons outside the study's age limits or geographic catchment area, and persons who asked not to be studied, 420,095 cellular telephone subscribers remained and formed the exposed cohort. All other Danish citizens during the study years became the non-exposed cohort. The list of personal identification numbers for exposed-group members was then matched to the nationwide cancer registry. The resulting data allowed calculation of cancer incidence rates for the exposed and unexposed cohorts. Overall, 3,391 cancers had occurred among cellular telephone subscribers, compared to 3,825 cases expected based on the age, gender, and calendar-year distribution of their person-time at risk. In particular, no excess risk was found for cancers of the brain, nervous system, salivary glands, or leukemia, which had been identified a priori as key outcomes. Much of the overall deficit of cases was in lung cancer and other smoking-related cancers.

A key feature of the Danish study is that the cancer cases of interest *had already occurred* by the time the study got underway in the late 1990s. Referring again to Figure 5–4, the study was conceived and begun at a time corresponding to the marker on the lower right. The investigators' work was to reconstruct from existing records a cohort study that, in effect, had already taken place. They were "looking back" at past events, which is why the term *retrospective* fits their design. Yet it was still a cohort study, because the initial step was to form exposed and non-exposed cohorts by looking even farther back in time to classify people's cellular telephone use before determining whether they went on to develop cancer.

Cohort studies have several generic strengths:

- Because they involve monitoring people over time for disease occurrence, cohort studies provide estimates of the absolute incidence of disease in exposed and non-exposed persons. For example, Table 5–1 showed that the incidence of cancer of the body of the uterus was several times higher in women who never used oral contraceptives than among ever-users, but the results also showed that this form of cancer was still quite rare among never-users, at 6 cases per 100,000 woman-years. This information could be helpful to women who are deciding whether to use oral contraceptives, and to the physicians who advise them.

- Like intervention trials, cohort studies also facilitate studying multiple outcomes. In both examples, the incidence of many different cancer types—and, for that matter, of other non-malignant diseases—could be compared between the same exposed and non-exposed groups without complicating the basic study design.

- By design, exposure status is determined and recorded before disease has been identified in any subjects. In most instances, this feature provides unambiguous information about whether exposure preceded disease, as required for a causal inference.

- Cohort studies are well suited to studying rare exposures. This is because the relative number of exposed and non-exposed persons in the study need not necessarily reflect true exposure prevalence in the population at large. In the oral-contraception study, for example, two equal-sized groups of oral contraceptive users and never-users were chosen at the outset, even though the population prevalence of oral contraceptive use among age-eligible women was probably much less than 50% at the time. Oral contraceptive users were deliberately oversampled. At the extreme, *all* available exposed persons can be studied—such as those with a rare occupational exposure—while only a fraction of many available non-exposed persons are studied.

Like intervention trials, prospective cohort studies are an inefficient way to study rare outcomes or outcomes that appear only long after exposure. These problems can be overcome with very large study populations or by monitoring disease occurrence in them for a prolonged period. The oral-contraception example shows that this strategy is possible, given sufficient resources and time. But even then, so few cases of some cancers (such as ovarian cancer) occurred that the study could not determine for certain whether the risk of developing such cancers varies importantly in relation to oral contraceptive use.

When a retrospective cohort study is possible, it can sometimes provide a way around these limitations. As the Danish cellular-telephone study illustrates, retrospective cohort studies depend critically on being able to get good exposure and outcome data, usually from pre-existing sources. Without computerized telephone company records and a population-based cancer registry, such a study would have been almost impossible. With them, almost everyone in Denmark became a subject in a huge, multi-year observational study that could be completed relatively quickly and at low cost.

Yet, while a prospective cohort study may involve opportunities to gather new data from study subjects on potential confounding factors, retrospective cohort

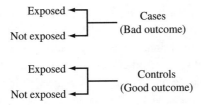

Figure 5–5. Case-Control Study Design.

studies are much more limited to available data. In the Danish study, for example, the paucity of lung cancer and other smoking-related cancers among cellular-telephone users raised the possibility that smoking was less common among users, but there was no ready way to assess or adjust for this potential confounding factor from data available in telephone-company billing records.

Case-control studies

A *case-control study* involves comparing the frequency of past exposure between *cases* who develop the disease (or other outcome of interest) and *controls* chosen to reflect the frequency of exposure in the underlying population at risk from which the cases arose. Often, the controls are simply persons who do not have the disease being studied. Figure 5–5 shows a diagram of the case-control design, which is discussed more fully in Chapter 15.

Example: Muscat and colleagues (2000) sought to test the hypothesis that cellular telephone use affects the risk of brain cancer. From 1994 to 1998, at five academic medical centers in the U.S., they recruited 469 cases aged 18 to 80 years with newly diagnosed cancer originating in the brain. Controls ($n = 422$) were inpatients without brain cancer at those hospitals, excluding patients with leukemia or lymphoma. Controls were sampled to match the cases on age, sex, race, and month of admission. Each case and control was then interviewed about any past subscription to a cellular telephone service. Those who had subscribed were asked about years of use, hours of use per month, brand of telephone used, and other details. During the first study year, interviews were conducted with a proxy respondent if the case or control could not be interviewed. Overall, 14.1% of cases and 18.0% of controls reported ever having had a subscription for cellular telephone service. After adjusting for age, sex, race, education, study center, month and year of interview, and whether a proxy respondent was interviewed, the risk of developing brain cancer in a cellular-telephone user was estimated to be 0.85 times as great as in a non-user (95% confidence interval, 0.6–1.2). Neither were any notable associations found between case/control status and years of use, hours of use per month, or cumulative hours of use.

At first, a case-control study may appear to be attacking the problem backwards by proceeding from effect to cause. The paradox can be resolved, however, by noting that two different time sequences are at play. One is the causal chain of events leading to the disease or other outcome. As always, to qualify as a cause, the exposure must precede the outcome in a subject's lifetime. In the above example, the investigators asked only about cellular telephone use that had occurred prior to the diagnosis of brain cancer in cases, or for a similar time period in controls.

The other time sequence to consider is the order in which information is gathered on exposure and disease in the process of carrying out the study. Here the first step is to ascertain a subject's status on the outcome, in order to determine whether he or she qualifies as a case or control. Often cases are scarce while potential controls are plentiful, so all eligible cases may be included but only a fraction of potential controls. The second step is then to gather information about past exposure for each case and control.

Newcomers to epidemiologic study designs sometimes wonder how case-control studies differ from retrospective cohort studies, inasmuch as both designs consider exposure-outcome associations involving cases that have already occurred. The distinction between them concerns how subjects are sampled to form the comparison groups:

- In a retrospective cohort study, the first step is to form comparison groups according to *exposure*. Then disease frequency is ascertained and compared between the exposed and non-exposed groups. The relative sizes of the exposed and non-exposed groups can be chosen by the investigator and may or may not reflect the true frequency of exposure in the population at large. If the exposure of interest is rare, a reasonable choice may be to include all exposed persons and only a fraction of the many non-exposed persons.
- In a case-control study, the first step is to form comparison groups according to *outcome*—i.e., disease status in a study of disease etiology. Then exposure data are gathered and compared between the case and control groups. The relative sizes of the case and control groups can be chosen by the investigator and usually do not reflect the true frequency of disease in the population at large. In fact, many case-control studies include all available cases but only a small fraction of the many available non-cases.

To see this distinction in action, contrast the design of the two studies just described—one by Johansen et al. (2001), the other by Muscat et al. (2000)—which both investigated the possible association between cellular telephone use and brain cancer.

Case-control studies have several generic strengths:

- They are well suited to studying rare diseases. This is because a study's ability to detect an association between exposure and the risk of a rare disease is usually limited mainly by the small number of cases available. Under a case-control design, the investigator can start by casting a wide net for cases, perhaps through surveillance in a large population at risk or over a long time period. All qualifying cases that are found can then be included. But gathering exposure data on *all* non-cases in the source population over the same time period is seldom necessary and would, in fact, be a waste of resources. Once the number of cases is set, it can be shown statistically that little additional information is gained by increasing the number of controls much beyond about three or four times the number of cases.

  To illustrate this point, Figure 5–6 shows how statistical power (i.e., the probability that a true exposure effect of a given magnitude would be detected as statistically significant) increases as the control:case ratio increases from 1 : 1 to 10 : 1 in a hypothetical case-control study. Other design features that would affect power are held fixed at certain arbitrary

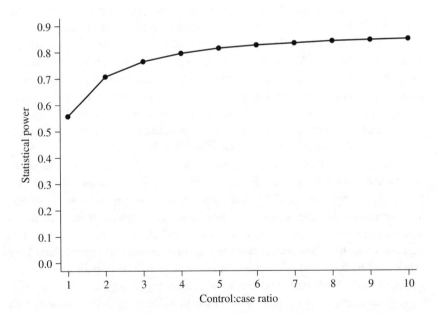

Figure 5–6. Statistical Power to Detect an Effect of Exposure in a Hypothetical Case-Control Study, as a Function of Control:Case Ratio. Assumptions: true odds ratio = 2.0, number of cases = 100, exposure prevalence in controls = 25%, two-tailed significance test at α = .05.

values. In this scenario, given 100 cases, studying 300 controls would yield almost as much statistical power to detect an exposure–disease association as studying 1000 controls or even 100,000 controls. Needless to say, gathering exposure data for 300 controls could be far less costly than gathering data for 100,000 controls. In short, the total number of study subjects—cases plus controls—may thus be quite modest under a case-control design.

- Case–control studies are also well suited to studying multiple exposures in relation to the same outcome. Once the case and control groups have been established, studying an additional exposure may be no more complicated than adding another question to an interview or another item to a data collection form.

- They can yield an answer relatively quickly even when exposure affects outcome only after a long time period—an advantage they share with retrospective cohort studies. The reason is that case-control studies begin by ascertaining the outcome, and by that time any long delay between exposure and outcome has already occurred.

Among their limitations, case-control studies do not directly yield information about the absolute risk of disease in exposed or unexposed persons. Instead, the frequency of disease *within the study population* merely reflects the investigator's choice of a control:case ratio, not the true frequency of disease in the population at large. As shown in Chapter 15, however, it is nearly always possible to estimate the *ratio* of risk in exposed persons to the risk in non-exposed persons directly from case-control data, even though neither the numerator nor the denominator of that ratio can itself be estimated. Moreover, external information about disease incidence often can be combined with results from a case-control study to estimate absolute risk in exposed and non-exposed individuals.

Many case-control studies, like that conducted by Muscat and colleagues on cellular telephone use and brain cancer, rely on interviews with cases and controls to ascertain past exposure status. In most instances, the cases are well aware that they have developed the disease, and this knowledge can influence their recall and/or reporting of past exposures. Cases may "ruminate" about the past in search of an explanation for their health misfortune and report an exposure that would have been overlooked or dismissed by a control. Alternatively, cases may purposefully deny a socially undesirable past exposure, such as a history of risky sexual behavior, if they are seeking to avoid blame. In either situation, differences in reporting of the same exposure by cases and controls is known as *recall bias*. Further discussion of recall bias, and of other sources of error in measuring exposure status in case-control studies, can be found in Chapter 15.

Cross-sectional studies

All of the analytic study designs described so far consider only exposures that precede the outcome in time. Intervention trials and cohort studies establish the exposure status of all subjects before any outcomes have occurred, while case-control studies limit themselves to exposures that occur prior to becoming a case.

In contrast, the distinguishing feature of a *cross-sectional study* is that exposure and outcome are ascertained as of the same point or period in time:

Figure 5–7

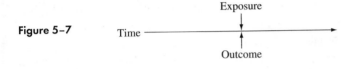

Example: Andersen and colleagues (1998) studied 4,063 children aged 8 to 16 years who had participated in the National Health and Nutrition Examination Survey to assess the relationship between television-watching and body-mass index, a measure of fatness. At a single examination session, each child was asked standardized questions about usual amount of television viewing. Height, weight, and other anthropometric measurements were also taken. Boys and girls who reported watching four or more hours of television per day had significantly greater mean body-mass indexes than boys and girls who reported watching fewer than two hours of television per day.

This study found an association between fatness and watching more television, but it was not designed to determine which came first. Causality could work in either direction: prolonged physical inactivity from watching television could lead to fatness, or fatness could make a child less inclined to engage in vigorous exercise and more inclined to watch television.

Potential ambiguity about the direction of causality is a common limitation of cross-sectional studies. But sometimes the causal arrow can only plausibly point in one direction—for example, if a cross-sectional study finds an association between a genetic marker and disease, it may not be possible that disease occurrence would have caused the genetic marker to appear or disappear.

Cross-sectional studies also characterize the exposure and disease status of study subjects as of a certain point in time or during the same short time interval. Cases thus found are *prevalent* cases, not incident cases. As noted in Chapter 4, this sampling scheme tends to cause cases of longer duration to be relatively over-represented. Hence an association found between exposure and disease in a cross-sectional study may actually represent an association with disease chronicity rather than with disease incidence.

Longitudinal studies

A longitudinal study involves measuring the exposure or the outcome repeatedly over time on study subjects.

Example: Yanovski and colleagues (2000) sought to test the common belief that the average American gains five pounds during the holiday period from Thanksgiving to New Year's Day. They recruited 195 adult volunteers and weighed each person four times over a period of several months: *(1)* in late September or early October, *(2)* in mid-November, *(3)* in early or mid-January, and *(4)* in late February or early March. A fifth weight was obtained one year after the initial weight on 165 subjects. Mean weight changes, in pounds, between consecutive observation times were: +0.4 (pre-holiday period), +0.8 (holiday period), −0.2 (post-holiday period), and +0.5 (March–September). They concluded that people may put on less weight over the holidays than previously thought, but that the weight gained is only partly shed after the holidays and probably contributes to the gradual increase in body weight that often occurs in adulthood.

In this example, "the holiday season" was the exposure. The outcome, weight gain, was compared on the same participants between exposed and non-exposed periods. There was no separate control group; subjects "served as their own controls." More elaborate longitudinal study designs may involve many more observations over time, or comparing patterns of change over time in one group with those in another group (Campbell and Stanley, 1966).

A pitfall with many longitudinal studies is that factors other than the exposure itself may be partly or fully responsible for observed differences in outcomes between exposed periods and non-exposed periods. This problem can be considered a form of confounding.

Other study designs

The study designs described above probably account for a large majority of epidemiologic research. Various other designs, however, are useful for specialized purposes. Three among many are noted here.

The *case-crossover* design can be used to study effects of transient exposures on risk of acute conditions, such as injury, stroke, or myocardial infarction (Maclure, 1991). The exposure status of cases at the time disease occurs is compared with their exposure status at one or more past reference times—e.g., the same day of the week and time of the day, but one week earlier. No disease-free control group is needed. The case-crossover design is discussed in more detail in Chapter 16.

The *case-cohort* design involves comparing the exposure status of cases with that of a random sample of people (the "subcohort") selected from the full population that generated the cases (Prentice, 1986). Unlike the case-control design, cases may also be members of the subcohort. This design permits comparison of several case groups to the same subcohort.

The *case-only* design can be useful for studying gene-environment interactions (Khoury and Flanders, 1996). Using data from cases only, the investigator examines the association between presence of a genetic marker and presence of an environmental exposure. If these two characteristics can be assumed to occur independently in the population at large, then their co-occurrence among cases (more than would be predicted from the frequency of each one alone among the cases) can be interpreted as evidence of gene–environment interaction. Other applications of the case-only design are described in Chapter 15.

EXERCISES

1. By the 1980s, several lines of evidence suggested that occurrence of a class of congenital abnormalities known as *neural tube defects* might be related to low intake of folic acid, a dietary vitamin, during pregnancy. Two studies that sought to test this hypothesis are described below:

   Milunsky and colleagues (1989) studied 22,776 pregnant mothers who were undergoing certain blood tests or amniocentesis about 16 weeks into the pregnancy. At that time, each woman completed a questionnaire about her use of vitamins or nutritional supplements during early pregnancy. Based on her responses, each woman was classified as exposed or not exposed to a multivitamin containing folic acid. All exposed and non-exposed women were then followed through the end of pregnancy, whether it ended with a live birth or with a spontaneous or induced abortion, to determine whether the offspring had a neural tube defect. The results showed that $39/11,944 = 3.3$ per 1000 babies had a neural tube defect among mothers who *had not* taken a folic acid supplement during the first six weeks of pregnancy, compared with $10/10,713 = 0.9$ per 1000 babies for women who *had* taken a folic acid supplement during the same period. The investigators estimated that the risk of having a baby with a neural tube defect was 73% lower for mothers who had taken a folic acid–containing multivitamin during the first six months of pregnancy, compared to never-users.

Mulinare and colleagues (1988) identified 347 babies with neural tube defects through a population-based birth defects registry in the Atlanta area. All had been born alive or stillborn during 1968–1980. Two comparison groups were used. The first was a sample of 2829 babies born without birth defects during the same years, identified through birth certificates for the study area. The second comparison group was a sample of babies born with birth defects other than a neural-tube defect. Telephone interviews were conducted with consenting mothers of babies in all three groups. They were asked about various pregnancy characteristics, including multivitamin use before and during pregnancy. The results showed that among mothers whose baby had a neural tube defect, 6.9% had taken multivitamins regularly during the three months before and three months after conception, compared to 14.5% among mothers of babies with no birth defect. They estimated that the risk of a neural tube defect was reduced by about 60% among mothers who used periconceptional multivitamins, compared to never-users. Findings using the second comparison group were similar.

(a) Identify the study design used in each study.

(b) What characteristics of neural tube defects made it attractive to study them with a case-control design? What characteristics made a cohort study design attractive?

(c) How did Milunsky et al. adapt their study to deal with the relatively low birth prevalence of NTDs?

(d) Which study was more susceptible to biased exposure assessment? What was done to deal with the problem?

(e) With regard to determining whether the association between use of folate/multivitamins and neural tube defects is causal, what key question is left unanswered by these two studies? Suggest a research design that could help resolve the issue.

2. During the years 1978–1983, 48 children with neonatal jaundice were born and treated at a hospital in Anchorage, Alaska. In 1987, an audiologist working at the hospital conducted a study comparing these children to others without neonatal jaundice. For each jaundiced baby, a comparison baby was chosen by selecting the next child of the same sex who had been born at the same hospital but who had not had neonatal jaundice. The audiologist then contacted the parents of children in both groups and arranged for each child to undergo a hearing test under the audiologist's supervision. The findings showed essentially no association between neonatal jaundice and diminished auditory acuity.

How would you classify this study design?

3. Cumming and colleagues (1997) reported results from a study of cataracts. All persons born before 1943 and residing in the Blue Mountains region near Sydney, Australia, were invited to make a single visit to a study clinic to undergo

a detailed eye examination. Over a two-year period, 3654 people did so. Lens photographs were used to detect and classify cataracts. During each person's visit to the study clinic, he/she was also asked about current use of inhaled corticosteroids, often used to treat asthma. Subcapsular cataracts proved to be 2.6 times more common among current users of these drugs than among non-users.

(a) How would you classify the study design?
(b) What limitations does this type of study design have for inferring whether use of inhaled corticosteroids causes cataracts?

ANSWERS

1. (a) The study by Milunsky and colleagues was a *prospective cohort study*. It was unusual because the frequency of the outcome (neural tube defect occurrence) was measured as prevalence at the time of pregnancy termination, rather than as incidence. The study by Mulinare and colleagues was a *case-control study*. It, too, was a bit unusual in that the investigators used two separate control groups.

(b) Neural tube defects are a fairly rare pregnancy outcome, making the case-control design a potentially efficient choice. But the time between exposure and outcome is short, which favors a cohort design.

(c) They used very large study population. They also used a fairly broad case definition that included not just cases discovered at birth (or stillbirth) but fetuses found to have an neural tube defect following an induced or spontaneous abortion.

(d) The Mulinare study was more susceptible to exposure measurement bias, which is a common problem in case-control studies. Because all case and control mothers knew at the time of the interview whether their infant had turned out to have a neural tube defect, they may have recalled perinatal vitamin use and dietary intake differently. The investigators therefore studied multivitamin use in a second control group, consisting of women whose infants had had other birth defects. Presumably any non-specific recall bias would influence exposure information in this second control group to a similar degree. The fact that the results were similar regardless of which control group was used provides reassurance that recall bias was not the sole basis for an association.

(e) Observational studies such as these leave open the possibility that some other characteristic of women who took folate, not the folate itself, accounted for the lower frequency of neural tube defects observed among their offspring. Probably the best way to settle this issue would be to conduct a randomized trial, giving folate to one group and placebo to the other. Under such a design, even unknown or difficult-to-measure factors other than folate that may affect risk should occur with nearly equal frequency in both groups. Although such a trial would probably be considered unethical now, one was already underway when these two studies were published. The participants were mothers who had previously borne a child with a neural tube defect and who were contemplating becoming pregnant again (MRC Vitamin Study Research Group, 1991). The findings confirmed those of the observational studies, showing a 72% decrease in neural tube defect occurrence in folate users.

2. This was a retrospective cohort study. Neonatal jaundice was the exposure; hearing impairment was the outcome of interest.

3. *(a)* This was a cross-sectional study. Each patient was observed only once, not over a period of time. Current exposure status and current disease status were both ascertained as of the time of each person's clinic visit.

   (b) i. We cannot be sure that exposure preceded disease onset.

   ii. From these data it would not be possible to disentangle a potential association between asthma and subcapsular cataracts from one between inhaled corticosteroids and subcapsular cataracts.

ACKNOWLEDGMENT

Parts of this chapter were adapted from Koepsell (2001).

REFERENCES

Andersen RE, Crespo CJ, Bartlett SJ, Cheskin LJ, Pratt M. Relationship of physical activity and television watching with body weight and level of fatness among children. Results from the Third National Health and Nutrition Examination Survey. JAMA 1998; 279:938–42.

Beral V, Hannaford P, Kay C. Oral contraceptive use and malignancies of the genital tract. Results from the Royal College of General Practitioners' Oral Contraception Study. Lancet 1988; 2:1331–35.

Campbell DT, Stanley JC. Experimental and quasi-experimental designs for research. New York: Rand McNally, 1966.

Carey JC, Klebanoff MA, Hauth JC, Hillier SL, Thom EA, Ernest JM, et al. Metronidazole to prevent preterm delivery in pregnant women with asymptomatic bacterial vaginosis. N Engl J Med 2000; 342:534–40.

Cumming RG, Mitchell P, Leeder SR. Use of inhaled corticosteroids and the risk of cataracts. N Engl J Med 1997; 337:8–14.

Johansen C, Boice J Jr, McLaughlin J, Olsen J. Cellular telephones and cancer—a nation-wide cohort study in Denmark. J Natl Cancer Inst 2001; 93:203–37.

Khoury MJ, Flanders WD. Nontraditional epidemiologic approaches in the analysis of gene–environment interaction: case-control studies with no controls! Am J Epidemiol 1996; 144:207–13.

Koepsell TD. "Selecting a study design for injury research." Chapter 7 in: Rivara FP, Cummings P, Koepsell TD, Grossman DC, Maier RV. Injury control: a guide to research and program evaluation. New York: Cambridge University Press, 2001.

Luepker RV, Rastam L, Hannan PJ, Murray DM, Gray C, Baker WL, et al. Community education for cardiovascular disease prevention. Morbidity and mortality results from the Minnesota Heart Health Program. Am J Epidemiol 1996; 144:351–62.

Maclure M. The case-crossover design: a method for studying transient effects on the risk of acute events. Am J Epidemiol 1991; 133:144–53.

Milunsky A, Jick H, Jick SS, Bruell CL, MacLaughlin DS, Rothman KJ, et al. Multivitamin/folic acid supplementation in early pregnancy reduces the prevalence of neural tube defects. JAMA 1989; 262:2847–52.

MRC Vitamin Study Research Group. Prevention of neural tube defects: results of the Medical Research Council Vitamin Study. Lancet 1991; 338:131–7.

Mulinare J, Cordero JF, Erickson JD, Berry RJ. Periconceptional use of multivitamins and the occurrence of neural tube defects. JAMA 1988; 260:3141–5.

Muscat JE, Malkin MG, Thompson S, Shore RE, Stellman SD, McRee D, et al. Handheld cellular telephone use and risk of brain cancer. JAMA 2000; 284:3001–7.

Prentice RL. A case-cohort design for epidemiologic cohort studies and disease prevention trials. Biometrika 1986; 73:1–11.

Schwarz DF, Grisso JA, Miles CG, Holmes JH, Wishner AR, Sutton RL. A longitudinal study of injury morbidity in an African-American population. JAMA 1994; 271:755–60.

Trivier JM, Caron J, Mahieu M, Cambier N, Rose C. Fatal aplastic anemia associated with clopidogrel. Lancet 2001; 357:446.

Will RG, Ironside JW, Zeidler M, Cousens SN, Estibeiro K, Alperovitch A, et al. A new variant of Creutzfeld-Jakob disease in the U.K. Lancet 1996; 347:921–25.

Williams T. Camino Real (Block Twelve). Norfolk, Conn.: New Directions, 1953.

Yanovski JA, Yanovski SZ, Sovik KN, Nguyen TT, O'Neil PM, Sebring NG. A prospective study of holiday weight gain. N Engl J Med 2000; 342:861–67.

6

SOURCES OF DATA ON DISEASE OCCURRENCE

Knowledge is of two kinds. We know a subject ourselves, or we know where we can find information upon it.

Samuel Johnson

Epidemiologists are often data scavengers. Using pre-existing data can allow a study to be done more cheaply, more quickly, and often on a larger scale than if new data collection were required.

As we have seen, most epidemiologic studies involve rates. All types of rates have a numerator and a denominator, which may come from different sources. Figure 6–1 gives an overview of several common sources through which disease cases can be identified. In other words, it shows sources of numerator data. The most suitable data source for a particular study depends partly on the nature of the disease: whether it is commonly fatal; whether it tends to occur only near the time of birth or later in life; whether it typically prompts victims to seek medical care, and if so, what kind of care is usually provided. It also depends on what kinds of pre-existing data are available in the study setting.

Denominator data for disease rates generally come from fewer sources. Sometimes the denominator can come from the same source that provides the numerator: for example, birth certificates can be used both to identify cases of some perinatal diseases and to characterize the population at risk. Otherwise, for geographically defined populations, such as residents of a city or state, census data or intercensal estimates are often available from the U.S. Census Bureau or from state or local government agencies. For administratively defined populations, such as enrollees of a health insurance plan or employees of a company, membership lists are usually available.

The problem with pre-existing information is that it was not necessarily collected with the researcher's needs in mind. Hence dealing with data limitations is often an important part of conducting and interpreting epidemiologic research. This chapter considers strengths and weaknesses of several commonly used kinds of pre-existing data, as well as some techniques for assessing and dealing with data limitations. It focuses mainly on data resources available in the United States.

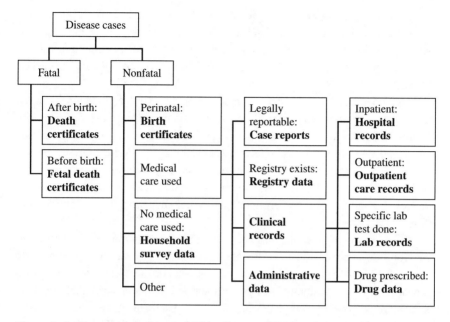

Figure 6-1. Common Data Sources for Identification of Disease Cases.

Use of pre-existing data in epidemiology has been revolutionized by rapid growth in information technology. Information once found only in reference libraries and obscure government publications is becoming almost instantly available over the Internet from almost anywhere in the world. The World Wide Web has become the first place to look for many kinds of health statistics, with traditional paper sources serving as a backup. The content and the specific location of information on the Web change often. Appendix 6A provides URLs for a few key Web sites that are likely to remain stable and that can be used as starting points for exploration.

NUMERATOR DATA

Death Records

Death and epidemiologic research have long gone hand-in-hand. John Graunt began analyzing parish "bills of mortality" in seventeenth century London, calling attention to what could be learned by tracking the number of deaths due to plague and other causes from year to year. Two centuries later, William Farr, as medical statistician for England and Wales, began compiling and disseminating cause-specific mortality statistics. Farr's system for organizing causes of death became the basis for the International Classification of Diseases (Thacker, 1994).

In modern times, a great deal of epidemiologic research continues to be based on mortality statistics. Some conditions, such as homicide and suicide, are fatal by definition. For some other diseases, the case fatality rate is very high—pancreatic cancer and amyotrophic lateral sclerosis, for example—rendering mortality a good approximation to incidence. Even for diseases that may or may not cause death, the fatal cases may arguably be those of greatest public health impact and those that we most want to prevent. As Farr put it, "Stone cold hath no fellow." (Fredrickson, 1968)

Registration of all deaths has been required by law in most developed countries for many years. A death certificate is also needed by survivors to claim life insurance, Social Security payments to next of kin, and other benefits. Hence, files of death certificates maintained by government offices in the developed world are believed to be virtually complete, and the data can span many decades.

In the U.S., the National Center for Health Statistics (NCHS) makes available a model death certificate that is used with minor modifications by all states and local jurisdictions in the United States. Its content and format are revised periodically; a near-final draft of the version intended for use in 2003 and beyond is shown in Appendix 6B. Personal information about the decedent is gathered and recorded by whoever is responsible for disposition of the body, usually the funeral director (National Center for Health Statistics, 1987). Cause-of-death information normally comes from the physician in attendance at the time of death. If there is any suspicion of foul play or suicide, if death occurred accidentally, or if no physician was in attendance, the case must legally be referred to a medical examiner (a physician, often a forensic pathologist) or coroner (a public official who is not necessarily a physician). The medical examiner or coroner decides whether an autopsy is necessary.

Cause-of-death information is recorded in a hierarchy that works back from immediate cause to underlying cause. For example, this section of the death certificate might contain *septic shock;* due to or as a consequence of *pneumococcal pneumonia;* due to or as a consequence of *bronchogenic carcinoma*. The last-listed cause in the sequence—here, bronchogenic carcinoma—is considered the *underlying* cause of death and used for compiling mortality statistics. Public-use data are also available that retain all causes listed in the hierarchy, which lessens the chance that a disease of interest is missed due to inconsistencies in how death certificates are completed or coded. Space is also provided for recording other significant coexisting medical conditions at the time of death.

The training and motivation of physicians in assigning cause of death is un-even (Messite and Stellman, 1996), and the certifying physician may not have com-plete medical knowledge of the case. Autopsies are rarely performed nowadays, and even when they are, the cause of death listed on the death certificate may not necessarily be updated to reflect autopsy results (Kircher et al., 1985). One fairly large study of 272 deaths with autopsy in Connecticut found a "major dis-agreement" between autopsy findings and the death certificate as to underlying cause of death for 29% of deaths (Kircher et al., 1985). Unfortunately, no widely used routine mechanism is in place to check the listed cause of death against other clinical information. For these reasons, cause-of-death data must be as-sumed to be subject to misclassification, the extent of which can vary by disease, reporting jurisdiction, or other factors (Gittelsohn and Royston, 1982). Validation substudies, as discussed below, are one way to gauge the extent of misclassifica-tion. Nonetheless, much useful knowledge has been gleaned even from imperfect death certificate data, so that an error in cause of death need not necessarily be a "fatal" flaw.

Coding and grouping of causes of death follows the International Classifica-tion of Diseases (ICD), discussed in Chapter 10. The ICD is revised about every 10 years by the World Health Organization (World Health Organization, 1992).

In the U.S., death certificates are filed with city and county health depart-ments, who check them for completeness and consistency and retain copies for local use. They are then forwarded to state vital statistics offices, where they are checked again and archived. States transmit death certificate data electron-ically to the National Center for Health Statistics. National mortality data are available to epidemiologists from NCHS in several forms, including traditional printed volumes (National Center for Health Statistics, 1993) and electronic me-dia containing a data record for each death but lacking personal identifiers. Custom tables of U.S. mortality statistics by age, sex, race, geographic area, and calendar year can be obtained over the Internet from CDC's WONDER system (Friede et al., 1993). Mortality data are also often available from state and local health departments.

NCHS established the National Death Index in 1979 (National Center for Health Statistics, 1997). Researchers can use it to determine who within a set of study subjects has died anywhere in the U.S. The user sends identifying information about subjects, such as name, date of birth, gender, or Social Security number to NCHS, then receives information about probable and possible matches to the National Death Index, including date of death, state of death, and (at extra cost) cause of death. Ascertainment of deaths by this means has been found to be nearly complete (Boyle and Decoufle, 1990). Other sources of vital status data are also available for selected populations, such as U.S. veterans (Boyko et al., 2000) and Social Security recipients (Boyle and Decoufle, 1990).

Example: Speizer and colleagues (1968) examined deaths due to asthma in England and Wales for the years 1952–1966. In contrast to trends in other countries, where asthma mortality had been stable or declining, rates in England and Wales had increased steadily after about 1960. Figure 6–2 shows that the rise had been especially marked among children aged 10 to 14. The researchers also noted that:

- Asthma in younger children can often be hard to distinguish from bronchiolitis, and asthma in adults can be confused with chronic obstructive pulmonary disease, but asthma among 10–14-year-olds would be less likely to be misclassified as another disease.
- The increase in deaths from asthma was not accompanied by a decrease in deaths from bronchitis, chronic respiratory disease, or pneumonia, as might be expected if shifts in diagnosis assignment or coding were the only explanation.
- There had been no concurrent increase in visits to physicians for asthma, suggesting that the rise in mortality was more likely due to increased case fatality than to increased incidence.
- The increase corresponded in time to rapid increases in sales of high-potency sympathomimetic aerosols as treatment for asthma.

Later research raised further concerns about the side effects of high-potency inhalers and led to greater caution in their therapeutic use. Even at its peak, asthma mortality in the highest-risk age group was only about 2.5 deaths per 100,000

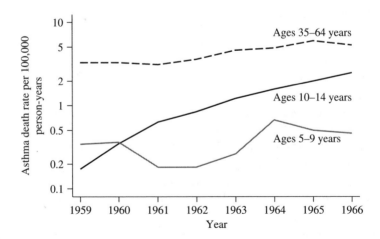

Figure 6–2. Death Rates from Asthma, by Age: England and Wales, 1959–1969 (based on Speizer et al., 1968).

person-years, making it extremely unlikely that an individual physician would see enough asthma deaths to notice the increase. But tracking deaths on a large-population scale made it possible to detect the epidemic.

Birth Records

Registration of births is also legally required in most developed countries. NCHS provides a model birth certificate, revised periodically, that is used with minor modifications by all U.S. states. A near-final draft of the version intended for use in 2003 and beyond is shown in Appendix 6C.

The upper *public* part of the model birth certificate contains identifying and demographic information about the baby and parents. The lower *confidential* part is retained by vital statistics offices, which publish statistics and make the data available for approved research. The lower part contains many items of interest to epidemiologists, including parents' race, education, and marital status; mother's pregnancy history; baby's birth weight, gestational age, and birth order; medical and behavioral factors for the current pregnancy; labor and delivery complications; obstetric procedures; complications affecting the newborn; and the presence of congenital anomalies.

Demographic information and mother's pregnancy history are recorded by the physician or midwife or by hospital personnel in consultation with the mother. These data are generally quite complete, except for items about the father if the mother is unmarried (Ventura et al., 2000). The physician or midwife records medical information in the confidential part, mostly by marking checkboxes. Unfortunately, an unmarked checkbox can mean either that the corresponding characteristic, procedure, or outcome was not present, or that the form was not thoroughly filled out. Validation studies have found considerable under-reporting on these items (Buescher et al., 1993). For example, of the estimated 4000 new cases of anencephaly or spina bifida in the U.S. in 1998, only about 30% were so identified on the birth certificate (Centers for Disease Control and Prevention, 2000a). Despite these data limitations, birth certificate data have been a rich information resource for epidemiologic research on maternal and infant health.

Example: Health authorities in Massachusetts wondered why the birth prevalence of low birth weight (under 2500 grams) was gradually rising in their state during the 1990s, even though maternal smoking during pregnancy, the teen birth rate, and infant mortality were all declining (Centers for Disease Control and Prevention, 1999a). Analysis of Massachusetts birth certificate data, summarized in Table 6–1, suggested an explanation. During the years 1989–1996, an increasing proportion of births were multiple births, such as twins and triplets.

Table 6–1. Birth Prevalence of Low Birth Weight (LBW), by Year and Plurality: Massachusetts, 1989–1996

YEAR	NO. OF BIRTHS	% LBW	Singletons % OF BIRTHS	% LBW	Twins % OF BIRTHS	% LBW	Triplets-Plus % OF BIRTHS	% LBW
1989	91,314	5.9	97.5	4.8	2.4	45.8	0.1	87.7
1990	92,460	5.8	97.4	4.7	2.5	46.5	0.1	88.9
1991	88,176	5.9	97.3	4.7	2.6	47.2	0.1	84.3
1992	87,202	5.9	97.2	4.7	2.7	45.3	0.2	87.2
1993	84,627	6.2	97.0	4.8	2.8	46.7	0.2	86.8
1994	83,758	6.4	96.9	5.0	2.8	47.7	0.3	92.5
1995	81,562	6.3	96.8	4.9	3.0	46.5	0.2	90.4
1996	80,167	6.4	96.5	4.8	3.3	48.2	0.2	86.1

[*Source:* Centers for Disease Control and Prevention (1999a).]

Each infant in a multiple birth is much more likely to weigh under 2500 grams than is a singleton infant. Within each plurality category, however, the birth prevalence of low birth weight had remained essentially unchanged. Further analysis of the birth certificate data indicated that much of the increase in multiple births had occurred among older, better-educated mothers, many of whom had used fertility drugs or assisted-reproduction technologies.

Fetal Death Records

Most states require registration of fetal deaths if the fetus had reached a gestational age of at least 20 weeks. (Some states mandate reporting of all fetal deaths regardless of gestational age.) NCHS issues a model fetal death certificate, which captures demographic and medical data as on the model birth certificate and cause-of-death data as on the model death certificate. Registration of fetal deaths is much less complete than registration of live births or of deaths that occur after birth, especially for fetal deaths that occur at earlier gestational ages (Harter et al., 1986; Greb et al., 1987). Moreover, cause-of-death information is often nonspecific or incomplete and has been found to correspond poorly with autopsy reports (Lammer et al., 1989). Accordingly, fetal death certificates have so far been less used for epidemiologic research than have other vital records.

Disease Reports

By state and local laws, certain diseases must be reported to health authorities by any care provider who encounters a new case (Centers for Disease Control and

Prevention, 2002b). The list of reportable diseases varies slightly among jurisdictions, but it generally includes infectious diseases for which timely information on case occurrence is needed for disease prevention and control. Some conditions, such as polio, syphilis, and tuberculosis, are transmissible from person to person. Reporting of individual cases can trigger public health efforts aimed at protection of other individuals who may already have been in contact with the reported case, or those who might have future contact. Other diseases, such as botulism or paralytic shellfish poisoning, occur after some environmental exposure such as contaminated food, and reporting can trigger a public health response to prevent others from being so exposed.

Laws and regulations often require more rapid notification of authorities for diseases that pose an immediate threat to others of potentially fatal or disabling illness. For example, in Washington State, a new case of rabies must be reported immediately, whereas seven working days are allowed for reporting a new case of nongonococcal urethritis.

Passive reporting of this kind is thought to be fairly complete for rare, clinically severe diseases of clear public health importance, such as rabies or plague (Centers for Disease Control and Prevention, 2002b). But for many other legally reportable diseases, underascertainment of cases is a serious problem (Marier, 1977; Wharton and Vogt, 1994). Some conditions, such as hepatitis A or salmonellosis, can be clinically mild and may never result in a medical care encounter. If care is sought but the illness is non-specific, the necessary diagnostic tests may not be done and the diagnosis may be missed. For example, a study of passive reporting for shigellosis in the U.S. estimated that of every 100 cases, 76 were symptomatic, 28 consulted a physician, 9 had a stool culture, and 7 had a positive stool culture (Rosenberg et al., 1977).

Even when a reportable disease is diagnosed, physicians often fail to submit a case report. One survey found that non-reporting physicians were unaware that they had this responsibility or that the particular disease was legally reportable, were unfamiliar with reporting forms or procedures, were concerned about patient confidentiality, or were unmoved by the incentives or sanctions in place (Konowitz et al., 1984).

For all of these reasons, the reported cases of many notifiable infectious diseases probably represent only a fraction of all truly occurring cases. Several approaches have been used to enhance ascertainment:

- *Sentinel physicians* are currently used for influenza surveillance in most states. Physician volunteers agree in advance to report all visits for influenza-like illnesses on a weekly basis (Centers for Disease Control and Prevention, 1999b). A sentinel system is also used to track certain occupational diseases (Baker, 1989). This approach to case identification sacrifices comprehensive population coverage for more complete ascertainment among patients of relatively motivated care providers.

- *Active surveillance* involves outreach to identify cases who would be missed by passive reporting. It was an important part of the successful program to eradicate smallpox—a disease spread only person-to-person and for which an effective vaccine has long been available (Foege et al., 1971). In the late 1960s, smallpox persisted in eight West and Central African nations where full vaccination of the population was practically impossible to achieve. Fortunately, full vaccination also proved unnecessary. The smallpox eradication team instead carried out early detection and aggressive control of local outbreaks. Their active-surveillance approach used newspapers, radio, teachers, mail carriers, village and area chiefs, and regular contacts with health care providers and volunteer agencies to identify cases not captured by the passive smallpox reporting system. As incidence declined, a larger and larger proportion of cases were identified only through active surveillance. The final push was timed to coincide with the seasonal dip in incidence. By mid-1969, the disease was completely wiped out from the region. Because of the added cost and effort, active surveillance is most often used only temporarily and locally as part of special programs for disease control or research.

- *Laboratory-based reporting* is an option when a specific test is routinely done to diagnose the disease. For example, rotavirus infections cause gastroenteritis in infants and young children and can be diagnosed by antigen-detection tests or electron microscopy on stool specimens (Centers for Disease Control and Prevention, 1998b). CDC's National Respiratory and Enteric Virus Surveillance System has used 66 clinical laboratories in 41 states to report weekly on the number of specimens tested and the number positive for rotavirus. This network was used to track the effects of a newly approved vaccine against rotavirus. Active laboratory surveillance, involving regular inquiries to clinical laboratories rather than passive reporting by laboratories, has also been used to study the incidence of foodborne illnesses (Centers for Disease Control and Prevention, 2000b).

Using case-report data contributed voluntarily by states, CDC compiles statistics for a list of nationally notifiable diseases. Case counts are received electronically, reported weekly in the *Morbidity and Mortality Weekly Report,* and summarized annually (Centers for Disease Control and Prevention, 2002b).

Disease Registries

Registries gather data from multiple sources on individual cases of disease. Linkage across sources prevents duplicate counting of the same cases. Here are some examples of diseases for which well-developed registries exist:

- *Cancer.* The National Cancer Institute funds population-based cancer registries in 11 different areas of the U.S. as part of the Surveillance, Epidemiology, and End Results (SEER) program. Collectively, they cover about 14% of the U.S. population and identify about 170,000 new cancer cases annually. Cases are identified from review of records of hospital discharges and pathology laboratories. Pathology reports are also used to classify tumors by histologic type, and medical records are abstracted to obtain demographic and clinical information, including stage at diagnosis and type of treatment. Survivorship is tracked through state vital records and the National Death Index. Cancer cases identified through SEER are regularly used in case-control studies of cancer etiology. SEER registries capture nearly all cancer cases in their geographically defined populations, which become sampling frames for selection of controls.
- *Birth defects.* The Metropolitan Atlanta Congenital Defects Program, begun in 1967, seeks to identify all birth defects among the approximately 50,000 infants born annually in five counties comprising greater Atlanta (Centers for Disease Control and Prevention, 2002a). Case-finding uses birth and death certificates, hospital and physician records, and genetics laboratory test results, which collectively are thought to capture about 87% of cases (Honein and Paulozzi, 1999). The Atlanta program has been used as a model for less extensive systems in other areas.
- *Trauma.* Population-based registries for trauma have been established in several areas, chiefly by gaining the cooperation of all area hospitals that treat trauma victims to contribute uniform data on each trauma patient (Mock, 2001). For example, Husberg and colleagues (1998) studied work-related injuries in Alaska, a state whose occupational mortality rate was five times the U.S. average, using data from the Alaska Trauma Registry. All 24 acute-care hospitals in the state reported to the registry on admissions for injury. During 1991–1995, the greatest *numbers* of injury admissions involved workers from the fishing (n = 390 admissions), construction (n = 365), and logging (n = 215) industries. But because the registry was population-based, the researchers could use denominator data obtained from industry, state, and federal employment statistics to account for differences in workforce size among industries. Examined in this way, the *incidence* of injury requiring hospitalization per 100 worker-years was found to be more than four times greater among loggers (2.50) than among construction workers (0.63) or fishermen (0.45).

Because of the extra expense of active surveillance and of data linkage and maintenance, most registries are limited in their geographic scope. Not all are population-based; some hospital- or clinic-based registries are set up mainly to create a list of potential participants for clinical research and are thus of more limited use to epidemiologists for lack of a denominator.

Health Care Utilization Data

For illnesses that prompt the use of health care, information generated in the process of providing that care can be valuable for epidemiologic research.

- *Clinical records* are a rich source of patient-specific data from clinical examinations, diagnostic tests, and procedures. In most settings, medical records remain largely paper-based, and extracting the information for epidemiologic research involves coping with several challenges. These include protecting patient confidentiality; coping with the possibility that a patient received care from more than one source, each of which maintains its own medical record; accessing the records, which may not be archived indefinitely; and dealing with the uneven organization, completeness, and legibility of the records themselves. Some of these difficulties are being lessened by growth of computer-based medical records.
- *Administrative data* that are generated as a byproduct of clinical care are technically easier than clinical records to access and to use. The data are typically computerized and in a standardized format. When care is provided on a fee-for-service basis, each service typically appears on a billing claim containing a patient identifier and the date, provider, and nature of the service. The patient's disease may be implicit in the service itself, as with coronary artery bypass grafting; most claim formats also include one or more diagnosis codes to justify delivery of the service.

  In some care settings, no bill is generated because the care is not paid for on a fee-for-service basis. Examples include Health Maintenance Organizations (HMOs), veterans hospitals, and military hospitals. Nonetheless, these organizations often track utilization for their own administrative purposes. An internal record may thus document each delivery of a service, containing much the same data as might otherwise have appeared on a billing claim.

  Epidemiologists must keep in mind that administrative data do not exist primarily to support epidemiologic research and may be prone to both random and systematic errors. The data systems themselves and the meaning of information in them can also change over time. For example, Helms (1987) described a "pseudo-epidemic" of septicemia among Medicare patients in Iowa hospitals during 1980–1986 that, strangely, did not appear to be localized to any particular hospital or due to any specific organism. The time course of the increase in cases coincided, however, with introduction of a new reimbursement system for Medicare patients based on Diagnosis-Related Groups (Cohen et al., 1987). The new payment system created financial incentives for hospitals to increase reporting of septicemia on billing claims, which may have occurred either through more complete reporting or by shifts in how diagnoses were coded.

Inpatient care

Some diseases, such as appendicitis, hip fracture, or meningitis, are almost always initially treated in a hospital. For these conditions, hospital discharge data can be a valuable resource for identifying cases. Discharge abstract data typically include at least demographic information, date and length of hospitalization, diagnoses, surgical procedures, and vital status on discharge.

The usefulness of such data for epidemiologic purposes is greatest if the hospitals involved provide essentially all inpatient care for a defined population, allowing calculation of incidence rates. This situation is fully or nearly satisfied in several U.S. states, in which all hospitals contribute records of discharges to a statewide database. In Washington State, for example, the state's Comprehensive Hospital Abstract Reporting System (CHARS) captures data for all patients in non-federal hospitals in the state (Washington State Department of Health, 2002). Nationally, NCHS has conducted the National Hospital Discharge Survey since 1965, based on a probability sample of about 500 non-federal, short-stay U.S. hospitals that currently account for about 300,000 discharges annually (National Center for Health Statistics, 2002).

Population-based hospital discharge data are also available for several kinds of administratively defined populations. Inpatient care for an estimated 95% of the U.S. population over age 65 years is covered by Medicare (Lauderdale et al., 1993), albeit with some variation in coverage by age and race (Fisher et al., 1990). Medicare data have been used, for example, to study the incidence and case fatality of hip fracture among New England Medicare beneficiaries (Fisher et al., 1991).

The Department of Veterans Affairs (VA) operates about 172 hospitals that provide care for U.S. veterans (Boyko et al., 2000). It has captured computerized discharge data on all hospitalizations since 1970. Use of the Social Security number as the primary patient identifier is a special advantage, facilitating linkage across hospitalizations, across facilities, or with other VA data. The population base for these data is less clear, however, because many veterans receive part or all of their health care outside the VA system. Linkage of VA and Medicare data may strengthen the epidemiologic research potential of both by enhancing completeness of case ascertainment for veterans aged 65 years or older (Fleming et al., 1992). Several large HMOs also maintain extensive computerized databases on health care use by their members, including hospitalizations (Selby, 1997; Psaty et al., 1991).

Outpatient care

Many diseases routinely result in health care but seldom require hospitalization—for example, rheumatoid arthritis, migraine headache, and urinary tract infection. Medically treated cases of these illnesses must therefore be sought using ambulatory-care medical records or administrative data that pertain to outpatient care.

For geographically defined populations, few settings have an ongoing mechanism in place to identify all cases of diseases treated on an outpatient basis. The Rochester Epidemiology Project in Rochester, Minnesota, is one such place, where medical records at the Mayo Clinic and at offices of a few independent care providers are regularly reviewed to capture diagnostic information community-wide (Melton, 1996). For example, this resource has been used to study the incidence, prevalence, and descriptive epidemiology of rheumatoid arthritis (Linos et al., 1983) and of epilepsy (Hauser et al., 1993), both of which are treated mainly outside the hospital.

Nationally, NCHS conducts two main ongoing surveys of ambulatory care (National Center for Health Statistics, 2002). The National Ambulatory Medical Care Survey studies a probability sample of approximately 30,000 outpatient visits each year to about 3000 U.S. physicians in office-based practice, capturing data on patient demographics, diagnoses, and treatments. A complementary activity, the National Hospital Ambulatory Medical Care Survey, captures similar data on about 50,000 outpatient visits annually to about 600 hospital-associated clinics or emergency departments nationwide. Other NCHS data systems capture information on outpatient surgery, nursing home care, and home and hospice care, as described on the extensive NCHS World Wide Web site (Appendix 6A). These systems yield reasonably precise national and regional estimates but generally include too few observations from any one state or community to yield stable state or local estimates. Ability to link repeated encounters by the same person over time is also limited.

Community-wide surveillance of outpatient records is sometimes organized specifically to meet the needs of an epidemiologic study. For example, the Northeastern Ohio Trauma Study (Barancik et al., 1983) arranged for regular review of emergency-department logs at all hospitals in the greater Cleveland, Ohio, area in order to study the frequency and distribution of medically treated trauma, including cases treated without hospitalization.

Billing claims or other administrative data on outpatient care can also be used for case identification. For example, the prevalence of diabetes among Alaska Natives and American Indians has been studied by counting the number of individuals who had received care for diabetes at Indian Health Service clinics, as recorded in a computerized database of all clinic encounters (Centers for Disease Control and Prevention, 1998c). Medicaid billing claims have also been used to study medically treated illness and injury among enrollees in Medicaid (Johnston et al., 2000; Ray et al., 1987; Turner et al., 1999). Medicaid data have also been especially useful for pharmacoepidemiologic research, because exposure to a prescription drug can be ascertained from billing claims in settings where the Medicaid program covers them (Ray and Griffin, 1989). Some HMOs also include diagnosis codes on computerized outpatient encounter data (Selby, 1997).

Pharmacy records

Besides providing a source of data on exposure to prescription drugs, computerized pharmacy data can also be used to identify cases of a disease linked to a particular drug. For example, records of prescriptions for insulin can be used to identify people with diabetes.

Health Surveys

Some nonfatal illnesses rarely result in a medical care encounter—for example, minor injuries, headaches, upper respiratory infections, and chronic fatigue. Although they may be medically less severe, many such diseases are very common and, in the aggregate, can constitute a significant public health burden. Yet the data sources listed above may not be adequate for case identification. Obtaining more complete population-based data on their occurrence often requires a health survey: that is, sampling persons from the target population and gathering data about them by mail, telephone, face-to-face contact, or other means not dependent on their use of medical care. Three large ongoing national surveys that use different methods of data collection exemplify this approach to obtaining disease frequency data.

- The *National Health Interview Survey,* conducted by NCHS, is a continuous survey of the civilian, non-institutionalized U.S. population. It currently involves about 40,000 households comprising about 100,000 individuals each year (National Center for Health Statistics, 2002). Households are selected using multi-stage probability sampling, with oversampling of blacks and Hispanics. Data are collected by in-person interview with an adult household member about household and family characteristics. In addition, one adult and one child (if applicable) are randomly sampled in each study household to gather more information on personal health characteristics. A core set of questions covers sociodemographics, family structure, income, acute and chronic conditions, injuries, overall health status, activity limitations, health behavior, immunizations, insurance status, health care use, and other topics. This core set of questions is supplemented by others on special topics that change from year to year, such as use of preventive services or cancer (National Center for Health Statistics, 2000).

Example: Guo and colleagues (1999) studied the frequency of back pain among 30,074 working adult respondents in the 1988 National Health Interview Survey, which included an occupational health supplement. Some 4.6% of workers reported having had back pain every day for a week or more during the year. Because of the national representativeness of the sample, the researchers were able to estimate that about 102 million days of work had been missed due to back pain in the U.S. in 1988, resulting in an estimated $14 billion in lost productivity.

Households in the National Health Interview Survey also form the sampling frame for certain other federal health surveys, including the Medical Expenditure Panel Survey conducted by the Agency for Healthcare Research and Quality. This survey monitors health care use and payments for health care over time in participating families (Cohen, 1997).

- The *National Health and Nutrition Examination Survey,* now conducted annually by NCHS, uses mobile examination centers to carry out standardized in-person interviews, physical examinations, nutritional assessments, and diagnostic tests on a probability sample of about 5000 people annually throughout the U.S. Blacks, Mexican Americans, persons over 60 years old, and adolescents are oversampled. This survey can yield estimates of the prevalence of undiagnosed, often asymptomatic conditions, such as diabetes, hypertension, osteoporosis, and iron-deficiency anemia (National Center for Health Statistics, 2002).

Example: Alter and colleagues (1999) studied the prevalence of hepatitis C virus infection in the U.S. Hepatitis C infection can be asymptomatic for many years but is associated with greatly increased risk of eventual liver failure and liver cancer. Antibody and viral RNA tests were performed on blood samples obtained from 21,241 participants in the National Health and Nutrition Examination Survey during 1988–1994. From the results, the investigators estimated that about 1.8% of the U.S. population, or about 3.9 million people, had been infected by hepatitis C virus, as demonstrated by a positive antibody test, and that 74% of them (2.7 million people) were chronic carriers who could transmit the virus to others.

- The *Behavioral Risk Factor Surveillance System,* conducted by CDC, involves telephone interviews with a probability sample of people aged 18 years or older in all states. In 2000, state-specific sample sizes ranged from about 1700 to about 8100, for a total of over 184,000 respondents. The survey focuses on health-related behaviors, such as smoking, alcohol use, immunizations, and use of screening tests. It also obtains information on selected health conditions including hypertension, diabetes, dental disease, obesity, and HIV/AIDS. Core questions are asked of all respondents, and states may add questions of their own devising or from optional "modules" that cover other health topics.

Example: Diez-Roux and colleagues (2000) used data from the Behavioral Risk Factor Surveillance System to investigate whether the extent of inequality in the distribution of income within U.S. states was associated with hypertension. Self-reported data on each respondent's hypertension status, family income, and other personal characteristics were drawn from the survey, while data on the income distribution in each state were drawn from the U.S. census. Multilevel statistical modeling was then used to account simultaneously for the effects of both individual-level and state-level factors. Even after adjustment for individual income, hypertension was found to be significantly more common among respondents living in states with more unequal income distributions—an association felt to represent a possible contextual effect of income inequality on health. Such a study would have been difficult or impossible without survey data on a large number of participants in each state.

Details on these surveys are obtainable from the World Wide Web sites of the respective agencies (Appendix 6A), including copies of survey instruments, data collection protocols, sampling details, and guidance on proper data analysis. All three surveys yield fairly precise estimates for the entire U.S. and for large geographic regions. Samples sizes in the Behavioral Risk Factor Surveillance System are generally large enough to yield fairly precise state-specific estimates as well. All three surveys involve complex sampling schemes that require the use of specialized analysis methods to obtain valid confidence limits and significance tests (Korn and Graubard, 1991, 1999).

DENOMINATOR DATA

Denominator data for geographically defined populations in the U.S. are usually based directly or indirectly on the decennial census. Counts from the most recent

Table 6–2. Selected Commonly Used Types of Census Areas

AREA TYPE	DESCRIPTION	NO. IN 2000
Nation	—	1
Region	Combination of states	4
Division	Combination of states	9
State or equivalent	—	57
County	—	3,219
Census tract	Small area within a county, usually with about 2500–8000 residents and boundaries that follow visible features	66,438
Block group	Area with about 250–550 housing units, averaging 1/4 of a census tract	211,827
Block	Small area bounded by streets, streams, or other natural or legal boundaries	8,269,131

census are available by age, gender, race/ethnicity, and sociodemographic characteristics at various levels of aggregation. Several of the most commonly used area types are summarized in Table 6–2 (U.S. Bureau of the Census, 2000). Other types sometimes used include ZIP codes, metropolitan areas, urban areas, voting districts, and county subdivisions.

The Census Bureau also prepares population estimates for calendar years between censuses by age, gender, and race for counties and larger areas, and total population counts for certain areas smaller than a county. These intercensal estimates use information from births, deaths, number of federal tax returns and Medicare enrollees, and immigration statistics. Many state and local governments supplement Census Bureau statistics with their own intercensal estimates.

Census data can be obtained in printed form from many reference libraries, purchased on computer media from the Census Bureau, or downloaded from the Census Bureau's own extensive World Wide Web site or from CDC WONDER (Friede et al., 1993).

Although other sources of error may be more important in epidemiologic applications, "raw" census counts have been found to underestimate population size. The extent of undercounting varies among population subgroups. Table 6–3 shows the Census Bureau's own estimates of degree of undercounting in the 1990 census, based on independent post-enumeration surveys. The proportion undercounted tended to be greater among minorities and younger people.

For administratively defined populations, a list of enrollees or population members almost always exists and may be continuously updated. For populations such as employee work forces, insurance plan enrollees, and school students, detailed data may also be available on member characteristics and each person's

Table 6–3. Estimated Degree of Underenumeration in the 1990
U.S. Census, by Race/Ethnicity and Age Group

	Percent Missed	
RACE/ETHNICITY	ALL AGES	AGE UNDER 18 YEARS
Total population	1.6%	3.2%
White	0.9%	2.2%
Black	4.4%	7.1%
Asian/Pacific Islander	2.3%	3.2%
American Indian/Alaska Native	4.5%	6.2%
Other	5.2%	5.1%
Hispanic	5.0%	5.0%

membership history, often in computerized form. These records can allow the epidemiologist to estimate accurately the number of people or amount of person-time at risk.

USES OF MULTIPLE DATA SOURCES

When information on disease occurrence is available from two or more sources for the same population, epidemiologists may be able to exploit them to obtain more accurate estimates of disease frequency. One data source can be used to evaluate, and sometimes to circumvent, limitations of another.

Excluding Ineligible Cases

A common problem is "false positives"—that is, persons identified as cases by a primary data source who do not actually qualify under the study's case definition. The problem can occur in various ways, including diagnostic errors, coding errors, or having insufficient data to judge eligibility. Sometimes it can be addressed by a validation substudy that uses a secondary data source with more detailed or accurate information. The secondary data source may be checked for all cases initially identified or for a sample. Because medical records contain relatively detailed clinical information, they are often used as a secondary source for validation.

Example: Jiang and colleagues (1995) sought to measure the incidence of Guillain-Barré syndrome (GBS), a rare form of ascending paralysis, in southwest Stockholm, Sweden, using a population-based registry that relied chiefly on hospital discharge records. They expected that patients with GBS diagnosis codes—those labelled as "Guillain-Barré polyradiculitis" or "Acute inflammatory polyneuropathy (Guillain-Barré syndrome)"—should qualify. But they were also concerned that some qualifying cases might be coded as "non-specific polyneuropathy," even though this catch-all category could also include patients with a variety of other neurologic conditions. Accordingly, they conducted a validation study. A neurologist reviewed the medical records for 83 of the 103 patients discharged with a diagnosis code indicating GBS during 1973 to 1991, and for 40 patients discharged with non-specific polyneuropathy, using published criteria for GBS developed by the U.S. National Institutes of Health. They found that 83% of patients discharged with a GBS diagnosis code indeed met the diagnostic criteria for GBS, while no patients with non-specific polyneuropathy met them. As a result, the investigators reported a lower incidence estimate for GBS than the registry data alone suggested. They were also able to report that very few cases were missed through miscoding as non-specific polyneuropathy.

Estimating the Number of Missed Cases

The opposite problem can be thought of as "false negatives"—persons who meet the case definition but who are missed by a data source. Population-based registries often try to minimize underascertainment by seeking cases through two or more data sources, recognizing that no one source captures them all.

   Perhaps surprisingly, having multiple data sources available for case identification can make it possible not only to estimate the number of cases missed by each source but also to estimate indirectly the number of cases missed by all sources combined. The statistical methods for doing so are based on *capture-recapture sampling* (Hook and Regal, 1995). The basic idea can be illustrated by considering just two data sources, which are assumed to cover the same base population over the same time period. Cases may be captured by both sources, by source no. 1 only, by source no. 2 only, or by neither source, as summarized in Table 6–4. The counts a, b, and c are thus known, while d is unknown. Yet d can be estimated if the probability of capturing a case in source no. 1 is assumed to be independent of the probability of capture in source no. 2. This independence assumption would imply that $a/(a + c) = b/(b + d)$. Solving this equation for the one unknown quantity, $\hat{d} = bc/a$ is an estimate of the number of cases missed by both sources.

Table 6–4. Sample Data Layout when Cases can be Identified from Two Sources

		Captured by Source No. 2?	
		YES	NO
Captured by source No. 1?	YES	a	b
	NO	c	d

Example: McCarty and colleagues (1993) used this method to estimate the incidence of childhood diabetes in Madrid, Spain. Using hospital discharge data, they found 432 cases during 1985–1988 who met eligibility criteria on diagnosis, residence, and age. Recognizing that this data source could miss cases who were never hospitalized or who resided in Madrid but were hospitalized elsewhere, cases were also sought through the Spanish Diabetes Association. This second source identified 138 eligible children, of whom 119 also appeared in the hospital-discharge list. From these data, the investigators estimated that $(432 - 119) \times (138 - 119)/119 = 50$ cases had been missed by both sources. Adding these 50 missed cases to those captured in one or both of the sources at hand, they estimated that the total number of cases was about $432 + 138 - 119 + 50 = 501$. Note that this corrected total was about 11% greater than the 451 cases actually identified.

Independence of case ascertainment between data sources is a fairly strong assumption and one not easily checked. Extensions of the capture-recapture method allow this assumption to be relaxed, however, particularly if there are three or more data sources (Hook and Regal, 1995).

Reducing Misclassification

A data source used chiefly for case ascertainment may also contain other information that allows cases to be classified on demographic or other characteristics, such as race, socioeconomic status, or residence. Often the goal is to estimate disease frequency in certain population subgroups. As we have seen, the data needed to assign each case to the proper subgroup may be incomplete or inaccurate in vital records, disease reports, or other sources. Better data may be available by linking to a second source.

Example: Sugarman and colleagues (1993) sought to determine the incidence of injury resulting in hospitalization or death among American Indians in Oregon. During 1989–1990, 301 injury cases were found in the statewide trauma registry who had been coded as American Indian. Suspecting possible misclassification of race in the registry data, the investigators linked them to patient registration data for the Indian Health Service (IHS) clinics in Oregon. Eligibility for care in IHS clinics required verification of tribe membership and blood quantum. They found an additional 89 trauma victims who had been coded in the registry as not being American Indians but who actually were American Indians according to IHS records. Additional American Indians were probably missed in the registry data, because only about half the number of American Indians counted in the census had registered at an IHS clinic. The investigators concluded that the true incidence of injury among American Indians in the state was probably about 69% higher than would have been determined from trauma registry data alone.

Expanded Opportunities for Research Through Data Linkage

More broadly, a very wide range of epidemiologic research questions can be addressed by linking data on disease occurrence from one data source with exposure data drawn from another source. For example, by linking birth certificate data with hospital discharge data, Lydon-Rochelle and colleagues (2000) found that the risk of postpartum rehospitalization, often for infection, was significantly increased among mothers whose babies were delivered by caesarean section or assisted vaginal delivery compared with those who had undergone a spontaneous vaginal delivery. Data on method of delivery (the exposure) and other data came from birth certificates, while data on postpartum rehospitalization (the outcome) came from hospital discharge records; no direct contact with patients was required.

CONCLUSION

This brief tour of data on disease occurrence has not been exhaustive. Many other specialized or localized resources are available, such as data from armed-forces-intake examinations, screening programs, school or workplace absenteeism records, employer or union records, law enforcement and regulatory agency records, and so on. More extensive lists of data resources and additional information about them can be found in several good references on disease surveillance (Teutsch and Churchill, 1994; Halperin et al., 1992; Thacker and Berkelman, 1988) and in review articles by Graubard and Korn (1999) and by Gable (1990).

APPENDIX 6A

Selected World Wide Web Sites

ORGANIZATION	URL
Centers for Disease Control and Prevention	www.cdc.gov
CDC WONDER data retrieval system	wonder.cdc.gov
National Center for Health Statistics	www.cdc.gov/nchs
U.S. Census Bureau	www.census.gov
World Health Organization	www.who.int

APPENDIX 6B. Draft Model Death Certificate for Adoption in 2003: Figure 6–3

DRAFT 02/05/2002

U.S. STANDARD CERTIFICATE OF DEATH

LOCAL FILE NO.   **STATE FILE NO.**

NAME OF DECEDENT____
For use by physician or institution

To Be Completed/Verified By: FUNERAL DIRECTOR

1. DECEDENT'S LEGAL NAME (Include AKA's if any) (First, Middle, Last)

2. SEX

3. SOCIAL SECURITY NUMBER

4a. AGE-Last Birthday (Years) | 4b. UNDER 1 YEAR — Months | Days | 4c. UNDER 1 DAY — Hours | Minutes | 5. DATE OF BIRTH (Mo/Day/Yr) | 6. BIRTHPLACE (City and State or Foreign Country)

7a. RESIDENCE-STATE | 7b. COUNTY | 7c. CITY OR TOWN

7d. STREET AND NUMBER | 7e. APT. NO. | 7f. ZIP CODE | 7g. INSIDE CITY LIMITS? ☐ Yes ☐ No

8. EVER IN US ARMED FORCES? ☐ Yes ☐ No

9. MARITAL STATUS AT TIME OF DEATH ☐ Married ☐ Married, but separated ☐ Widowed ☐ Divorced ☐ Never Married ☐ Unknown

10. SURVIVING SPOUSE'S NAME (If wife, give name prior to first marriage)

11. FATHER'S NAME (First, Middle, Last)

12. MOTHER'S NAME PRIOR TO FIRST MARRIAGE (First, Middle, Last)

13a. INFORMANT'S NAME | 13b. RELATIONSHIP TO DECEDENT | 13c. MAILING ADDRESS (Street and Number, City, State, Zip Code)

14. PLACE OF DEATH (Check only one: see instructions)

IF DEATH OCCURRED IN A HOSPITAL: ☐ Inpatient ☐ Emergency Room/Outpatient ☐ Dead on Arrival

IF DEATH OCCURRED SOMEWHERE OTHER THAN A HOSPITAL: ☐ Hospice facility ☐ Nursing home/Long term care facility ☐ Decedentis home ☐ Other (Specify):

15. FACILITY NAME (If not institution, give street & number) | 16. CITY OR TOWN, STATE, AND ZIP CODE | 17. COUNTY OF DEATH

18. METHOD OF DISPOSITION: ☐ Burial ☐ Cremation ☐ Donation ☐ Entombment ☐ Removal from State ☐ Other (Specify):____

19. PLACE OF DISPOSITION (Name of cemetery, crematory, other place)

20. LOCATION—CITY, TOWN, AND STATE

21. NAME AND COMPLETE ADDRESS OF FUNERAL FACILITY

22. SIGNATURE OF FUNERAL SERVICE LICENSEE OR OTHER AGENT | 23. LICENSE NUMBER (Of Licensee)

To Be Completed By: MEDICAL CERTIFIER

ITEMS 24-28 MUST BE COMPLETED BY PERSON WHO PRONOUNCES OR CERTIFIES DEATH

24. DATE PRONOUNCED DEAD (Mo/Day/Yr) | 25. TIME PRONOUNCED DEAD

26. SIGNATURE OF PERSON PRONOUNCING DEATH (Only when applicable) | 27. LICENSE NUMBER | 28. DATE SIGNED (Mo/Day/Yr)

29. ACTUAL OR PRESUMED DATE OF DEATH (Mo/Day/Yr) (Spell Month) | 30. ACTUAL OR PRESUMED TIME OF DEATH | 31. WAS MEDICAL EXAMINER OR CORONER CONTACTED? ☐ Yes ☐ No

CAUSE OF DEATH (See instructions and examples)

Approximate interval: Onset to death

32. PART I. Enter the chain of events—diseases, injuries, or complications—that directly caused the death. DO NOT enter terminal events such as cardiac arrest, respiratory arrest, or ventricular fibrillation without showing the etiology. DO NOT ABBREVIATE. Enter only one cause on a line. Add additional lines if necessary.

IMMEDIATE CAUSE (Final disease or condition ———➤ resulting in death) a.____
Due to (or as a consequence of):

Sequentially list conditions, if any, leading to the cause listed on line a. Enter the **UNDERLYING CAUSE** (disease or injury that initiated the events resulting in death) **LAST**
b.____
Due to (or as a consequence of):
c.____
Due to (or as a consequence of):
d.____

PART II. Enter other significant conditions contributing to death but not resulting in the underlying cause given in PART I.

33. WAS AN AUTOPSY PERFORMED? ☐ Yes ☐ No

34. WERE AUTOPSY FINDINGS AVAILABLE TO COMPLETE THE CAUSE OF DEATH? ☐ Yes ☐ No

35. DID TOBACCO USE CONTRIBUTE TO DEATH? ☐ Yes ☐ Probably ☐ No ☐ Unknown

36. IF FEMALE: ☐ Not pregnant within past year ☐ Pregnant at time of death ☐ Not pregnant, but pregnant within 42 days of death ☐ Not pregnant, but pregnant 43 days to 1 year before death ☐ Unknown if pregnant within the past year

37. MANNER OF DEATH ☐ Natural ☐ Homicide ☐ Accident ☐ Pending Investigation ☐ Suicide ☐ Could not be determined

38. DATE OF INJURY (Mo/Day/Yr) (Spell Month) | 39. TIME OF INJURY | 40. PLACE OF INJURY (e.g., Decedent's home; construction site; restaurant; wooded area) | 41. INJURY AT WORK? ☐ Yes ☐ No

42. LOCATION OF INJURY: State: | City or Town: — Street & Number: | Apartment No.: | Zip Code:

43. DESCRIBE HOW INJURY OCCURRED:

44. IF TRANSPORTATION INJURY, SPECIFY: ☐ Driver/Operator ☐ Passenger ☐ Pedestrian ☐ Other (Specify)

45. CERTIFIER (Check only one):
☐ Certifying physician-To the best of my knowledge, death occurred due to the cause(s) and manner stated.
☐ Pronouncing & Certifying physician-To the best of my knowledge, death occurred at the time, date, and place, and due to the cause(s) and manner stated.
☐ Medical Examiner/Coroner-On the basis of examination, and/or investigation, in my opinion, death occurred at the time, date, and place, and due to the cause(s) and manner stated.

Signature of certifier:____

46. NAME, ADDRESS, AND ZIP CODE OF PERSON COMPLETING CAUSE OF DEATH (Item 32)

47. TITLE OF CERTIFIER | 48. LICENSE NUMBER | 49. DATE CERTIFIED (Mo/Day/Yr) | 50. **FOR REGISTRAR ONLY**- DATE FILED (Mo/Day/Yr)

To Be Completed By: FUNERAL DIRECTOR

51. DECEDENT'S EDUCATION-Check the box that best describes the highest degree or level of school completed at the time of death.
☐ 8th grade or less
☐ 9th - 12th grade; no diploma
☐ High school graduate or GED completed
☐ Some college credit, but no degree
☐ Associate degree (e.g., AA, AS)
☐ Bachelor's degree (e.g., BA, AB, BS)
☐ Master's degree (e.g., MA, MS, MEng, MEd, MSW, MBA)
☐ Doctorate (e.g., PhD, EdD) or Professional degree (e.g., MD, DDS, DVM, LLB, JD)

52. DECEDENT OF HISPANIC ORIGIN? Check the box that best describes whether the decedent is Spanish/Hispanic/Latino. Check the "No" box if decedent is not Spanish/Hispanic/Latino.
☐ No, not Spanish/Hispanic/Latino
☐ Yes, Mexican, Mexican American, Chicano
☐ Yes, Puerto Rican
☐ Yes, Cuban
☐ Yes, other Spanish/Hispanic/Latino
(Specify) ____

53. DECEDENT'S RACE (Check one or more races to indicate what the decedent considered himself or herself to be)
☐ White
☐ Black or African American
☐ American Indian or Alaska Native (Name of the enrolled or principal tribe) ____
☐ Asian Indian
☐ Chinese
☐ Filipino
☐ Japanese
☐ Korean
☐ Vietnamese
☐ Other Asian (Specify) ____
☐ Native Hawaiian
☐ Guamanian or Chamorro
☐ Samoan
☐ Other Pacific Islander (Specify) ____
☐ Other (Specify) ____

54. DECEDENT'S USUAL OCCUPATION (Indicate type of work done during most of working life. DO NOT USE RETIRED.)

55. KIND OF BUSINESS/INDUSTRY

APPENDIX 6C. Draft Model Birth Certificate for Adoption in 2003: Figure 6–4

U.S. STANDARD CERTIFICATE OF LIVE BIRTH

LOCAL FILE NO.   BIRTH NUMBER:

CHILD

1. CHILD'S NAME (First, Middle, Last, Suffix)		2. TIME OF BIRTH (24hr)	3. SEX	4. DATE OF BIRTH (Mo/Day/Yr)

5. FACILITY NAME (If not institution, give street and number)	6. CITY, TOWN, OR LOCATION OF BIRTH	7. COUNTY OF BIRTH

MOTHER

8a. MOTHER'S CURRENT LEGAL NAME (First, Middle, Last, Suffix)   8b. DATE OF BIRTH (Mo/Day/Yr)

8c. MOTHER'S NAME PRIOR TO FIRST MARRIAGE (First, Middle, Last, Suffix)   8d. BIRTHPLACE (State, Territory, or Foreign Country)

9a. RESIDENCE OF MOTHER-STATE	9b. COUNTY	9c. CITY, TOWN, OR LOCATION

9d. STREET AND NUMBER	9e. APT. NO.	9f. ZIP CODE	9g. INSIDE CITY LIMITS? ☐ Yes ☐ No

FATHER

10a. FATHER'S CURRENT LEGAL NAME (First, Middle, Last, Suffix)	10b. DATE OF BIRTH (Mo/Day/Yr)	10c. BIRTHPLACE (State, Territory, or Foreign Country)

CERTIFIER

11. CERTIFIER'S NAME: _____

TITLE: ☐ MD ☐ DO ☐ HOSPITAL ADMIN. ☐ CNM/CM ☐ OTHER MIDWIFE
☐ OTHER (Specify)_____

12. DATE CERTIFIED ___/___/___ MM DD YYYY	13. DATE FILED BY REGISTRAR ___/___/___ MM DD YYYY

INFORMATION FOR ADMINISTRATIVE USE

MOTHER

14. MOTHER'S MAILING ADDRESS: ☐ Same as residence, or: State: City, Town, or Location:

Street & Number: Apartment No.:   Zip Code:

15. MOTHER MARRIED? (At birth, conception, or any time between) ☐ Yes ☐ No

IF NO, HAS PATERNITY ACKNOWLEDGMENT BEEN SIGNED IN THE HOSPITAL? ☐ Yes ☐ No

16. SOCIAL SECURITY NUMBER REQUESTED FOR CHILD? ☐ Yes ☐ No

17. FACILITY ID. (NPI)

18. MOTHER'S SOCIAL SECURITY NUMBER: 19. FATHER'S SOCIAL SECURITY NUMBER:

INFORMATION FOR MEDICAL AND HEALTH PURPOSES ONLY

MOTHER

20. MOTHER'S EDUCATION (Check the box that best describes the highest degree or level of school completed at the time of delivery)	21. MOTHER OF HISPANIC ORIGIN? (Check the box that best describes whether the mother is Spanish/Hispanic/Latina. Check the "No" box if mother is not Spanish/Hispanic/Latina)	22. MOTHER'S RACE (Check one or more races to indicate what the mother considers herself to be)
☐ 8th grade or less	☐ No, not Spanish/Hispanic/Latina	☐ White
☐ 9th - 12th grade, no diploma	☐ Yes, Mexican, Mexican American, Chicana	☐ Black or African American
☐ High school graduate or GED completed	☐ Yes, Puerto Rican	☐ American Indian or Alaska Native (Name of the enrolled or principal tribe)____
☐ Some college credit but no degree	☐ Yes, Cuban	☐ Asian Indian
☐ Associate degree (e.g., AA, AS)	☐ Yes, other Spanish/Hispanic/Latina	☐ Chinese
☐ Bachelor's degree (e.g., BA, AB, BS)	(Specify)_____	☐ Filipino
☐ Master's degree (e.g., MA, MS, MEng, MEd, MSW, MBA)		☐ Japanese
☐ Doctorate (e.g., PhD, EdD) or Professional degree (e.g., MD, DDS, DVM, LLB, JD)		☐ Korean
		☐ Vietnamese
		☐ Other Asian (Specify)_____
		☐ Native Hawaiian
		☐ Guamanian or Chamorro
		☐ Samoan
		☐ Other Pacific Islander (Specify)____
		☐ Other (Specify)_____

DRAFT 11/09/2001

FATHER

23. FATHER'S EDUCATION (Check the box that best describes the highest degree or level of school completed at the time of delivery)	24. FATHER OF HISPANIC ORIGIN? (Check the box that best describes whether the father is Spanish/Hispanic/Latino. Check the "No" box if mother is not Spanish/Hispanic/Latino)	25. FATHER'S RACE (Check one or more races to indicate what the father considers himself to be)
☐ 8th grade or less	☐ No, not Spanish/Hispanic/Latino	☐ White
☐ 9th - 12th grade, no diploma	☐ Yes, Mexican, Mexican American, Chicano	☐ Black or African American
☐ High school graduate or GED completed	☐ Yes, Puerto Rican	☐ American Indian or Alaska Native (Name of the enrolled or principal tribe)____
☐ Some college credit but no degree	☐ Yes, Cuban	☐ Asian Indian
☐ Associate degree (e.g., AA, AS)	☐ Yes, other Spanish/Hispanic/Latino	☐ Chinese
☐ Bachelor's degree (e.g., BA, AB, BS)	(Specify)_____	☐ Filipino
☐ Master's degree (e.g., MA, MS, MEng, MEd, MSW, MBA)		☐ Japanese
☐ Doctorate (e.g., PhD, EdD) or Professional degree (e.g., MD, DDS, DVM, LLB, JD)		☐ Korean
		☐ Vietnamese
		☐ Other Asian (Specify)_____
		☐ Native Hawaiian
		☐ Guamanian or Chamorro
		☐ Samoan
		☐ Other Pacific Islander (Specify)____
		☐ Other (Specify)_____

Mother's Name   Mother's Medical Record No.

26. PLACE WHERE BIRTH OCCURRED (Check one) ☐ Hospital ☐ Freestanding birthing center ☐ Home Birth: Planned to deliver at home? ☐ Yes ☐ No ☐ Clinic/Doctor's office ☐ Other (Specify)_____	27. ATTENDANT'S NAME, TITLE, AND NPI NAME: _____ NPI: _____ TITLE: ☐ MD ☐ DO ☐ CNM/CM ☐ OTHER MIDWIFE ☐ OTHER (Specify)_____	28. MOTHER TRANSFERRED FOR MATERNAL MEDICAL OR FETAL INDICATIONS FOR DELIVERY? ☐ Yes ☐ No IF YES, ENTER NAME OF FACILITY MOTHER TRANSFERRED FROM: _____

138

Draft Model Birth Certificate, Page 2

MOTHER

29a. DATE OF FIRST PRENATAL CARE VISIT	29b. DATE OF LAST PRENATAL CARE VISIT	30. TOTAL NUMBER OF PRENATAL VISITS FOR THIS PREGNANCY
___/___/_____ ☐ No Prenatal Care MM DD YYYY	___/___/_____ MM DD YYYY	_____ (If none, enter "0".)

31. MOTHER'S HEIGHT	32. MOTHER'S PREPREGNANCY WEIGHT	33. MOTHER'S WEIGHT AT DELIVERY	34. DID MOTHER GET WIC FOOD FOR HERSELF
_____ (feet/inches)	_____ (pounds)	_____ (pounds)	DURING THIS PREGNANCY? ☐ Yes ☐ No

35. NUMBER OF PREVIOUS LIVE BIRTHS (Do not include this child)	36. NUMBER OF OTHER PREGNANCY OUTCOMES (spontaneous or induced losses or ectopic pregnancies)	37. CIGARETTE SMOKING BEFORE AND DURING PREGNANCY	38. PRINCIPAL SOURCE OF PAYMENT FOR THIS DELIVERY

37. For each time period, enter either the number of cigarettes or the number of packs of cigarettes smoked. IF NONE, ENTER "0".
Average number of cigarettes or packs of cigarettes smoked per day.

	# of cigarettes	# of packs
Three Months Before Pregnancy	_____	OR _____
First Three Months of Pregnancy	_____	OR _____
Second Three Months of Pregnancy	_____	OR _____
Last Three Months of Pregnancy	_____	OR _____

38. PRINCIPAL SOURCE OF PAYMENT FOR THIS DELIVERY
☐ Private Insurance
☐ Medicaid
☐ Self-pay
☐ Other (Specify) _____

35a. Now Living Number _____ ☐ None	35b. Now Dead Number _____ ☐ None	36a. Other Outcomes Number _____ ☐ None

35c. DATE OF LAST LIVE BIRTH ___/_____ MM YYYY	36b. DATE OF LAST OTHER PREGNANCY OUTCOME ___/_____ MM YYYY	39. DATE LAST NORMAL MENSES BEGAN ___/___/_____ MM DD YYYY	40. MOTHER'S MEDICAL RECORD NUMBER

MEDICAL AND HEALTH INFORMATION

41. RISK FACTORS IN THIS PREGNANCY (Check all that apply)

Diabetes
☐ Prepregnancy (Diagnosis prior to this pregnancy)
☐ Gestational (Diagnosis in this pregnancy)

Hypertension
☐ Prepregnancy (Chronic)
☐ Gestational (PIH, preeclampsia, eclampsia)

☐ Previous preterm birth

☐ Other previous poor pregnancy outcome (Includes, perinatal death, small-for-gestational age/intrauterine growth restricted birth)

☐ Vaginal bleeding during this pregnancy prior to the onset of labor

☐ Pregnancy resulted from infertility treatment

☐ Mother had a previous cesarean delivery
If yes, how many _____

☐ None of the above

42. INFECTIONS PRESENT AND/OR TREATED DURING THIS PREGNANCY (Check all that apply)

☐ Gonorrhea
☐ Syphilis
☐ Herpes Simplex Virus (HSV)
☐ Chlamydia
☐ Hepatitis B
☐ Hepatitis C
☐ None of the above

43. OBSTETRIC PROCEDURES (Check all that apply)
☐ Cervical cerclage
☐ Tocolysis
External cephalic version:
☐ Successful
☐ Failed
☐ None of the above

44. ONSET OF LABOR (Check all that apply)
☐ Premature Rupture of the Membranes (prolonged, >12 hrs.)
☐ Precipitous Labor (<3 hrs.)
☐ Prolonged Labor (>20 hrs.)
☐ None of the above

45. CHARACTERISTICS OF LABOR AND DELIVERY (Check all that apply)

☐ Induction of labor

☐ Augmentation of labor

☐ Non-vertex presentation

☐ Steroids (glucocorticoids) for fetal lung maturation received by the mother prior to delivery

☐ Antibiotics received by the mother during labor

☐ Clinical chorioamnionitis diagnosed during labor or maternal temperature ≥38°C (100.4°F)

☐ Moderate/heavy meconium staining of the amniotic fluid

☐ Fetal intolerance of labor such that one or more of the following actions was taken: in-utero resuscitative measures, further fetal assessment, or operative delivery

☐ Epidural or spinal anesthesia during labor

☐ None of the above

46. METHOD OF DELIVERY

A. Was delivery with forceps attempted but unsuccessful?
☐ Yes ☐ No

B. Was delivery with vacuum extraction attempted but unsuccessful?
☐ Yes ☐ No

C. Fetal presentation at birth
☐ Cephalic
☐ Breech
☐ Other

D. Final route and method of delivery (Check one)
☐ Vaginal/Spontaneous
☐ Vaginal/Forceps
☐ Vaginal/Vacuum
☐ Cesarean
If cesarean, was a trial of labor attempted?
☐ Yes
☐ No

47. MATERNAL MORBIDITY (Check all that apply) (Complications associated with labor and delivery)

☐ Maternal transfusion
☐ Third or fourth degree perineal laceration
☐ Ruptured uterus
☐ Unplanned hysterectomy
☐ Admission to intensive care unit
☐ Unplanned operating room procedure following delivery
☐ None of the above

NEWBORN INFORMATION

NEWBORN

48. NEWBORN MEDICAL RECORD NUMBER:

49. BIRTHWEIGHT (grams preferred, specify unit)
_____ ☐ grams ☐ lb/oz

50. OBSTETRIC ESTIMATE OF GESTATION:
_____ (completed weeks)

51. APGAR SCORE:
Score at 5 minutes: _____
If 5 minute score is less than 6,
Score at 10 minutes: _____

52. PLURALITY - Single, Twin, Triplet, etc.
(Specify) _____

53. IF NOT SINGLE BIRTH - Born First, Second, Third, etc. (Specify)
_____

54. ABNORMAL CONDITIONS OF THE NEWBORN (Check all that apply)

☐ Assisted ventilation required immediately following delivery

☐ Assisted ventilation required for more than six hours

☐ NICU admission

☐ Newborn given surfactant replacement therapy

☐ Antibiotics received by the newborn for suspected neonatal sepsis

☐ Seizure or serious neurologic dysfunction

☐ Significant birth injury (skeletal fracture(s), peripheral nerve injury, and/or soft tissue/solid organ hemorrhage which requires intervention)

☐ None of the above

55. CONGENITAL ANOMALIES OF THE NEWBORN (Check all that apply)

☐ Anencephaly
☐ Meningomyelocele/Spina bifida
☐ Cyanotic congenital heart disease
☐ Congenital diaphragmatic hernia
☐ Omphalocele
☐ Gastroschisis
☐ Limb reduction defect (excluding congenital amputation and dwarfing syndromes)
☐ Cleft Lip with or without Cleft Palate
☐ Cleft Palate alone
☐ Down Syndrome
  ☐ Karyotype confirmed
  ☐ Karyotype pending
☐ Suspected chromosomal disorder
  ☐ Karyotype confirmed
  ☐ Karyotype pending
☐ Hypospadias
☐ None of the anomalies listed above

56. WAS INFANT TRANSFERRED WITHIN 24 HOURS OF DELIVERY? ☐ Yes ☐ No IF YES, NAME OF FACILITY INFANT TRANSFERRED TO: _____	57. IS INFANT LIVING AT TIME OF REPORT? ☐ Yes ☐ No ☐ Infant transferred, status unknown	58. IS INFANT BEING BREASTFED? ☐ Yes ☐ No

Figure 6–4. *(Continued.)*

139

EXERCISES

1. For each of the following research topics, suggest a suitable source of existing data on disease occurrence:

   (a) Over the past 20 years, many technical advances have been made in prevention and treatment of coronary heart disease. To what extent has mortality from coronary heart disease declined in the U.S. since 1980, and which demographic subgroups have experienced the greatest changes in risk of dying of this disease?

   (b) It has been hypothesized that acute appendicitis may sometimes be initiated by an infectious agent. Many infectious diseases exhibit seasonal variations in incidence. How does the incidence of acute appendicitis vary by season of the year?

   (c) Relatively short intervals between pregnancies have been associated with increased risk of adverse birth outcomes. Health education and better access to family-planning services have been proposed as preventive strategies. To help guide resources toward women at highest risk, how does the frequency of short interpregnancy intervals vary in relation to maternal age, education, marital status, and Medicaid program participation?

   (d) A major goal of clinical care for diabetes mellitus is to prevent complications, including retinopathy, renal disease, and peripheral vascular disease. As an epidemiologist for the state of Minnesota, how can you estimate the annual incidence of lower-extremity amputation among older adults (age 65 years or older) with diabetes in your state?

   (e) Clinical liver-disease specialists have the impression that they are seeing more and more patients with hepatocellular carcinoma. Has the incidence of this malignancy actually risen in the past two decades?

   (f) Neural-tube defects, including spina bifida, are thought to be at least partially preventable by giving folic acid supplements to pregnant women. How has the birth prevalence of spina bifida changed over the past 15 years?

   (g) Despite economic prosperity in the U.S. during the 1990s, poverty has hardly been eliminated. How common is food insufficiency in contemporary America, and how does its prevalence vary by age, race, income, and employment status?

   (h) Randomized trials have shown that perinatal transmission of HIV can be significantly reduced by HIV testing during pregnancy and treatment of infected mothers with zidovudine (AZT) before delivery. The U.S. Public Health Service has recommended voluntary screening and AZT treatment since 1994. To what extent has the frequency of perinatally acquired AIDS declined since then?

(i) Infant mortality in New York City showed only slight declines (0.5% per year) from 1984 to 1989 but a much sharper drop (5.8% per year) from 1989 to 1992. To what extent was this steeper decline associated with a change in the distribution of birth weight and/or with changes in the survival of newborns within birth weight categories?

2. Jara et al. (2000) studied the incidence of AIDS in Massachusetts. New AIDS cases were to be reported to a statewide AIDS registry, which was notified of 7,834 AIDS cases between January 1, 1994, and May 1, 1996.

Massachusetts also had a Uniform Hospital Discharge Data Set (UHDDS) that recorded diagnostic information on all patients hospitalized in the state. For the same period, the UHDDS recorded 2,218 qualifying patients with AIDS, of whom 2,053 also appeared in the registry.

Estimate the total number of eligible AIDS cases occurring in Massachusetts during the study period.

ANSWERS

1. Each topic has been investigated in an epidemiologic study. The data sources that were actually used are noted. In some instances, other options would have been possible as well.

(a) CDC epidemiologists used death certificate data, obtainable from the National Center for Health Statistics (1992b).

(b) Addiss et al. (1990) used National Hospital Discharge Survey data.

(c) CDC epidemiologists used Utah birth certificate data (Centers for Disease Control and Prevention, 1998d).

(d) Because almost all adults aged 65 years or older in the U.S. are covered by Medicare, and because lower-extremity amputation is an inpatient procedure, the number of lower-extremity amputations among diabetics in Minnesota was obtained from Medicare hospital claims data (Centers for Disease Control and Prevention, 1998a).

Estimating the number of older adults with diabetes in the state was more difficult. The investigators used data from the CDC Behavioral Risk Factor Surveillance System's ongoing telephone survey of adults in each state.

(e) To address this question, El-Serag and Mason (1999) used data from the National Cancer Institute's Surveillance, Epidemiology, and End Results (SEER) system of regional cancer registries.

    (f) CDC epidemiologists used birth defects registry data from several state-wide birth defects monitoring systems, covering about 23.5% of the U.S. population (Centers for Disease Control and Prevention, 1992a).

    (g) Alaimo et al. (1998) addressed this question using data from the National Health and Nutrition Examination Survey.

    (h) Lindgren et al. (1999) used data from disease-reporting systems for AIDS surveillance in all U.S. states and territories, compiled by the CDC.

    (i) Kalter et al. (1998) used birth and death certificate data for New York City. Many state and local health departments, including New York City's, routinely link birth certificate and infant death records to support such analyses.

2. The data can be organized as follows:

		Registry +	Registry −	
UHDDS	+	2053	165	2218
	−	5781	?	
		7834		

A total of $2053 + 165 + 5781 = 7999$ cases were identified through the registry and UHDDS. But the fact that each source found cases that had been missed by the other source indicates that neither source captured them all, and there were almost certainly additional AIDS cases in Massachusetts that were not identified by *either* data source.

    Capture-recapture sampling methods were used to obtain an indirect estimate of the number of AIDS cases missed by both the registry and UHDDS. Under the assumption that the probabilities of capture by the registry and by UHDDS were independent, the lower-right cell was estimated as $5781 \times 165/2053 = 465$. Adding these 465 doubly missed cases to the three other cells yielded an estimated 8464 total cases.

    The assumption of independence of capture is not always true, and one must judge its plausibility from the research context. For example, if one were to treat inpatient records and outpatient records at the same hospital as two separate data sources, it is unlikely that a case's probabilities of appearance in each source would be independent. Unfortunately, the independence assumption cannot usually be tested with the data at hand. Note, however, that the alternative is usually worse: assuming that *no* cases were missed, even though the data themselves show that neither source offered complete capture.

REFERENCES

Addiss DG, Shaffer N, Fowler BS, Tauxe RV. The epidemiology of appendicitis and appendectomy in the United States. Am J Epidemiol 1990; 132:910–25.

Alaimo K, Briefel RR, Frongillo EA, Olson CM. Food insufficiency exists in the United States: Results from the Third National Health and Nutrition Examination Survey (NHANES III). Am J Public Health 1998; 88:419–26.

Alter MJ, Moran DK, Nainan OV, McQuillan GM, Gao F, Moyer LA, et al. The prevalence of hepatitis C virus infection in the United States, 1988 through 1994. N Engl J Med 1999; 341:556–62.

Baker EL. Sentinel event notification system for occupational risks (SENSOR): the concept. Am J Public Health 1989; 79S:18–20.

Barancik JI, Chatterjee BF, Greene YC, Michenzi EM, Fife D. Northeastern Ohio trauma study: I. Magnitude of the problem. Am J Public Health 1983; 105:746–51.

Boswell J. The life of Samuel Johnson. New York: Penguin, 1791.

Boyko EJ, Koepsell TD, Gaziano JM, Horner RD, Feussner JR. U.S. Department of Veterans Affairs medical care system as a resource to epidemiologists. Am J Epidemiol 2000; 151:307–14.

Boyle CA, Decoufle P. National sources of vital status information: extent of coverage and possible selectivity in reporting. Am J Epidemiol 1990; 131:160–68.

Buescher PA, Taylor KP, Davis MH, Bowling JM. The quality of the new birth certificate data: A validation study in North Carolina. Am J Public Health 1993; 83:1163–65.

Centers for Disease Control and Prevention. Spina bifida incidence [*sic*] at birth—United States, 1983–1990. MMWR 1992a; 41:497–500.

Centers for Disease Control and Prevention. Trends in ischemic heart disease mortality— United States, 1980–1988. MMWR 1992b; 41:548–49.

Centers for Disease Control and Prevention. Diabetes-related amputations of lower extremities in the Medicare population—Minnesota, 1993–1995. MMWR 1998a; 47: 649–52.

Centers for Disease Control and Prevention. Laboratory-based surveillance for rotavirus— United States, July 1997–June 1998. MMWR 1998b; 47:978–80.

Centers for Disease Control and Prevention. Prevalence of diagnosed diabetes among American Indians/Alaska Natives—United States, 1996. MMWR 1998c; 47:901–4.

Centers for Disease Control and Prevention. Risk factors for short interpregnancy interval— Utah, June 1996–June 1997. MMWR 1998d; 43:930–34.

Centers for Disease Control and Prevention. Impact of multiple births on low birthweight— Massachusetts, 1989–1996. MMWR 1999a; 48:289–92.

Centers for Disease Control and Prevention. Influenza activity—United States, 1999–2000 season. MMWR 1999b; 48:1039–42.

Centers for Disease Control and Prevention. Neural tube defect surveillance and folic acid intervention—Texas-Mexico border, 1993–1998. MMWR 2000a; 49:1–4.

Centers for Disease Control and Prevention. Preliminary FoodNet data on the incidence of foodborne illnesses—selected sites, United States, 1999. MMWR 2000b; 49:201–5.

Centers for Disease Control and Prevention. Metropolitan Atlanta Congenital Defects Program. Atlanta, Ga.: Centers for Disease Control and Prevention, 2002a.

Centers for Disease Control and Prevention. Summary of notifiable diseases, United States—2000. MMWR 2002b; 49:1–102.

Cohen BB, Pokras R, Meads MS, Krushat WM. How will diagnosis-related groups affect epidemiologic research? Am J Epidemiol 1987; 126:1–9.

Cohen J. Design and methods of the Medical Expenditure Panel Survey Household Component. MEPS Methodology Report No. 1. AHCPR Pub. No. 97-0026. Rockville, Md.: Agency for Healthcare Research and Quality, 1997.

Diez-Roux AV, Link BG, Northridge ME. A multilevel analysis of income inequality and cardiovascular disease risk factors. Soc Sci Med 2000; 50:673–87.

El-Serag HB, Mason AC. Rising incidence of hepatocellular carcinoma in the United States. N Engl J Med 1999; 340:745–50.

Fisher ES, Baron JA, Malenka DJ, Barrett J, Bubolz TA. Overcoming potential pitfalls in the use of Medicare data for epidemiologic research. Am J Public Health 1990; 80:1487–90.

Fisher ES, Baron JA, Malenka DJ, Barrett JA, Kniffin WD, Whaley FS, et al. Hip fracture incidence and mortality in New England. Epidemiology 1991; 2:116–22.

Fleming C, Fisher ES, Chang CH, Bubolz TA, Malenka DJ. Studying outcomes and hospital utilization in the elderly. The advantages of a merged data base for Medicare and Veterans' Affairs hospitals. Med Care 1992; 30:377–91.

Foege WH, Millar JD, Lane JM. Selective epidemiologic control in smallpox eradication. Am J Epidemiol 1971; 94:311–15.

Fredrickson DS. The field trial: some thoughts on the indispensable ordeal. Bull N Y Acad Med 1968; 44:985–93.

Friede A, Reid JA, Ory HW. CDC WONDER: A comprehensive on-line public health information system of the Centers for Disease Control and Prevention. Am J Public Health 1993; 83:1289–94.

Gable CB. A compendium of public health data sources. Am J Epidemiol 1990; 131:381–94.

Gittelsohn A, Royston PN. Annotated bibliography of cause-of-death validation studies, 1958–1980. National Center for Health Statistics. Vital and Health Statistics 2(89), 1982.

Graubard BI, Korn EL. Analyzing health surveys for cancer-related objectives. J Natl Cancer Inst 1999; 91:1005–16.

Greb AE, Pauli RM, Kirby RS. Accuracy of fetal death reports: comparison with data from an independent stillbirth assessment program. Am J Public Health 1987; 77:1202–6.

Guo HR, Tanaka S, Halperin WE, Cameron LL. Back pain prevalence in US industry and estimates of lost workdays. Am J Public Health 1999; 89:1029–35.

Halperin WE, Baker EL, Monson RR. Public health surveillance. New York: Van Nostrand Reinhold, 1992.

Harter L, Starzyk P, Frost F. A comparative study of hospital fetal death records and Washington State fetal death certificates. Am J Public Health 1986; 76:1333–34.

Hauser WA, Annegers JF, Kurland LT. Incidence of epilepsy and unprovoked seizures in Rochester, Minnesota: 1935–1984. Epilepsia 1993; 34:453–68.

Helms CM. A pseudo-epidemic of septicemia among Medicare patients in Iowa. Am J Public Health 1987; 77:1331–32.

Honein MA, Paulozzi LJ. Birth defects surveillance: assessing the "gold standard." Am J Public Health 1999; 89:1238–40.

Hook EB, Regal RR. Capture-recapture methods in epidemiology: methods and limitations. Epidemiol Rev 1995; 17:243–64.

Husberg BJ, Conway GA, Moore MA, Johnson MS. Surveillance for nonfatal work-related injuries in Alaska, 1991–1995. Am J Ind Med 1998; 34:493–98.

Jara MM, Gallagher KM, Schieman S. Estimation of completeness of AIDS case reporting in Massachusetts. Epidemiology 2000; 11:209–13.

Jiang GX, de Pedro-Cuesta J, Fredrikson S. Guillain-Barré syndrome in South-West Stockholm, 1973–1991. 1. Quality of registered hospital diagnoses and incidence. Acta Neurol Scand 1995; 91:109–17.

Johnston BD, Grossman DC, Connell FA, Koepsell TD. High-risk periods for childhood injury among siblings. Pediatrics 2000; 105:562–68.

Kalter HD, Na Y, O'Campo P. Decrease in infant mortality in New York City after 1989. Am J Public Health 1998; 88:816–20.

Kircher T, Nelson J, Burdo H. The autopsy as a measure of accuracy of the death certificate. N Engl J Med 1985; 313:1263–69.

Konowitz PM, Petrossian GA, Rose DN. The underreporting of disease and physician's knowledge of reporting requirements. Public Health Rep 1984; 99:31–35.

Korn EL, Graubard BI. Epidemiologic studies utilizing surveys: accounting for the sampling design. Am J Public Health 1991; 81:1166–73.

Korn EL, Graubard BI. Analysis of health surveys. New York: Wiley, 1999.

Lammer EJ, Brown LE, Anderka MT, Guyer B. Classification and analysis of fetal deaths in Massachusetts. JAMA 1989; 261:1757–62.

Lauderdale DS, Furner SE, Miles TP, Goldberg J. Epidemiologic uses of Medicare data. Epidemiol Rev 1993; 15:319–327.

Lindgren ML, Byers RH Jr, Thomas P, Davis SF, Caldwell B, Rogers M, et al. Trends in perinatal transmission of HIV/AIDS in the United States. JAMA 1999; 282: 531–38.

Linos A, Worthington JW, O'Fallon WM, Kurland LT. The epidemiology of rheumatoid arthritis in Rochester, Minnesota: a study of incidence, prevalence, and mortality. Am J Epidemiol 1983; 111:87–98.

Lydon-Rochelle M, Holt VL, Martin DP, Easterling TR. Association between method of delivery and maternal rehospitalization. JAMA 2000; 283:2411–16.

Marier R. The reporting of communicable disease. Am J Epidemiol 1977; 105:587–90.

McCarty DJ, Tull ES, Moy CS, Kwoh CK, LaPorte RE. Ascertainment of corrected rates: applications of capture-recapture methods. Int J Epidemiol 1993; 22:559–65.

Melton LJ. History of the Rochester Epidemiology Project. Mayo Clin Proc 1996; 71:266–74.

Messite J, Stellman SD. Accuracy of death certficate completion: the need for formalized physician training. JAMA 1996; 275:794–96.

Mock C. "Case series and trauma registries." Chapter 13 in Rivara FP, Cummings P, Koepsell TD, Grossman DC, Maier RV. Injury control: a guide to research and program evaluation. New York: Cambridge University Press, 2001.

National Center for Health Statistics. Funeral directors' handbook on death registration and fetal death reporting. DHHS Pub. No. (PHS) 87–1109. Hyattsville, Md.: National Center for Health Statistics, 1987.

National Center for Health Statistics. Vital statistics of the United States. Hyattsville, Md.: National Center for Health Statistics, 1993.

National Center for Health Statistics. National Death Index user's manual. Hyattsville, Md.: National Center for Health Statistics, 1997.

National Center for Health Statistics. 1998 National Health Interview Survey (NHIS) provisional data release. NHIS survey description. Hyattsville, Md.: National Center for Health Statistics, 2000.

National Center for Health Statistics. Programs and activities. DHHS Pub. No. (PHS) 2002–1200. Hyattsville, Md.: National Center for Health Statistics, 2002.

Psaty BM, Koepsell TD, Siscovick D, Wahl P, Logerfo JP, Inui TS, et al. An approach to several problems in using large databases for population-based case-control studies of the therapeutic efficacy and safety of anti-hypertensive medicines. Stat Med 1991; 10:653–62.

Ray WA, Griffin MR. Use of Medicaid data for pharmacoepidemiology. Am J Epidemiol 1989; 129:837–49.

Ray WA, Griffin MR, Schaffner W, Baugh DK, Melton LJ 3rd. Psychotropic drug use and the risk of hip fracture. N Engl J Med 1987; 316:363–69.

Rosenberg MJ, Gangarosa EJ, Pollard RA, Wallace M, Brolnitsky O. Shigella surveillance in the United States, 1975. J Infect Dis 1977; 136:458–60.

Selby JV. Linking automated databases for research in managed care settings. Ann Intern Med 1997; 127:719–24.

Speizer FE, Doll R, Heaf P. Observations on recent increase in mortality from asthma. BMJ 1968; 1:335–39.

Sugarman JR, Soderberg R, Gordon JE, Rivara FP. Racial misclassification of American Indians: its effect on injury rates in Oregon, 1989 through 1990. Am J Public Health 1993; 83:681–84.

Teutsch SM, Churchill RE. Principles and practice of public health surveillance. New York: Oxford, 1994.

Thacker S. "Historical development." Chapter 1 in: Teutsch SM, Churchill RE (eds.). Principles and practice of public health surveillance. New York: Oxford, 1994.

Thacker SB, Berkelman RL. Public health surveillance in the United States. Epidemiol Rev 1988; 10:164–90.

Turner BJ, Cocroft J, Hauck WW, Schwarz DF, Casey R. Frequency and predictors of medically attended injuries in HIV-infected children. Clin Pediatr 1999; 38:625–35.

US Bureau of the Census. Census 2000 geographic terms and concepts. Washington, D.C.: U.S. Department of Commerce, 2000.

Ventura SJ, Martin JA, Curtin SC, Mathews TJ, Park MM. Births: final data for 1998. National vital statistics reports; vol. 48 no. 3. Hyattsville, Md.: National Center for Health Statistics, 2000.

Washington State Department of Health. The Health of Washington State. Olympia, Wash.: Washington State Department of Health, 2002.

Wharton M, Vogt RL. "State and local issues in surveillance." Chapter 12 in: Teutsch SM, Churchill RE (eds.). Principles and practice of public health surveillance. New York: Oxford, 1994.

World Health Organization. International Statistical Classification of Diseases and Related Health Problems (10th revision). Geneva: World Health Organization, 1992.

7

PERSON, PLACE, AND TIME

I keep six honest serving-men
(They taught me all I knew);
Their names are What and Why and When
And How and Where and Who ...

Rudyard Kipling

If there were one idea that all epidemiologists could agree on, it would probably be: *diseases do not occur at random.* Virtually every form of human ill health exhibits variation in its frequency within populations, between populations, or over time that exceeds the play of chance.

The simple conceptual framework summarized by the title of this chapter has traditionally been used to organize the many factors with which disease frequency can be associated:

- *Person.* What kinds of people tend to develop the disease, and who tends to be spared? What's unusual about those people?
- *Place.* Where is the disease especially common or rare, and what's different about those places?
- *Time.* How does disease frequency change over time, and what other factors are temporally associated with those changes?

Even when these kinds of associations are not causal, knowledge of their presence can be informative. Sometimes just knowing where to look for a disease can provide helpful guidance for disease control. For example, knowing how the prevalence of occult breast cancer varies with age guides policy about the age at which women should start receiving screening mammography for breast cancer. But the greater challenge is to understand *why* the observed patterns are as they are. The more fully we understand why a disease strikes certain people, in certain places, and at certain times, the more likely it is that we can find opportunities to intervene and to prevent disease.

This chapter elaborates on the person-place-time framework and illustrates some of its uses through examples. Occasionally we will employ methods of comparison that have not yet been covered in detail, such as age-adjusted mortality rates. Rate adjustment is discussed in Chapter 11, and curious readers are welcome to peek ahead. For now, think of adjusted rates as the rates that would be observed in the groups being compared if they had identical compositions on the adjustment factor.

PERSON

People can be grouped or distinguished on a great many personal characteristics, and one might wonder where to start and where to stop. Often as a starting point in trying to understand the causes of a disease, we look to the pattern of its occurrence in relation to personal characteristics that are routinely ascertained and recorded in available data sources, as described in Chapter 6. The range of characteristics included in these sources is generally limited, often restricted to sociodemographic characteristics such as age, gender, race, and marital status. When additional information is present—perhaps birth order or maternal age on a birth certificate, or occupation on a death certificate—it can be considered as well.

Age

Nearly every known disease varies in frequency with age, many to a marked degree. A variety of underlying mechanisms can be responsible, producing quite different patterns of association. For example:

- *Immunity.* A few weeks or months after a baby is born, maternally derived antibodies dissipate and leave the infant susceptible to various common infectious diseases. Figure 7–1 shows how the incidence of acute respiratory infections was found to vary by age among children in the community of Tecumseh, Michigan, declining steadily with age (Monto and Ullman, 1974). Acute respiratory infections were characterized by very high incidence rates, up to 6.1 cases *per person-year* among children less than one year of age.
- *Human development.* Age can also indicate approximately where someone falls in the maturational sequence of physical, mental, and behavioral changes that normally occur over the human lifespan. Figure 7–2 shows how the mortality rate for drowning varied by age among children and young adults in the U.S. during 1999 (Hoyert et al., 2001). The rate was highest in toddlers (aged 1 to 4 years)—an age when children are mobile and curious about everything around them, even though they often do not understand the hazards of deep water or know how to survive if they fall in.

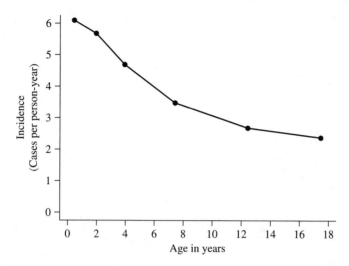

Figure 7-1. Incidence of Respiratory Infections by Age: Tecumseh, Michigan, 1969-1971 (based on Monto and Ullman, 1974).

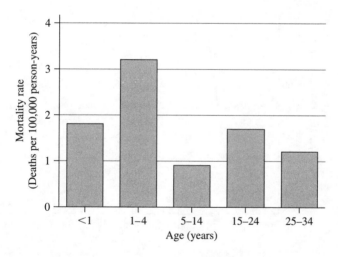

Figure 7-2. Mortality from Drowning by Age: U.S., 1999.

- *Slowly progressive diseases.* Atherosclerosis can begin at an early age, but it generally goes unrecognized until atherosclerotic plaques become large enough to reduce blood flow significantly in major arteries. Many factors influence how rapidly plaques grow—family history, smoking, blood pressure, and lipid levels among them—but the process typically requires several decades before disease becomes clinically apparent. Mortality rates for acute myocardial infarction, which almost always results from atherosclerosis of the coronary arteries, vary several–thousand-fold from childhood

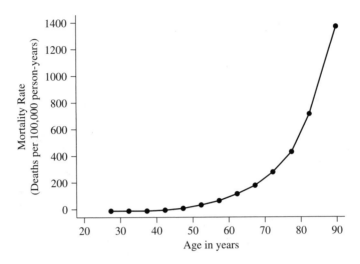

Figure 7–3. Mortality from Acute Myocardial Infarction by Age: U.S., 1998.

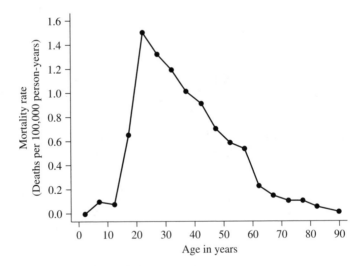

Figure 7–4. Mortality from Motorcycle Crashes by Age: U.S., 1999.

to old age in the U.S. (Figure 7–3) (Murphy, 2000)—a pattern that fits with a model of gradual disease pathogenesis.

- *Age-related variation in lifestyle.* Age is also strongly related to what activities people engage in and what exposures they encounter in daily life. For example, mortality rates from motorcycle collisions in the U.S. have been observed to peak in young adulthood (Figure 7–4) (Centers for Disease

Control and Prevention). This pattern fits with the ages at which people like to ride motorcycles and with how driving styles vary with age.

Besides being a personal characteristic, age can also be considered a time scale on which disease frequency can vary, as discussed later in this chapter.

Gender

Differences in disease frequency between the sexes are also the rule, not the exception. In broad terms, both biological and non-biological factors can be at play.

- *Biological.* At one extreme, most diseases of the reproductive system occur either only among men (e.g., prostate cancer) or only among women (e.g., uterine cancer, complications of childbirth). Even for some diseases of organs related to reproduction, however, the association with gender is not absolute. The age-adjusted incidence of invasive breast cancer among U.S. *males* in 1997 was 1.1 per 100,000 person-years, not zero (Ries et al., 2000). Yet this rate was only about 1% of the rate for U.S. females (115.4 per 100,000 person-years), and it is reasonable to assume that anatomic and hormonal differences between men and women account for a large part of this difference.

  Besides diseases of the reproductive system, many other diseases predominate in one gender or the other for reasons that are believed to be biological. Red-green color blindness is inherited as a recessive trait on the X-chromosome and for this reason appears almost entirely in males (Pokorny et al., 1979). In the U.S., the prevalence of osteoporosis has been found to be far higher in women than in men (Figure 7–5), which is thought to be explained in part by gender-related hormonal effects on bone physiology (Reeve, 2000).
- *Non-biological.* The major differences in social roles and health-related behavior between men and women undoubtedly underlie many gender differences in disease frequency. Gender serves as a marker for exposure to more proximate disease causes. For example, Table 7–1 compares U.S. age-adjusted mortality rates between males and females for three causes of death: chronic liver disease and cirrhosis, chronic obstructive pulmonary disease, and cancer of the lung and intrathoracic organs. As a group, men were at much higher risk of dying of these diseases than were women, which is almost certainly due to the higher prevalence of heavy alcohol use and tobacco smoking among men.

Table 7–1. Age-Adjusted Mortality Rates for Three
Causes of Death, by Gender: U.S., 1998

| | Mortality Rate[a] | |
	MALES	FEMALES
Chronic liver disease and cirrhosis	10.3	4.4
Chronic obstructive pulmonary disease	25.9	18.1
Cancer of lung and intrathoracic organs	51.7	27.6

[a] Deaths per 100,000 person-years.
[*Source:* National Center for Health Statistics (2000).]

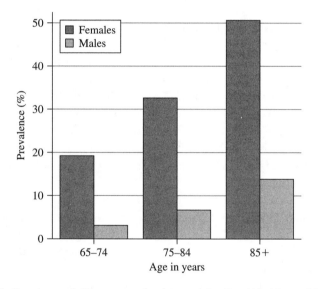

Figure 7–5. Prevalence of Osteoporosis by Age and Gender: U.S. National Health and Nutrition Examination Study, 1988–1994 (National Center for Health Statistics, 1998b).

Even larger gender differences have prevailed for firearm injury deaths, as shown in Figure 7–6. At ages 20 to 24 years, firearm mortality in 1998 was more than eight times greater in males than in females.

Curves with two or more peaks, such as that in Figure 7–6, sometimes suggest that what is being treated as a single condition may be divided into two or more component subtypes, each of which has a different descriptive epidemiologic profile. In this instance, the peak in firearm deaths among younger men consists chiefly of homicides, while the peak in older men consists chiefly of suicides.

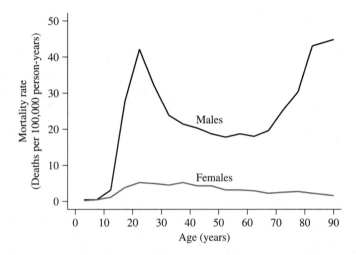

Figure 7-6. Mortality Rates from Firearm Injury by Age and Gender: U.S., 1998 (National Center for Health Statistics, 2000).

Race and Ethnicity

Race and *ethnicity* refer to self-perceived membership in groups defined by skin color, ancestral place of residence, language, cultural heritage, and related factors. There is no consensus that they reflect fundamental biological characteristics as age and gender do (Lin and Kelsey, 2000; Williams, 1997). Nonetheless, the frequency of many diseases varies strongly by race and ethnicity, and knowledge of this variation can provide clues as to disease etiology.

Some race–disease associations almost certainly are biologically based. For example, in 1993–1997, the age-adjusted incidence of invasive malignant melanoma in the SEER cancer registries was 13.8 cases per 100,000 person-years for whites vs. 0.8 for blacks—a 17-fold difference (Ries et al., 2000). This form of skin cancer has been associated with prolonged or intense exposure to sunlight, and dark natural skin pigmentation probably protects deeper skin layers from potentially carcinogenic ultraviolet radiation (Armstrong and English, 1996). Various genetic markers that affect disease susceptibility are also associated with race—for example, the hemoglobin S gene, which causes sickle-cell anemia, is found predominantly in blacks (Ashley-Koch et al., 2000).

However, race and ethnicity are also associated with socioeconomic status, living conditions, dietary habits, cultural background, health behaviors, exposure to discrimination, access to health care, and other factors that can themselves be linked to disease risk. Moreover, classification and misclassification of race or ethnicity in data commonly used for epidemiologic research are a greater problem than for most

Table 7–2. Selected Birth and Infant Health Characteristics
by Race/Ethnicity of Mother: U.S., 1997

CHARACTERISTIC	Non-Hispanic WHITE	Non-Hispanic BLACK	HISPANIC	AMERICAN INDIAN OR ALASKA NATIVE	ASIAN OR PACIFIC ISLANDER
Infant mortality rate[a]	6.0	13.7	6.0	8.7	5.0
Percent of babies weighing <2500 grams	6.5	13.1	6.4	6.8	7.2
Percent of live births with:					
Mother aged <18 years	3.2	9.8	7.2	8.6	2.0
Unmarried mother	21.5	69.4	40.9	58.7	15.8
No prenatal care, or only in third trimester	2.4	7.3	6.2	8.6	3.8

[a]Deaths in first year of life per 1000 births.
[*Source:* National Center for Health Statistics (2000).]

other sociodemographic characteristics (Hahn et al., 1992; Hahn, 1992). Hence, describing race–disease associations is often much easier than understanding what they mean.

For example, Table 7–2 compares infant mortality rates and the prevalence of low birth weight across five racial and ethnic groups in the U.S. in 1997. To put the observed differences in context, the prevalences of three risk factors related to pregnancy outcomes and infant health are also shown, derived from birth certificate data. Infant mortality and low birth weight were most common in blacks. The data also suggest possible contributing factors at which prevention programs might be directed to help reduce the observed racial disparities in birth outcomes.

Probing more deeply, however, calculation and interpretation of race-specific infant mortality rates is not straightforward. One problem is defining the baby's race when the parents are of different races. Before 1989, the National Center for Health Statistics used a complex algorithm, classifying a baby as white only if both parents were white (National Center for Health Statistics, 2000). Since 1989, the baby's race has been defined simply as the race of the mother—a change that affects comparability of statistics over time (National Center for Health Statistics, 1994).

Another problem is classification of the race of an infant who dies. Race as recorded on the death certificate (usually by the funeral director) can disagree with race as recorded on the birth certificate. Hahn and colleagues (1992) found that coding inconsistencies were rare for blacks or whites, but that many infants of other races who died were coded as white on the death certificate. Unless this misclassification were to be corrected by linking birth and death certificates and drawing better race data from the birth certificate, the excess in infant mortality rates among American Indians and Alaska Natives could go undetected.

Lastly, widely used race and ethnicity groupings such as those shown in Table 7–2 can obscure large differences within them. For example, within the Asian/Pacific Islander category, the infant mortality rate varied nearly threefold among Asians of different nationalities, from 3.1 among Chinese to 9.0 among Hawaiians.

Socioeconomic Status

Example: In 1914, a team headed by Dr. Joseph Goldberger of the U.S. Public Health Service was commissioned to investigate pellagra, which had become common in parts of the southeastern United States (Goldberger et al., 1920). Pellagra is characterized by symmetrical skin eruptions; in advanced cases, gastrointestinal and nervous-system symptoms also appear. Earlier small studies had suggested an association between pellagra and poverty.

The research team decided to study seven small cotton-mill villages in South Carolina, each with 500 to 800 residents, where pellagra was thought to be prevalent. Although local doctors were cooperative, it was felt—and later shown—that many cases would be missed by relying solely on their records to identify people with pellagra. Hence, for several months, biweekly visits were made to every home in which a white cotton-mill worker resided. The field worker sought to identify and count pellagra cases according to a standard case definition and to gather data on household composition, income, living conditions, and diet.

Family income information for the preceding half-month was obtained from the housewife or other responsible family member, supplemented by data from the local cotton mill's payroll. Almost all households proved to have annual family incomes of $700 to $1000. But the researchers recognized that the same family income could result in different standards of living depending on household size and composition, which were quite variable. Because at least half of most families' income went for food, they chose a measure of family size that weighted each family member according to a previously published scale of food requirements according to age and gender. The weights assigned ranged from 1.0 for an adult male to 0.3 for a child under two years of age. Family size was thus measured in "adult male units."

Table 7–3 shows how the period prevalence of pellagra and the consumption of selected food items varied by economic status, measured as half-monthly family income per adult male unit. A striking increase in the frequency of pellagra was found with decreasing economic status. Poorer households were also found to consume more salt pork and corn meal but fewer eggs and fresh meats. The

Table 7–3. Period Prevalence of Pellagra and Relative Consumption of
Selected Foodstuffs in Seven South Carolina Cotton-Mill Villages

HALF-MONTHLY FAMILY INCOME PER ADULT MALE UNIT	PELLAGRA CASES	PERSONS	CASES PER 1000 PERSONS[a]	Relative Consumption[a]			
				SALT PORK	CORN MEAL AND GRITS	EGGS	FRESH MEATS
$14.00 and over	1	291	3.4	100	100	100	100
$10.00–$13.99	3	736	4.1	126	121	97	68
$8.00–$9.99	10	784	12.8	138	120	75	64
$6.00–$7.99	27	1037	26.0	144	138	64	45
Under $6.00	56	1312	42.7	138	134	56	40

[a]Relative amount purchased per adult male unit (100 = amount in households with highest economic status).
[*Source:* Goldberger et al. (1920).]

researchers concluded that poverty was associated with pellagra in this setting and suggested that the association might be due to inability to buy food needed for a balanced diet.

Goldberger and colleagues (1923) went on to conduct intervention studies in orphanages and sanitariums which suggested that pellagra could be prevented by a diet with adequate protein in the form of milk, eggs, or meats. Years later, the condition was finally found to result from niacin deficiency. The body can synthesize niacin from the amino acid tryptophan in high-protein foods (Goldsmith, 1965), but the low-protein, high-cornmeal diet that was common among poor Southern cotton-mill workers did not provide enough tryptophan.

Goldberger's studies focused on per-capita family income, which remains a commonly used index of socioeconomic status. Income, education, and occupational classification (e.g., white collar, blue collar, service, farm) are often used individually as measures of socioeconomic status, each with its own strengths and weaknesses (National Center for Health Statistics, 1998a). Summary indices of socioeconomic status have also been developed that combine information from two or more of these variables (Miller, 1991; Krieger et al., 1997).

An individual's own income, education, and/or occupation can influence his or her disease risk through many mechanisms, probably often acting in combination, including safety of housing and mode of transportation, financial access to health care, awareness and practice of healthy behaviors, exposure to health hazards on the job, and others. These associations can be strong, highlighting the importance of socioeconomic-status indicators as potential confounding factors in etiologic studies. For example, Table 7–4 shows that age-adjusted mortality

Table 7–4. Age-Adjusted Mortality[a] among Adults Aged 25–64 Years:
United States, 1998

	Years of School Completed		
CAUSE OF DEATH	<12	12	13+
All causes	562	466	224
Chronic and non-communicable diseases	425	363	181
Injury	95	75	32
Communicable diseases	42	28	11
HIV infection	17	12	4
Other	24	17	7

[a]Deaths per 100,000 person-years.
[*Source:* National Center for Health Statistics (2001).]

rates for working-age U.S. adults in 1998 varied more than 2.5-fold in relation to education in three broad categories, and by an even larger ratio for such selected causes such as HIV infection.

Indicators of socioeconomic status can also have *contextual* effects. That is, a person's risk of disease may be influenced not only by his or her own education or income, but also by the education or income of others with whom he or she interacts. For example, as Goldberger and colleagues realized, household income should be interpreted in relation to household size and composition. Average income or education levels in the community may be informative as indicators of the physical and social environment in which an individual lives or works (Krieger et al., 1997; Von Korff et al., 1992). The amount of *dispersion* in income within a social group—income inequality—may also be associated with differences in health for reasons not yet well understood (Lynch et al., 2000). They may relate to perceptions of disadvantage and/or to deeper features of social structure that favor one subgroup over another (Kaplan et al., 1996).

Marital Status

Marital status, too, can be associated with disease occurrence for many reasons. The incidence of cervical cancer has been found to be lower in unmarried women than in married women (Leck et al., 1978)—an association now thought to be related to differences in women's likelihood of exposure to sexually transmitted viral agents involved in the etiology of cervical cancer (Koutsky, 1997).

A mother's marital status is routinely captured on the birth certificate and has proven valuable in perinatal epidemiology. For example, infant mortality in the U.S. during 1997 was 10.5 per 1000 liveborn infants among babies of unmarried mothers, vs. 5.6 per 1000 among babies of married mothers, an association that also held within racial/ethnic groups (MacDorman and Atkinson, 1999). In this context, marital status may reflect social support within the household, or instrumental male support in the form of income and sharing child care.

Marital status has often been found associated with the frequency of mental illnesses. For example, mortality from suicide has been found to be sharply higher among divorced or separated men compared to married men; interestingly, these associations appear to be much weaker in women (Kposowa, 2000; Baker et al., 1992).

PLACE

Example: In the late summer of 1854, a particularly terrible outbreak of cholera struck in London, England, with over 500 cholera deaths in ten days (Snow, 1936). What caused cholera epidemics was unknown at that time, but studies during previous outbreaks had suggested an association with living at low elevations. This association spawned various theories about how a person contracted cholera, including a "miasma" hypothesis positing that cholera came from breathing foul air that collected in low-lying areas.

British physician John Snow, who noted that cholera was primarily a gastrointestinal disease, suspected that it might instead arise from ingesting contaminated water, which he thought might be more common in low-elevation areas. He interrupted other studies of this theory to investigate the 1854 outbreak. Having obtained from the General Register Office a list of the first 83 deaths ascribed to cholera during the epidemic, he went to the neighborhood where most deaths had occurred. He soon found that nearly all of the fatal cases had lived within a short distance of a public, hand-operated water pump located on Broad Street near the corner of Cambridge Street. In his words:

> There were only ten deaths in houses situated decidedly nearer to another street pump. In five of these cases the families of the deceased persons informed me that they always sent to the pump in Broad Street, as they preferred the water to that of the pump which was nearer. In three other cases, the deceased were children who went to school near the pump in Broad Street. Two of them were known to drink the water; and the parents of the third think it probable that it did so. The other two deaths, beyond the district which this pump supplies, represent only the amount of mortality from cholera that was occurring before the irruption took place....
>
> The result of the inquiry, then, was that there had been no particular outbreak or increase of cholera, in this part of London, except among the persons who were in the habit of drinking the water of the above-mentioned pump-well.
>
> I had an interview with the Board of Guardians of St. James's parish on the evening of Thursday, 7th September, and represented the above circumstances to them. In consequence of what I said, the handle of the pump was removed on the following day....

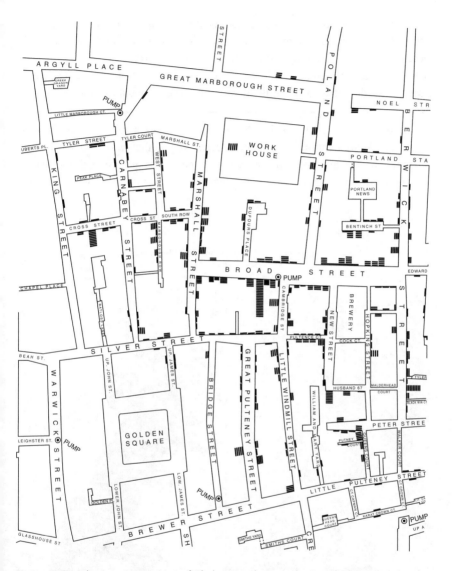

Figure 7-7. John Snow's Spot Map of Cholera Deaths Near the Broad Street Pump: London, 1854 (Snow, 1936).

Later that year, Snow illustrated the results of his outbreak investigation using a *spot map* of the area on which each fatal case was shown as a small black bar (Figure 7–7) (Brody et al., 2000). Geographical clustering of cases near the Broad Street pump was clearly evident.

Spot maps like the one Snow constructed remain a useful tool even today in outbreak investigation to suggest spatial clusters of cases by visual inspection. But because they involve simply plotting the place of occurrence of each case, they have much the same limitation as counts do as a measure of disease frequency; namely, they do not account for the distribution of the population at risk.

Example: Variant Creutzfeld-Jakob disease (vCJD) is a rare human nervous-system disease thought to be due to the infectious agent that causes bovine spongiform encephalopathy ("mad cow disease"). As described in Chapter 5, the disease was first reported in 1996. Figure 7–8 shows two maps of Great Britain on which

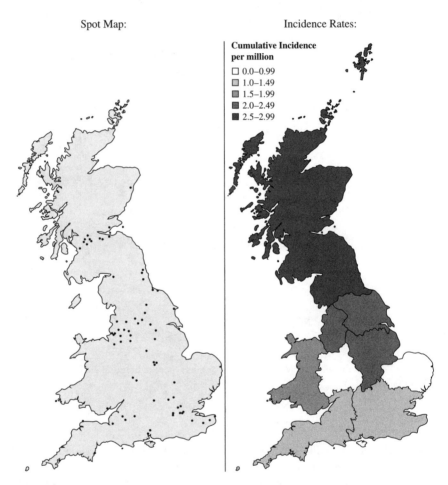

Figure 7-8. Geographic Distribution of Variant Creutzfeld-Jakob Disease in Great Britain, 1996–2000 (from Cousens et al., 2001).

the geographic distribution of vCJD is displayed, from a report by Cousens and colleagues (2001). The left panel is a spot map showing the place of occurrence of all 84 qualifying cases that had been reported through November 10, 2000. Most cases resided in southern, and especially southeastern, England. The right panel is a map showing population-based incidence rates of vCJD for ten regions, based on the same 84 cases and census data. In fact, vCJD incidence was greater in Scotland and northern England once the size of the population at risk in each region had been taken into account.

Geographic variability in disease frequency can be due to variations in the physical environment. For example, Figure 7–9 shows age-adjusted mortality rates for malignant melanoma in U.S. white males, 1950 to 1994. Higher rates in the sunnier, warmer southern states agree well with the theory that greater unprotected exposure to sunlight increases the risk of this form of skin cancer (Armstrong and English, 1996). Lyme disease, which results from a spirochetal infection acquired through an *Ixodes scapularis* tick bite, occurs only in parts of the country where environmental conditions favor survival and reproduction of this tick species (Walker, 1998).

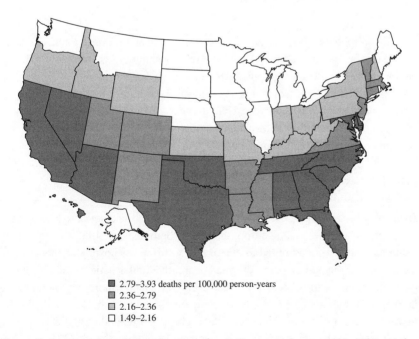

■ 2.79–3.93 deaths per 100,000 person-years
▨ 2.36–2.79
▢ 2.16–2.36
□ 1.49–2.16

Figure 7–9. Age-Adjusted Mortality Rates for Malignant Melanoma: U.S. White Males, 1950–1994.

Table 7–5. Comparison of Mortality from Selected Diseases (1998), and Prevalence of Selected Behavioral Risk Factors (1997): Utah and Nevada

	UTAH	NEVADA
Age-adjusted mortality[a]		
All causes	404.5	539.1
Cancer	93.5	133.9
Heart disease	87.4	139.7
Chronic obstructive pulmonary disease	17.3	32.1
Chronic liver disease and cirrhosis	6.6	12.6
Motor-vehicle collisions	18.3	20.0
Suicide	16.6	21.2
Homicide	3.1	10.6
Firearm injury	11.7	21.1
Risk factor prevalence[b]		
Current smoking	13.8%	28.0%
Binge drinking	7.7%	19.2%
Chronic drinking	1.7%	4.7%

[a] Deaths per 100,000 person-years
[b] Among persons aged 18 years or older
[*Sources:* Murphy (2000), Nelson (1998).]

Geographic location can also be just a proxy for spatial variation in exposure to disease risk factors that may have little relationship to the natural environment but may instead reflect geographic differences in sociocultural milieu or behavior. For example, Table 7–5 compares selected mortality rates and the prevalence of smoking and alcohol use between Utah and Nevada, two neighboring states that have generally similar climates and topography. The observed disparities almost certainly reflect differences in lifestyle, not in physical environment.

Lastly, variation in disease incidence by place can provide clues about important differences in medical practice.

Example: Ignaz Semmelweis was an obstetrician and teacher at a large public maternity hospital in Vienna during the 1840s (Semmelweis, 1988). At that time, women in labor were admitted to one of two wards at the hospital, depending on the day of the week. For years, despite apparently similar patients, deaths due to puerperal (childbirth-related) fever had been consistently more common among mothers and infants on Ward no. 1, where Semmelweis worked. He calculated that in 1846, the cumulative incidence of fatal childbirth-related complications was $459/4010 = 11.4\%$ among mothers on Ward no. 1, compared to $105/3754 = 2.8\%$ among mothers on Ward no. 2.

Semmelweis noted that medical students received their training on Ward no. 1, while midwives trained on Ward no. 2. The medical students and their teachers often participated in autopsies as part of their study of anatomy. When a pathologist was accidentally cut in the finger during an autopsy of a puerperal fever victim and went on to die of a clinically similar disease himself, Semmelweis suspected that transmission of "cadaverous particles" via the hands of students and teachers might be involved in puerperal fever. He noted that this hypothesis also fitted other epidemiologic observations, such as rarity of the condition among women who had delivered en route to the hospital and among those who had delivered in past years before the educational emphasis on learning from autopsies. He initiated a policy of regular hand-washing with a chlorinated solution after autopsies and between clinical examinations. It was followed by a sharp reduction in the cumulative incidence of fatal complications on Ward no. 1 to $56/1841 = 3.0\%$ over the next seven months.

Advances in computing technology and statistics have led to growing use of geographic information systems for epidemiologic research (Moore and Carpenter, 1999; Glass et al., 1995; Becker et al., 1998). These systems produce customized maps showing the spatial distribution of disease and permit visual pattern recognition. Some systems also include statistical tools to test for area-level associations between disease frequency and other factors, or to detect clustering of cases in space and time.

TIME

Secular Trends

Patterns of change in disease frequency over periods of calendar time are termed *secular trends*. Figure 7–10 depicts the rise and fall of age-adjusted mortality rates for coronary heart disease in the U.S. from 1950 to 2000, by race and sex (National Heart, Lung, and Blood Institute, 2002). It shows that mortality peaked in the late 1960s and has been declining ever since—a decline thought to be due to a combination of better control of preventable risk factors and the advent of more effective treatments (Goldman and Cook, 1984). The figure also shows steeper recent declines in whites than in blacks, narrowing the gap in rates between black and white men and reversing its direction in women. Note the three vertical lines, which indicate when new versions of the International Classification of Diseases (ICD) came into use. These changes must be taken into account when interpreting trends that straddle the boundaries between ICD versions.

An *epidemic* is said to occur when the frequency of a disease exceeds the expected level (Last, 2000). This definition is not very specific, and there is no

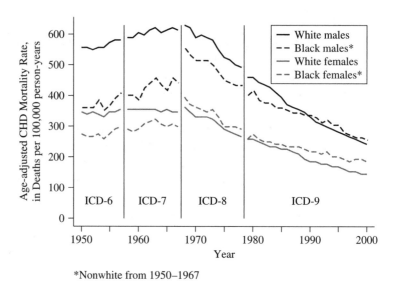

Figure 7–10. Secular Trend in Coronary Heart Disease Mortality: U.S., 1950-1998 (adapted from National Heart, Lung, and Blood Institute, 2002).

universal method for determining what level is "expected." Often the expected level is simply the historically observed level, and in that sense any steady rise in disease incidence can qualify as an epidemic. Because the term *epidemic* often has dire connotations, however, the term *outbreak* is sometimes preferred in an acute situation to avoid causing needless alarm. Short-term disease outbreaks are discussed in Chapter 19.

Cyclical Variation

The incidence of many diseases exhibits a recurring pattern of variation over time periods of a certain length.

- *Pneumonia and influenza deaths,* which are often combined for analysis to minimize the effect of diagnostic misclassification, have historically peaked in the U.S. during winter and fallen to lower levels in summer (Figure 7–11). Thus, in order to gauge whether an epidemic of pneumonia/influenza has occurred, the proportion of deaths due to these diseases must be compared to seasonally adjusted expected levels. On this basis, an epidemic was deemed to have occurred in the 1988–1989 season and the 1989–1990 season, but not in the 1990–1991 season (Centers for Disease Control and Prevention, 1993).

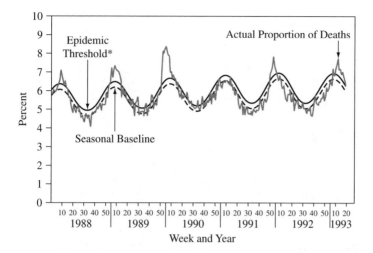

Figure 7-11. Proportion of Deaths Due to Pneumonia and Influenza, by Week: U.S., 1988-1991 (based on Centers for Disease Control and Prevention, 1993).

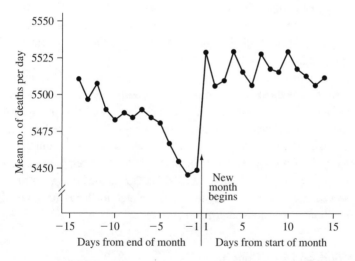

Figure 7-12. Mean Daily Deaths by Days Before and After the First Day of a Month: U.S., 1973-1988 (based on Phillips et al., 1999).

- *Deaths* in the U.S. have been observed to vary to small degree in a monthly cycle (Figure 7–12). Phillips and colleagues (1999) found that deaths due to substance abuse accounted for much of the monthly periodicity and hypothesized an association with the timing of benefit checks from government programs.

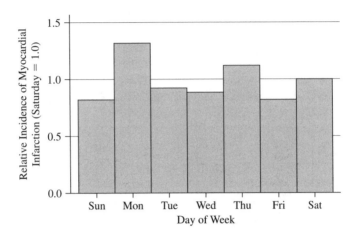

Figure 7–13. Relative Incidence of Acute Myocardial Infarction by Day of Week among Working Persons: Augsburg, Germany, 1985–1990 (based on Willich et al., 1994).

- *Myocardial infarction* occurrence has been seen in a European study to vary among the days of the week, particularly among working people (Figure 7–13) (Willich et al., 1994). It seems there is an empirical basis for loathing of Mondays!
- *In-hospital mortality* among patients who were admitted to a hospital with a serious medical condition on a weekend has been found to exceed that among patients admitted on a weekday—an association that may relate to lower staffing levels in hospitals on weekends (Bell and Redelmeier, 2001).
- *Sudden Infant Death Syndrome (SIDS)* cases have been found to be most likely to occur—or at least to be discovered—between 6:00 A.M. and noon (Figure 7–14) (Bergman et al., 1972). This association with time of day served as a clue to investigate factors related to sleep, including sleeping position, as possible contributing causes.

Age, Period, and Birth Cohort

Consider Table 7–6, which shows mortality rates from lung cancer by age group among U.S. women in 1975, 1985, and 1995. From this typical arrangement of rates in rows and columns, two kinds of comparisons immediately come to mind. First, rates can be compared horizontally within each row to see how lung cancer mortality varied over time, keeping age fixed. Second, rates can be compared vertically within each column to see how they varied according to age, keeping calendar year fixed. The table thus allows associations with both age and time to be examined separately, by the simple expedient of making horizontal or vertical comparisons.

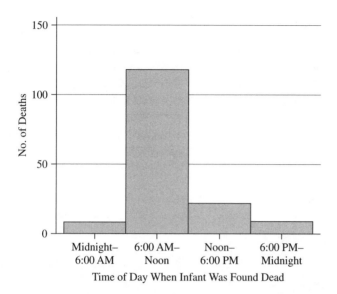

Figure 7–14. Incidence of Sudden Infant Death Syndrome by Time of Day When Infant Was Found Dead: King County, Washington, 1965–1968 (based on Bergman et al., 1972).

Table 7–6. Mortality from Lung Cancer among U.S.
Women by Age, in 1975, 1985, and 1995

AGE (YEARS)	Mortality Rate[a]		
	1975	1985	1995
35–44	7.3	5.7	5.1
45–54	28.1	36.0	30.0
55–64	58.3	94.3	104.5
65–74	67.6	144.9	204.5
75–84	70.8	134.9	244.5
85+	71.5	103.7	186.8

[a]Deaths per 100,000 person-years.

Figure 7–15 shows the same set of rates graphically, with lines connecting rates that were observed in the same calendar year. In this instance, a rather odd pattern emerges if we try to summarize how lung cancer mortality varied with age. In 1975, the rates rose steadily with age. In 1985, they peaked at ages 65 to 74 years and then declined for older women. In 1995, they kept climbing until ages 75 to 84 years and then fell among the oldest women. One might speculate that the observed fall in age-specific rates among the oldest women in 1985 and 1995

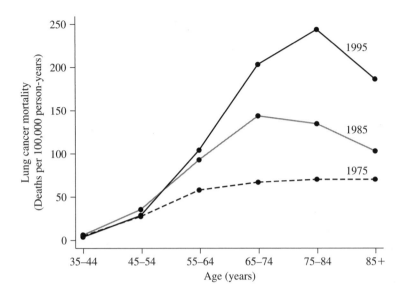

Figure 7-15. Lung Cancer Mortality Rates in U.S. Women, by Age and Calendar Year.

could represent "survival of the fittest": perhaps women who were most prone to lung cancer had already died before reaching very old age. Still, an explanation would be needed for why this phenomenon should take effect at different ages in different years.

But there is another, less obvious, factor at play. Note that the age groups in question were set up to be ten years apart—the same time interval that separates adjacent columns. As a result, the group of women who experienced the rate of 58.3 at ages 55 to 64 in 1975 were largely the same women who, a decade later, had a rate of 144.9 at ages 65 to 74 in 1985. Another decade later, their mortality rate from lung cancer was 244.5 at ages 75 to 84. All of these women were born during the ten-year period 1911–1920 and thus comprised a *birth cohort*. Their experience is chronicled along a diagonal path in Table 7–6. Other birth cohorts trace out other parallel diagonal paths in the table, either above or below that of the 1911–1920 birth cohort. For example, the 1921–1930 birth cohort contributed the rates in the diagonal path one row higher.

But why should a woman's year of birth matter at all here, when the rates being examined pertain to late adulthood? In actuality, year of birth is merely a convenient way to identify people who belong to a certain generation. For example, people born shortly after the end of World War II are often referred to as "baby boomers," some of their offspring as "Generation X," and so on. Members of the same generation march through history as a cohort, often sharing experiences by virtue of being about the same age when various world events and cultural shifts occur. Some of these common experiences can have long-lasting effects on their future risk of developing certain diseases.

For lung cancer, tobacco smoking is now known to be a strong risk factor, as several landmark epidemiologic studies in the 1950s and 1960s helped establish (Doll and Hill, 1950; Wynder and Graham, 1950; Doll and Hill, 1964). Among U.S. women, the prevalence of smoking increased steadily through most of the 20th century. Thus, at any given age, women in later birth cohorts were more likely to have adopted smoking than were their counterparts in earlier birth cohorts. For example, about 44% of women in the 1921–1930 birth cohort were current smokers by the time they reached age 25 years, compared with about 37% of the 1911–1920 birth cohort when *they* were 25, and only about 18% of the 1901–1910 birth cohort (Burns et al., 1997). The higher prevalence of smoking during early adulthood affected the incidence of lung cancer in later birth cohorts through the remainder of their adult lives, partly because smoking is a persistent habit and partly because it affects not only current risk but future risk of lung cancer in an individual.

Figure 7–16 shows the same set of lung cancer mortality rates as in Table 7–6 and Figure 7–15, but now connecting with lines the points that pertain to the same birth cohort. This way of looking at the data reveals a simple, regular pattern: at any age for which they can be compared, later birth cohorts had higher lung cancer mortality than did earlier birth cohorts.

Note also the pattern of change in lung cancer mortality in relation to age within birth cohorts in Figure 7–16. In each birth cohort, lung cancer mortality rose steadily with age. It did not peak at some age and then decline, as was the

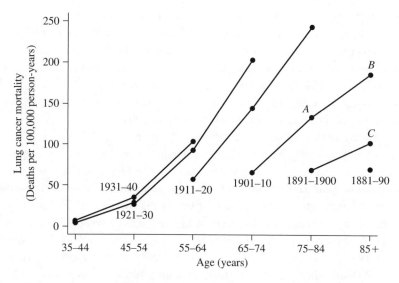

Figure 7–16. Lung Cancer Mortality Rates in U.S. Women, by Age and Birth Cohort.

impression first suggested by Figure 7–15. Thus it is no longer necessary to invoke a "survival of the fittest" hypothesis to explain such a decline, nor is there a need to embellish that hypothesis further to explain why the decline occurred at different ages in different years. In fact, if a selective-survival mechanism were the sole factor at play, a similar rise-and-fall curve shape would be expected within each birth cohort, which was not evident.

To understand why the relationship between age and lung cancer mortality appears different between Figures 7–15 and 7–16, consider point A in Figure 7–16. It pertains to the rate observed for women in the 1901–1910 birth cohort in calendar year 1985, at which time they were 75 to 84 years old. In Figure 7–16, point A is connected to point B, which pertains to the same birth cohort after they had aged another ten years. The rate for point B was observed in calendar year 1995. In Figure 7–15, point A was connected to point C, which pertains to the same calendar year as does point A—1985. But moving from point A to point C actually involves two changes: *(1)* women at point C were ten years older than those at point A, and *(2)* they were members of a different birth cohort. In this instance, the effect of "dropping down" to an earlier birth cohort outweighs the effect of "sliding up" to an older age group. An age effect is mixed with a cohort effect.

More broadly, age, birth cohort, and calendar year (often called *period*) are three conceptually separate time scales, each of which can influence disease frequency. But the three time scales are also intimately related, because:

$$\text{Calendar year} - \text{age} = \text{year of birth}.$$

Once any two of these quantities have been specified, the third is not free to vary but instead is fully determined. Among statisticians, this analytic problem is termed one of *non-identifiability*—it is impossible to fully disentangle the separate contributions of three factors when fixing any two of them automatically fixes the third (Holford, 1991; Clayton and Schifflers, 1987; Weinkam and Sterling, 1991). More details about the difficulties this poses for statistical modeling of age, period, and birth-cohort effects are discussed by Holford (1991).

Among epidemiologists, alternative ways of representing the same set of rates, often graphically, have proven helpful in the search for structure, simplicity, and agreement with other observations. For example, Figure 7–15 focuses on age and calendar year, leaving birth cohort in the background. Figure 7–16 focuses on age and birth cohort, leaving calendar year in the background. In this instance, the simplicity and regularity apparent in Figure 7–16 are compelling reasons to think of lung cancer mortality chiefly in terms of age and birth cohort. Tuberculosis (Frost, 1939), testicular cancer (Liu et al., 1999), and malignant melanoma (Dennis et al., 1993) are other diseases for which examining trends in mortality or incidence in terms of birth cohorts has provided new insights.

EXERCISES

1. *Streptococcus pneumoniae* is a common cause of community-acquired pneumonia, meningitis, and bacteremia. Vaccines have now been developed against many specific strains of *S. pneumoniae*. To help quantify the burden of disease caused by this pathogen on the U.S. population, Robinson and colleagues (2001) used data from a nine-state laboratory-based surveillance system to estimate the number of cases and deaths from invasive *S. pneumoniae* infection in the U.S. during 1998. Table 7–7 shows the distribution of these events by age. The mean age among all cases was approximately 43 years (median: 42 years).

    To what extent can the data in Table 7–7 be used to assess which age groups are burdened disproportionately by invasive *S. pneumoniae* in the U.S.?

2. Mortality from cardiovascular disease (CVD) in the state of Utah is among the lowest in the U.S. Lyon and colleagues (1978) studied CVD mortality within Utah, comparing rates in Mormons and non-Mormons. Such a study was possible because, since 1941, the Mormon Church maintained centralized records of all church members (alive or dead), which could be matched to Utah death records. Table 7–8 shows results for ischemic heart disease, which accounted for a large majority of CVD deaths, expressed in terms of *standardized mortality ratios* (SMRs). The SMR (to be covered in Chapter 11) can be interpreted here as the ratio of the CVD mortality rate *observed* in a particular study group to the rate that would be *expected* if the age- and sex-specific CVD mortality rates for the U.S. as a whole were applied to that study group, given its age and sex composition.

    (a) To what extent do these results appear to help explain why cardiovascular mortality rates in Utah were relatively low compared to the U.S. as a whole?

Table 7–7. Estimated Number of Cases and of Deaths from Invasive *Streptococcus pneumoniae* Infection: United States, 1998

AGE (YEARS)	CASES	DEATHS
<2	12,560	110
2–4	4020	0
5–17	1980	50
18–34	4740	210
35–49	10,150	1150
50–64	8840	1150
65–79	11,890	1890
80+	8660	1520

[*Source:* Robinson et al. (2001).]

Table 7–8. Standardized Mortality Ratios for Acute, Chronic, and All Ischemic Heart
Disease: Utah, 1969–1971

| | Standardized Mortality Ratio[a] | | |
CARDIOVASCULAR DISEASE TYPE	MORMONS	NON-MORMONS	ALL UTAH RESIDENTS
Ischemic heart disease	.644	.963	.737
Acute	.671	.942	.752
Chronic	.619	1.002	.727

[a]Relative to 1970 U.S. rates.
[*Source:* Lyon et al. (1978).]

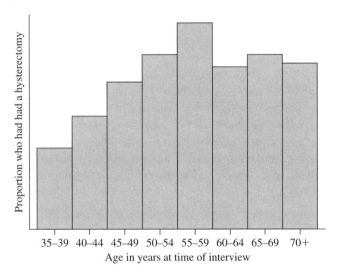

Figure 7–17. Hysterectomy Status of a Sample of King County, Washington, Women, by Age at Interview.

(b) What hypotheses might you advance to account for the difference in rates between Mormons and non-Mormons?

3. A random sample of women aged 35 years and over in King County, Washington, were asked a series of questions about their childbearing and reproductive history. (Their responses were later compared with answers provided by cases of a certain gynecological cancer.) One question concerned whether the respondent had undergone a hysterectomy prior to the interview. When hysterectomy status was analyzed in relation to age of respondent on the interview date, the pattern shown in Figure 7–17 was observed.

Table 7–9. Percentage of Women Who Reported Having
Had a Hysterectomy Prior to Attaining Age X, in
Relation to Age on Day of Interview

	Age on day of interview			
AGE X	40–49	50–59	60–69	70–79
35	11%	5%	6%	6%
40	18%	10%	11%	11%
45		22%	19%	17%
50		35%	26%	23%
55			33%	26%
60			37%	27%
65				31%
70				35%

Although one might expect *a priori* that the proportion of women with a prior hysterectomy would increase steadily with age (because a hysterectomy is not reversible), the data showed that in this sample of women the prevalence of prior hysterectomy peaked among women aged 55 to 59 years and was actually somewhat lower among older women.

Each woman who reported having undergone a hysterectomy was also asked how old she was when the operation was performed. From this information, Table 7–9 was constructed.

The table shows, for example, that 6% of those aged 70 to 79 on the interview day had undergone a hysterectomy by the time they were age 35; 11% of these women had undergone a hysterectomy by the time they were age 40; 17% had undergone a hysterectomy by the time they were age 45; etc.

Examine these results and use them to explain in words (no numbers needed) why the prevalence of prior hysterectomy declined after age 55 to 59 in the initial analysis.

ANSWERS

1. Table 7–7 shows only numerator data. It provides no information about the size of the population at risk in each age group. (The age groups also span different numbers of years.) When Robinson and colleagues combined this information with denominator estimates obtained from the census, the incidence rates shown in Table 7–10 were obtained. There was a clear U-shaped pattern of variation in incidence by age, with infants and older adults at far higher risk than were

Table 7–10. Incidence and Case Fatality from
Invasive *Streptococcus pneumoniae* Infection:
United States, 1998

AGE (YEARS)	INCIDENCE[a]	CASE FATALITY
<2	166.9	0.9%
2–4	35.2	0.0%
5–17	3.9	2.5%
18–34	7.4	4.4%
35–49	16.0	11.3%
50–64	23.0	13.0%
65–79	46.4	15.9%
80+	98.5	17.6%

[a]Cases per 100,000 person-years.
[*Source:* Robinson et al. (2001).]

older children or younger adults. Individuals in the age group that included the
mean and median age of cases were in fact at relatively low overall risk. This
illustrates how the mean or median age of cases can be misleading as guides to
which age group is most commonly affected.

On the other hand, the data in Table 7–7 are sufficient to allow calculation
of age-specific case fatality, a crude but useful measure of disease severity. As
shown in Table 7–10, older adults were much more likely to die of invasive
S. pneumoniae infection if they developed it, supporting the notion that the elderly may be a high-priority group for preventive efforts, including vaccination.

2. *(a)* The SMRs for Utah as a whole confirmed that ischemic heart disease mortality was indeed about 25%–27% lower in Utah than expected from U.S.
rates. Among non-Mormons, however, the SMRs were very close to 1.0,
suggesting that residence in Utah per se had little association with ischemic
heart disease mortality. Sharply lower SMRs were observed for all three
disease types among Mormons, which accounted for most of the overall
difference between Utah and U.S. rates.

(b) Lifestyle differences between Mormons and non-Mormons would be a
strong possibility. Cigarette smoking is a known strong risk factor for ischemic heart disease, and the Mormon church advocates abstention from
tobacco use. Differences in socioeconomic status, access to health care,
and other behavioral risk factors for heart disease could also play a role.

3. This is an example of a birth cohort effect. The graph shows the prevalence
of having had a hysterectomy in relation to age at the time of the interview.
But women who were in different age groups at the time of the interview were

also members of different birth cohorts. As such, they had reached any specific earlier age in different calendar years. For example, women who were 70 to 79 years old at the time of the interview would have achieved age 40 ten years earlier in history than did women who were 60 to 69 years old at the time of the interview. The likelihood of having undergone a hysterectomy as treatment for various gynecologic conditions, or for birth control, evidently increased steadily over the decades prior to the interview. This can be seen by reading across in any row of Table 7–9. At any given age, women who were younger at the time of the interview, and who were therefore members of later birth cohorts, were more likely to have had a hysterectomy by that age than were older women who were members of earlier birth cohorts.

The data in the table can be graphed by age at interview (= birth cohort) as shown in Figure 7–18. Note that the curves for different birth cohorts are not superimposed. Instead, the curve for each later birth cohort is shifted upward in relation to the curves of earlier birth cohorts. Because the age groupings differ between Table 7–9 and the original bar graph in Figure 7–17, we cannot directly identify women in the bar graph in particular cells of the table. But the thinner gray line in Figure 7–18 shows the pattern of variation in hysterectomy frequency by age in a cross-sectional look at data in the table, and it reveals the same pattern as the data in Figure 7–17.

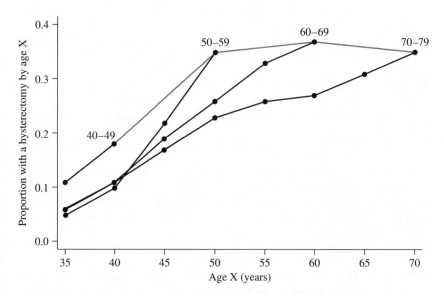

Figure 7–18. Proportion of Women with a Hysterectomy by Age X, in Relation to Age at Interview.

REFERENCES

Armstrong BK, English DR. "Cutaneous malignant melanoma." Chapter 59 in Schottenfeld D, Fraumeni JF Jr. Cancer epidemiology and prevention (2nd ed.). New York: Oxford University Press, 1996.

Ashley-Koch A, Yang Q, Olney RS. Sickle hemoglobin (HbS) allele and sickle cell disease: a HuGE review. Am J Epidemiol 2000; 151:839–45.

Baker SP, O'Neill B, Ginsburg MJ, Li G. The injury fact book (2nd ed.). New York: Oxford University Press, 1992.

Becker KM, Glass GE, Brathwaite W, Zenilman JM. Geographic epidemiology of gonorrhea in Baltimore, Maryland, using a geographic information system. Am J Epidemiol 1998; 147:709–16.

Bell CM, Redelmeier DA. Mortality among patients admitted to hospitals on weekends as compared with weekdays. N Engl J Med 2001; 345:663–68.

Bergman AB, Ray CG, Pomeroy MA, Wahl PW, Beckwith JB. Studies of the sudden infant death syndrome in King County, Washington. 3. Epidemiology. Pediatrics 1972; 49:860–70.

Brody H, Rip MR, Vinten-Johansen P, Paneth N, Rachman S. Map-making and myth-making in Broad Street: the London cholera epidemic, 1854. Lancet 2000; 356:64–68.

Burns DM, Lee L, Shen LZ, Gilpin E, Tolley HD, Vaughn J, et al. "Cigarette smoking behavior in the United States." Chapter 2 in: Burns DM, Garfinkel L, Samet JM (eds). Changes in cigarette-related disease risks and their implication for prevention and control. Bethesda, Md.: National Cancer Institute, 1997.

Centers for Disease Control and Prevention. http://wonder.cdc.gov, accessed 4/18/2001.

Centers for Disease Control and Prevention. Update: influenza activity—United States, 1992–93 season. MMWR 1993; 42:385–87.

Clayton D, Schifflers E. Models for temporal variation in cancer rates: I. Age-period and age-cohort models. Stat Med 1987; 6:449–67.

Cousens S, Smith PG, Ward H, Everlington D, Knight RSG, Zeidler M, et al. Geographical distribution of variant Creutzfeld-Jakob disease in Great Britain, 1994–2000. Lancet 2001; 357:1002–7.

Dennis LK, White E, Lee JAH. Recent cohort trends in malignant melanoma by anatomic site in the United States. Cancer Causes Control 1993; 4:93–100.

Doll R, Hill AB. Smoking and carcinoma of the lung: preliminary report. BMJ 1950; 2:739–48.

Doll R, Hill AB. Mortality in relation to smoking: ten years' observations of British doctors. BMJ 1964; 1:1399–410.

Frost WH. The age selection of mortality from tuberculosis in successive decades. Am J Hygiene 1939; 30:91–96.

Glass GE, Schwartz BS, Morgan JM, Johnson DT, Noy PM, Israel E. Environmental risk factors for Lyme disease identified with geographic information systems. Am J Public Health 1995; 85:944–48.

Goldberger J, Waring CH, Tanner WF. Pellagra prevention by diet among institutional inmates. Public Health Rep 1923; 38:2361–68.

Goldberger J, Wheeler GA, Sydenstricker E. A study of the relation of family income and other economic factors to pellagra incidence in seven cotton-mill villages of South Carolina in 1916. Public Health Rep 1920; 35:2673–714.

Goldman L, Cook EF. The decline in ischemic heart disease mortality rates. An analysis of the comparative effects of medical interventions and changes in lifestyle. Ann Intern Med 1984; 101:825–36.

Goldsmith GA. Niacin: antipellagra factor, hypocholesterolemic agent. Model of nutrition research yesterday and today. JAMA 1965; 194:167–73.

Hahn RA. The state of federal health statistics on racial and ethnic groups. JAMA 1992; 267:268–71.

Hahn RA, Mulinare J, Teutsch SM. Inconsistencies in coding of race and ethnicity between birth and death in U.S. infants. JAMA 1992; 267:259–63.

Holford TR. Understanding the effects of age, period, and cohort on incidence and mortality rates. Annu Rev Public Health 1991; 12:425–57.

Hoyert DL, Arias E, Smith BL, Murphy SL, Kochanek KD. Deaths: final data for 1999. National Vital Statistics Reports; vol. 49, no. 8. Hyattsville, Md.: National Center for Health Statistics, 2001.

Kaplan GA, Pamuk ER, Lynch JW, Cohen RD, Balfour JL. Inequality in income and mortality in the United States: analysis of mortality and potential pathways. BMJ 1996; 312:999–1003.

Kipling R. In: Rudyard Kipling's verse. Inclusive edition. London: Hodder and Stoughton, 1933.

Koutsky L. Epidemiology of genital human papillomavirus infection. Am J Med 1997; 102:3–8.

Kposowa AJ. Marital status and suicide in the National Longitudinal Mortality Study. J Epidemiol Community Health 2000; 34:254–61.

Krieger N, Williams DR, Moss NE. Measuring social class in U.S. public health research: concepts, methodologies, and guidelines. Annu Rev Public Health 1997; 18:341–78.

Last JM (ed.) A dictionary of epidemiology (4th edition). New York: Oxford, 2000.

Leck I, Sibary K, Wakefield J. Incidence of cervical cancer by marital status. J Epidemiol Community Health 1978; 32:108–10.

Lin SS, Kelsey JL. Use of race and ethnicity in epidemiologic research: concepts, methodological issues, and suggestions for research. Epidemiol Rev 2000; 22:187–202.

Liu S, Wen SW, Mao Y, Mery L, Rouleau J. Birth cohort effects underlying the increasing testicular cancer incidence in Canada. Can J Public Health 1999; 90:176–80.

Lynch JW, Smith GD, Kaplan GA, House JS. Income inequality and mortality: importance to health of individual income, psychosocial environment, or material conditions. BMJ 2000; 320:1200–4.

Lyon JL, Wetzler HP, Gardner JW, Klauber MR, Williams RR. Cardiovascular mortality in Mormons and non-Mormons in Utah, 1969–1971. Am J Epidemiol 1978; 108:357–66.

MacDorman MF, Atkinson JO. Infant mortality statistics from the 1997 period linked birth/infant death data set. National Vital Statistics Reports, vol. 47, no. 23. Hyattsville, Md.: National Cancer for Health Statistics, 1999.

Miller DC. Handbook of research design and social measurement (5th ed.). Newbury Park, Calif.: Sage Publications, 1991.

Monto AS, Ullman BM. Acute respiratory illness in an American community. The Tecumseh study. JAMA 1974; 227:164–69.

Moore DA, Carpenter TE. Spatial analytical methods and geographic information systems: use in health research and epidemiology. Epidemiol Rev 1999; 21:143–61.

Murphy SL. Deaths: final data for 1998. National Vital Statistics Reports; vol. 48, no. 11. Hyattsville, Md.: National Center for Health Statistics, 2000.

National Center for Health Statistics. Effect on mortality rates of the 1989 change in tabulating race. Vital Health Stat Series No. 21 (25), Pub. No. (PHS) 94-1853. Hyattsville, Md.: National Center for Health Statistics, 1994.

National Center for Health Statistics. Health, United States, 1998, with socioeconomic status and health chartbook. Hyattsville, Md.: National Center for Health Statistics, 1998a.

National Center for Health Statistics. Health, United States, 1999, with health and aging chartbook. Hyattsville, Md.: National Center for Health Statistics, 1998b.

National Center for Health Statistics. Health, United States, 2000, with adolescent chartbook. Hyattsville, Md.: National Center for Health Statistics, 2000.

National Center for Health Statistics. Health, United States, 2001, with urban and rural health chartbook. Hyattsville, Md.: National Center for Health Statistics, 2001.

National Heart, Lung, and Blood Institute. Morbidity & mortality: 2002, chart book on cardiovascular, lung, and blood diseases. Bethesda, Md.: National Heart, Lung, and Blood Institute, 2002.

Nelson DE. 1997 BRFSS summary prevalence report. Atlanta, Ga.: Centers for Disease Control and Prevention, 1998.

Phillips DP, Christenfeld N, Ryan NM. An increase in the number of deaths in the United States in the first week of the month. An association with substance abuse and other causes of death. N Engl J Med 1999; 341:93–98.

Pokorny J, Smith VC, Verriest G. "Congenital color defects." Chapter 7 in Pokorny J, Smith VC, Verriest G, Pinckers AJLG. Congenital and acquired color vision defects. New York: Grune & Stratton, 1979.

Reeve J. How do women develop fragile bones? J Steroid Biochem Mol Biol 2000; 74:375–81.

Ries LAG, Eisner MP, Kosary CL, Hankey BF, Miller BA, Clegg L, et al. SEER Cancer Statistics Review, 1973–1997. Bethesda, Md.: National Cancer Institute, 2000.

Robinson KA, Baughman W, Rothrock G, Barrett NL, Pass M, Lexau C, et al. Epidemiology of invasive *Streptococcus pneumoniae* infections in the United States, 1995–1998. JAMA 2001; 285:1729–35.

Semmelweis I. "The etiology, concept, and prophylaxis of childbed fever." In: Buck C, Llopis A, Najera E, Terris M (eds.). The challenge of epidemiology. Issues and selected readings. Washington, D.C.: Pan American Health Organization, 1988.

Snow J. Snow on Cholera. New York: Commonwealth Fund, 1936.

Von Korff M, Koepsell T, Curry S, Diehr P. Multi-level analysis in epidemiologic research on health behaviors and outcomes. Am J Epidemiol 1992; 135:1077–82.

Walker DH. Tick-transmitted infectious diseases in the United States. Annu Rev Public Health 1998; 19:237–69.

Weinkam JJ, Sterling TD. A graphical approach to the interpretation of age-period-cohort data. Epidemiology 1991; 2:133–37.

Williams DR. Race and health: basic questions, emerging directions. Ann Epidemiol 1997; 7:322–33.

Willich SN, Lowel H, Lewis M, Hormann A, Arntz HR, Keil U. Weekly variation of acute myocardial infarction. Increased Monday risk in the working population. Circulation 1994; 90:87–93.

Wynder EL, Graham EA. Tobacco smoking as a possible etiologic factor in bronchogenic carcinoma: a study of six hundred and eighty-four proved cases. JAMA 1950; 143:329–36.

8

INFERRING A CAUSAL RELATION BETWEEN EXPOSURE AND DISEASE

Epidemiologists not only measure the occurrence of disease, they seek to identify the causes of disease by interpreting observed patterns of variation in disease occurrence. Epidemiologic research is valued primarily because the causal inferences it generates can inform decisions about prevention of illness. These decisions are faced by:

1. *Individuals on their own.* For example, a middle-aged American man may consider adopting a diet that is relatively low in saturated fat and cholesterol, or high in seafood, with an eye to reducing his risk of a heart attack. Or a pregnant Kenyan woman who has learned she is seropositive for HIV must decide whether or not to nurse her newborn, balancing the benefits of breast feeding against an increased risk of her child's becoming infected with HIV.

2. *Health care providers on behalf of their patients.* Part of the job of a health-care provider is to advise patients about what they can do to prevent disease. In addition, these providers may have interventions that they can offer directly to reduce disease occurrence. For example, for that same middle-aged man who seeks advice about dietary modification of fat intake, a physician might prescribe a cholesterol-lowering medication.

3. *Society as a whole.* Decisions about the prevention of illness and injury are often made collectively. For instance, many communities have chosen to fluoridate their water supplies in an effort to reduce the burden of dental caries. Other communities have not done so, concerned that there may be untoward consequences of fluoridation that would outweigh this benefit.

The information most relevant to these decisions, whoever is making them, is whether a particular exposure (e.g., dietary modification) does or does not give rise to an altered occurrence of illness or injury, and, if so, by how much. These decision-makers wish to know whether the exposure in question leads to an increase in risk; that is, but for the presence of the exposure, would some cases of illness or injury not occur (is exposure causal)? Or they may wish to know whether the exposure leads to some cases not occurring (is exposure protective?). However, epidemiologists may be able to indicate only whether the incidence of illness or injury differs in relation to the presence of a given exposure; i.e., whether an *association* is present. Associations can be observed in data collected to address a specific question, such as whether the incidence of lung cancer is greater in cigarette smokers than in nonsmokers, or whether the prevalence of dental caries is higher in populations whose water supply is not fluoridated than in populations that receive fluoridated water. But not all observed associations between an exposure or characteristic and disease are causal ones.

Example: Scurvy had long been recognized as being common among seafarers. Those with scurvy who returned to port often recovered relatively quickly. We now know that these associations were due to the lack of vitamin C in the diets of sailors. Prior to the identification of vitamin C, however, all that was known was that there was something about leaving land that predisposed sailors to scurvy, and something about returning to port that somehow led to its cure. Epidemics of scurvy were not restricted to sailors; they could occur any time there was nutritional deprivation. One such outbreak occurred during the California gold rush, at the Sonora mining camp, where "in November of 1849 they established a hospital for the destitute sick, of which there were large numbers, with land scurvy being the most prominent disease" (Carpenter, 1986). It was not terribly surprising that scurvy was common then, because the miners' diet "seemed to consist of stewed beans and flapjacks 21 times per week, though the latter was occasionally replaced by flour dumplings and molasses." To address the problem, "some miners resorted to the old treatment of burial up to the neck in earth. The whole camp would do it at once, except a few who remained out to keep out grizzlies and coyotes." Apparently, "... these miners would try to maximize the effect of land by immersing themselves in it." We would not have expected that immersion in land had any influence on the natural history of scurvy (we know of no studies of the efficacy of this treatment!) since the association between not being in proximity to land and the development of scurvy need not be a causal one.

When we are trying to judge whether an association represents a causal influence of an exposure, we run into an immediate impediment: We don't actually observe causes. We do observe associations, and perhaps an apparent temporal sequence of events, but we must infer causes. For instance, most of us have inferred that we can cause a car to start by turning its key in the ignition. How have we made that inference? First, there is a very strong association: Almost all of the time, when we turn the key, the car will promptly start, and rarely if ever will it do so when they key is not turned in the ignition. Second, there is a very reasonable mechanism, in terms of the way the car has been built, that underlies this association and would predict that it would be a causal one. Nonetheless, we have not *seen* causation. Rather, we have noted events, and in our minds we have drawn a connection.

When we attempt to make an inference regarding causes of disease, we have several handicaps that were not present in our automotive example. First, exposure may occur long before disease appears. Taking up cigarette smoking as a teenager probably has little effect on one's risk of lung cancer until well into adulthood. This means that our observations may have to span years, or even decades, depending on the nature of the disease and how its occurrence is influenced by the exposure. Also, our ability to infer causation may be impaired by the fact that the same illness can occur due to causes other than the one we happen to be investigating. Smoking may be a cause of lung cancer, but since this disease can occur even in the absence of smoking, as a result of other etiologic factors, the association between smoking and lung cancer will be diluted in proportion to the frequency of these other factors.

Finally, the lack of a perfect correspondence between a particular exposure and the occurrence of a particular disease arises when the exposure can exert its influence only in the presence of another factor. Cigarette smoking by itself will not cause lung cancer; most people who smoke cigarettes never develop lung cancer. Whether it is the presence of a genetic characteristic or some other environmental exposure, there have to be reasons why only the occasional cigarette smoker becomes ill with this disease and other smokers do not.

In epidemiology, as in other sciences, we make observations and try to draw inferences from these observations. The inferences take the shape of judgments about the likelihood of the truth or falsity of hypotheses regarding cause and effect. A given hypothesis can stimulate us to make additional observations to test its validity. Some of the hypotheses that are generated, if unrefuted by additional observations, are sufficiently plausible that they are tentatively accepted as valid, and so serve as a guide to decisions about prevention. As an example, the increasing incidence of cancers of the respiratory tract in the first half of the 20th century in Europe and North America followed an increase in cigarette consumption in these populations. This temporal correlation, and the fact that the respiratory tract receives a large, direct exposure to inhaled cigarette smoke, were compatible with the hypothesis that cigarette smoking could cause cancers at this site. This hypothesis has been tested many times in epidemiologic studies, most notably through comparisons of the incidence of respiratory cancer in smokers and nonsmokers who appeared to be similar otherwise. Those comparisons typically have revealed a strikingly higher incidence among smokers. Non-epidemiologic studies have gone on to identify many substances in cigarette smoke whose administration to laboratory animals resulted in an increased incidence of cancer. To most of us, the causal hypothesis remains unrefuted, and so we are willing to tally an increased risk of respiratory cancer as a consequence of cigarette smoking when deciding on the desirability of preventing or modifying cigarette smoking behavior.

EVIDENCE USED TO DRAW CAUSAL INFERENCES

Beginning in the middle of the twentieth century, stimulated by the accumulating data pointing to a possible causal influence of cigarette smoking on lung cancer and other diseases, specific types of evidence have been identified that bear on the plausibility of a causal relation between an exposure and a disease (U.S. Public Health Service, 1964; Hill, 1965). Our version of these types of evidence—they differ slightly from epidemiologist to epidemiologist—is contained in Table 8–1.

Results from Randomized Controlled Trials

First, we ask if an association has been observed in one or more randomized controlled trials. As discussed in Chapter 13, trials of this sort involve recruitment of study participants who allow the investigator to allocate them, using some form of random process, either to receive or not receive an intervention (or one of several possible interventions). Thus, a difference in the incidence of illness or death between intervention groups, especially a large difference, cannot be readily attributed to other characteristics of persons who received or failed to receive the intervention; on average, those other characteristics will be present to the same extent in both groups. As an example, it was observed that among men with very high diastolic blood pressure (115–129 mm Hg) who were assigned at random

Table 8–1. Sources of Support for the Hypothesis That a Given Exposure Is a Cause of Disease or Injury in Human Beings

---

1. Data from randomized studies in human beings show an association between the presence of the exposure and disease occurrence
2. Data from non-randomized studies in human beings show an association, and:
   (a) The suspected cause precedes the presence of the disease
   (b) The association is strong
   (c) There is:
      i. No plausible non-causal explanation that would account for the (entirety of the) association; and
      ii. A plausible explanation for the association's being a causal one
   (d) The magnitude of the association is strongest when it is predicted to be so

---

to receive antihypertensive treatment had a lower rate of complications of cardio-vascular disease than similarly hypertensive men assigned to receive a placebo (Veterans Administration Cooperative Study Group on Antihypertensive Agents, 1967). The study was large enough that the probability of a difference in rates of the observed magnitude or greater occurring by chance, given no true influence of therapy, was extremely small. Because of randomization, the treatment and placebo groups would be expected to be similar with regard to mortality and hypertensive complications if treatment conferred no benefit, so there is no plausible explanation for the association other than a beneficial influence of antihypertensive therapy.

Unfortunately, not every potential causal relationship can be evaluated by a randomized trial. Let us say we are interested in the question of whether an induced abortion can predispose a woman to developing breast cancer later in life. One of the ways we would *not* go about studying this is to ask pregnant women who are considering having an abortion to allow themselves to enter a study in which the luck of the draw would dictate who among them would indeed have the abortion and who would attempt to carry her pregnancy to term! Similarly, no randomized trials have been conducted to examine whether cigarette smoking is an etiologic factor in the occurrence of lung cancer. To address potential causal relations such as these, it is necessary to obtain the results of non-randomized studies.

Inferences from Non-randomized Studies

When the only data available to guide a causal inference come from non-randomized studies, it is necessary to tread particularly carefully to sidestep errors that might lead us to make a causal inference when no causation is present; or the reverse. Just as with randomized trials, an association between exposure and illness must be evident in order to even consider the possibility of a cause–effect relationship. Often there will be more than one study available by which to judge whether an association is or is not present. In this situation, the results of each study (along with its size and perceived quality) need to be taken into account so that an overall assessment can be made.

Temporal sequence of events

Of course, an association between exposure and disease can only be attributed to the causal influence of the exposure if it is clear that the exposure precedes the disease in time. From the epidemiologic studies in which these associations have emerged, it will generally be straightforward whether the exposure or disease occurred first. For example, an excess risk of lung cancer among cigarette smokers is not observed until at least a decade after smoking has been initiated. Thus, it is hard to imagine that in some way a person's lung tumor had influenced him or her to begin to smoke cigarettes 10 or more years before it was diagnosed. Nonetheless, the sequence of events may not be so obvious, and special efforts in the study's design and analysis may be needed to clarify the situation.

Example: Reye's syndrome (RS) is a childhood condition characterized by damage to the liver and central nervous system. The damage may be transient, but in many instances the disease leads to death or retardation. RS typically develops following a bout of chickenpox or influenza, and it was suspected that the use of aspirin to treat the symptoms of these infections predisposed a child to getting RS. The results of an epidemiologic study indicating an increased incidence of RS in children who took aspirin for fever, relative to children in general, could be interpreted in one of two ways:

1. Aspirin use predisposes to RS; or
2. Early in its course, and before it is diagnosed as such, RS gives rise to fever that leads to aspirin use. The association observed may thus reflect the causal influence of RS on aspirin use, rather than the reverse.

Anticipating this possible ambiguity, some epidemiologic studies (Halpin et al., 1982; Hurwitz et al., 1987; Forsyth et al., 1989) confined their study populations to children with a recent episode of chickenpox or flu. Their observation of a substantially higher risk of RS in children with one of these conditions who received aspirin, relative to other children with a similar recent infection who did not, argues strongly against the second interpretation above, and strongly in favor of the notion that aspirin use did in fact precede the presence of RS.

Strength of the association

The larger the association between an exposure and the occurrence of illness or injury, the more likely it is that the association reflects a causal influence of the exposure. This is because the larger the association, the less likely it is that errors in the study, or the presence of other risk factors for the disease that tend to co-exist with the one in question, could be responsible for the whole of the association. For example, one of the arguments in support of a causal relationship between cigarette smoking and lung cancer is that the incidence of lung cancer in smokers and nonsmokers is markedly different. In order for one of the correlates of smoking behavior (e.g., alcohol consumption, socioeconomic status, occupation) to entirely explain that large association, it would have to be associated with lung cancer to at least that degree and also be highly correlated with cigarette smoking.

The strength of an association is generally quantified as the ratio of the incidence of disease between exposed and non-exposed individuals; for example, we would describe the strength of the association between smoking and lung cancer by saying that smokers have about a tenfold greater risk than nonsmokers. A relative rather than absolute measure is used to characterize "strength," since it is expected that the sources of bias encountered in epidemiologic studies tend to be present to a similar relative degree, whether an association is present or absent, strong or weak. One way to think of this is to imagine that we are trying to estimate the passage of time without using a timepiece. If we erred by one second after the first ten had elapsed, then after 60 seconds it is more likely that we would misestimate that duration by six seconds (one in 10) than by just one second (one in 60). By the same token, absolute measures of the size of an association—the difference in incidence between exposed and non-exposed persons—are strongly influenced by the underlying frequency of the disease being studied, and so do not serve as well as ratios for judging whether an association is present beyond the influence of error.

Plausibility of causal and non-causal hypotheses

The stronger the basis for suspecting that an exposure *ought* to cause a disease or injury, the stronger will be the inference that an association between that exposure and disease or injury is a causal one. Conversely, a compelling alternative explanation can argue against causation. Many different types of evidence, epidemiologic and non-epidemiologic, can provide a basis for suspicion. Cigarette smoke contains many substances that are carcinogenic in the laboratory; it comes into direct contact with the bronchi when inhaled; and the incidence of cancers of the bronchi and lung from population to population, and over time within one population, has paralleled the prevalence of cigarette smoking. All of the foregoing facts strengthen an inference of a causal connection when one is seeking to interpret an observed association within a population between cigarette smoking and the incidence of cancers of the bronchi and lung. Similarly, it might be expected that wearing a helmet can provide structural protection against head injury in a bicycle crash, or that wearing a condom can provide a physical barrier against HIV transmission. Because of this, an association between helmet use and a reduced risk of head injury, or between condom use and a reduced risk of acquiring HIV, is widely interpreted as indicating at least some degree of protection.

Many studies of possible exposure/disease associations are able to gather information to assess the plausibility of at least some non-causal explanations for any association that is observed.

Example: In a multi-center study in Europe (de Vicenzi, 1994), heterosexual couples in whom only one member had been infected with HIV were followed for approximately two years. The incidence of a new HIV infection in the previously negative partner was monitored in relationship to whether or not the couple consistently used a condom during sexual intercourse in those two years. Of 124 couples who consistently used a condom, no instances of transmission occurred, whereas 12 of the 121 previously uninfected members of couples who did not consistently use condoms became HIV-positive.

The investigators sought to uncover other characteristics of couples who did and did not consistently use condoms that might have been responsible for this difference. For example, the efficiency of transmission of HIV is known to be relatively greater from men to women than from women to men. Did the condom-using couples tend to have a relatively low proportion of men as the initially infected partner? No, at least not to any appreciable degree: in 61 percent of the condom-using couples, the index partner was male, in contrast to 67 percent of the other couples. Did the condom-using couples simply have sexual intercourse relatively less frequently, and for this reason have a low rate of transmission? No, their median frequency of sexual intercourse during the follow-up period actually was higher (twice per week) than that of the other couples (once per week). The distribution of other potential risk factors for HIV transmission similarly did not suggest that anything other than consistent condom use itself was responsible for the observed difference in the occurrence of HIV.

Pattern of variation in the strength of the association

Often, the risk of a disease among exposed persons is seen to rise steadily as the intensity of exposure increases. In some of these instances, our knowledge of the basis underlying the induction of the disease is complete enough to have predicted the steady rise. For example, we know that exposure to carbon monoxide (CO) gives rise to hypoxia because this molecule competes with oxygen for hemoglobin transport, and so we would predict that the occurrence of hypoxic signs and symptoms would rise with increasingly high CO concentrations in inspired air.

Even when our knowledge of the mechanism underlying disease occurrence is less precise, we tend to use the presence of such a "dose–response" relationship as supporting a causal hypothesis. Early in the course of research on this subject, the observed rise in the risk of lung cancer with an increasing number of cigarettes smoked each day was viewed as supporting the hypothesis of a causal influence of smoking on the incidence of this disease.

The intensity of an exposure is only one of several characteristics that can be examined for its possible impact on disease incidence. The risk of endometrial cancer among postmenopausal women who have taken estrogens unopposed by a progestogen appears to be heavily influenced by the duration and recency of use: the longer and more recent the use, the higher the risk of this cancer. In other instances, the interval from the time the exposure first was encountered has a substantial bearing on risk. For example, the inference that receipt of A/New Jersey influenza (swine flu) vaccine predisposed to the occurrence of Guillain-Barré syndrome was enhanced when it was observed that the high risk of this disease was largely confined to the second and third weeks following vaccination (Marks and Halpin, 1980). Since it takes one to two weeks for primary immune responses to be mounted, the observed temporal pattern of increased risk is compatible with the hypothesis that, in some way, an immune response to the vaccine was responsible—just as an immune response to various infectious illnesses had been suspected as being responsible for many prior cases of Guillain-Barré syndrome in unvaccinated persons.

A steady rise in risk with increasing intensity or duration of exposure does not mean that a causal relation must be present. One or more factors might be strongly associated with both exposure and disease to give rise to a pattern of this sort without there being any causal connection between them. For example, while a woman's age at which she first nurses a baby may be directly related to breast-cancer risk in a graded way, this association would probably be the result of the strong relationship between age at first birth (whether the woman had breast-fed or not) and both age at first breast-feeding and breast-cancer risk. Furthermore, some causal relations are threshold in nature: Squeezing the trigger of a gun can lead to a homicide, but, beyond a certain intensity of squeezing, the risk stays constant!

Yet another way to examine variation in the strength of an association between exposure and disease is according to the presence of other characteristics or other exposures that might be predicted to have an influence. The restriction of the association of tetracycline use to the development of discolored teeth to children under five years of age argues in support of a causal connection, since:

- Tetracyclines chelate with calcium ions; and
- Only in children under five are the crowns of teeth still undergoing calcification.

Similarly, the hypothesis that long-term estrogen use is a cause of endometrial cancer is supported by the observation that such use is strongly associated with cancer risk only when it is not accompanied by a progestogen, since progestogens are known to counter estrogen-stimulated proliferation of endometrial tissue.

In summary, a causal inference is strengthened when the size of an association between exposure and disease varies in a way that could be predicted from other knowledge. The variation may be on the basis of some feature of the exposure itself (e.g., intensity, duration, or recency), or of another characteristic or exposure altogether (Weiss, 1981).

The pattern of associations between a given exposure and *different* outcomes occasionally can inform a causal inference as well (Weiss, 2002). For example, we believe that screening sigmoidoscopy (endoscopic evaluation of the rectum and lower colon) leads to reduced mortality from tumors arising in the rectum and lower colon because screened persons have: *(1)* a sharply reduced death rate from those tumors; and *(2) no* reduced death rate from tumors arising in the upper colon, beyond the reach of the sigmoidoscope (Selby et al., 1992). Similarly, a causal inference is strengthened if several related exposures have been evaluated with respect to the occurrence of a single disease, and an association is observed only for the one (or ones) for which an association had been predicted. Thus, the inference that the observed association between the presence of ovarian endometriosis and the subsequent occurrence of ovarian cancer represents a causal relationship is supported by the absence of a similar association for extra-ovarian endometriosis (Brinton et al., 1997). In contrast, the increased risk of stomach cancer in users of cimetidine and of antacids (Schumacher et al., 1990) argues more strongly that as-yet-undiagnosed stomach cancer (or an antecedent of stomach cancer) leads to use of the treatments for peptic disease than it does for both agents' acting to cause stomach cancer.

APPLICATION OF THE GUIDELINES

A tentative inference regarding the presence or absence of a causal relationship between exposure and disease—such an inference is always tentative, pending the presence of additional data—is made by a subjective process in which one judges how many of the above features are present and (especially) the degree to which they are present. In some instances, the process is straightforward—all the evidence supports a causal hypothesis—and nearly all persons considering the issue arrive at the same conclusion; e.g., that cigarette smoke is a cause of lung cancer. In other instances, little or none of the evidence argues in support of causation—perhaps, in the case of occupational exposure to magnetic fields and cancer, or of silicone breast implants and scleroderma—and most observers feel it is not appropriate to infer an etiologic connection when considering action to modify or remove the exposure in question. Since it is impossible to rule out completely the existence of an effect of exposure on disease occurrence that is weak enough to be below the limits of detection in epidemiologic studies, it is also not surprising that some debate continues regarding the safety of such exposures as occupational magnetic fields and silicone breast implants.

Some of the underpinnings of a particular causal hypothesis may be stronger than others. Years ago, in laboratory studies, aflatoxin (the toxic product of the mold *Aspergillus flavus*) had been found to be an extremely potent carcinogen, but at that time the only relevant data in humans consisted of correlations of liver cancer mortality rates across national populations with differences in estimated aflatoxin intake. While the interpretation of the positive correlations seen in these studies was ambiguous—the populations with the highest rates no doubt differed in relevant ways other than their consumption of aflatoxin—the strength of the laboratory evidence served as a basis for a (very) tentative causal inference. Later, stronger epidemiologic data became available to further support the hypothesis (Qian et al., 1994; Wang et al., 1996). In contrast, the enormously strong association between aspirin and Reye's syndrome observed in epidemiologic studies, along with the lack of any such association with other analgesics (Halpin et al., 1982; Hurwitz et al., 1987; Forsyth et al., 1989), served as an adequate basis for discouraging aspirin use in children in the absence of any precise knowledge of the means by which aspirin use might have caused the occasional child with flu or chickenpox to develop this complication.

COMMON MISPERCEPTIONS OF THE NATURE OF CAUSES OF ILLNESS AND INJURY

There Are Direct and Indirect Causes of Disease, and the Direct Causes Are More Important

If we accept the definition of a cause of disease as that given previously—but for the presence of an exposure, some additional cases of disease would not occur—then for purposes of causal inference it is not critical that we know where in the sequence of events leading to disease a given exposure has taken place. The psychological and sociological forces that give rise to and sustain cigarette-smoking behavior are just as much causes of lung cancer as smoking itself, if it is inferred that in the absence of these forces some persons would not become or remain cigarette smokers, and thus would not develop lung cancer. Other cultural and economic forces that have led men to become asbestos miners or women to become commercial sex workers are also causes of asbestosis or AIDS, if it is judged that some additional cases of these illnesses occurred as a result of having worked in those occupations.

In any event, our labeling of a causal agent as "direct" may be due only to our ignorance of the "downstream" consequences of the actions of that agent. For example, cigarette smoking would no longer be considered a "direct" cause of lung cancer once we understood the biochemical and molecular changes produced by the carcinogens in cigarette smoke. The accuracy with which we label cigarette smoking as acting directly or indirectly is not relevant to whether its presence truly does give rise to lung cancer in some individuals.

In Order To Be Considered a Cause of Disease, an Exposure Must Be Present in Every Case

If the illness or injury in question is defined by the presence of a particular causal agent—e.g., staphylococcal pneumonia, or motor vehicle injury—then of course that causal factor must be present in every case. But many illnesses or injuries are defined by a particular manifestation—e.g., myocardial infarction, or a fracture of the femur—that allows for the possibility of two or more separate pathways that can lead to that disease or injury. The fact that a particular exposure is not a necessary cause of a disease in no way detracts from its potential causal role. Excessive alcohol consumption is not the cause of every motor vehicle injury, but it surely is a cause of some such injuries.

In Order To Be Considered a Cause of Disease, an Exposure Must Be Capable of Producing that Disease on Its Own

Clearly, the capability to independently produce a disease cannot be considered appropriate as a criterion: We acknowledge that infection with the tubercle bacillus is a cause of tuberculosis, but also that only some infected persons—particularly those who are malnourished or consume excessive amounts of alcohol—develop the disease. Nonetheless, the issue is at the heart of a controversy exemplified by the question, "Do guns kill people, or do people kill people?" A gun by itself cannot commit a homicide; it needs an assailant to pull the trigger. Does the need for an assailant detract from the hypothesis that the availability of a gun is a cause of homicide? No, as long as there is evidence to suggest that, because of the presence of a gun, some homicides occurred that otherwise would not. The nature of such evidence may take the forms described earlier in the chapter—an association between gun availability and homicide occurrence, and non-epidemiologic data regarding possible differences in the ability or inclination of potential assailants to commit a homicide using a gun or using another weapon.

CAUSAL INFERENCE IN PRACTICE: THE EXAMPLE OF SLEEPING POSITION AND SUDDEN INFANT DEATH SYNDROME (SIDS)

In North America and Europe, SIDS (otherwise known as crib death or cot death) is a relatively common cause of death among infants beyond the first several weeks of life. Until a few years ago, the mortality rate from SIDS had been relatively stable in most parts of the world. Research had been done for several decades to try to determine what the causes were, but little progress was made until the late 1980s and early 1990s, when studies examined the possibility that the sleeping position of the infant was somehow involved.

The initial studies (see Guntheroth and Spiers, 1992; Dwyer and Ponsonby, 1996, for a summary) were conducted in Australia, New Zealand, and several parts of Europe. All but one used a case-control design—that is, a comparison of the last or usual sleeping position between infants who died of SIDS and a control group of healthy infants. In each of the case-control studies, there was a higher proportion of SIDS cases who had been put to sleep in the prone position. From these results, it was possible to estimate (through means described in Chapter 9) that there was at least a several-fold increase in the incidence of SIDS associated with the prone sleeping position. The temporal sequence of events underlying this consistently observed and strong association was compatible with a causal role of sleeping position. One additional study addressed the (unlikely) possibility that recall bias had been responsible for the positive association seen in the case-control studies— that parents of recently deceased infants and parents of healthy children had not furnished information about sleeping position with the same degree of accuracy. These Australian investigators (Dwyer et al., 1991) queried parents of some 3,000 five-week old healthy infants regarding the position in which they laid the child down to sleep. Infants who had usually been put to sleep prone subsequently had a threefold increase in the risk of SIDS relative to other infants. Since the magnitude of the increase in risk associated with sleeping prone observed in this study was well within the range of those observed in the case-control studies, the possibility of differential recall between parents of cases and parents of controls as the entire basis for the association could largely be dismissed.

Is there a plausible means by which sleeping prone can lead to SIDS? There are several candidates, including oropharyngeal or nasal obstruction and thermal imbalance. Yet when the results of the initial epidemiologic studies appeared, these were no more than candidate hypotheses.

Despite the uncertainty about why sleeping prone might be hazardous, most observers made the inference that it indeed was hazardous, at least regarding the risk of SIDS. For example, in 1992 the American Academy of Pediatrics Task Force on Infant Positioning recommended (AAP Task Force on Infant Positioning and SIDS, 1992) that "healthy infants, when being put down for sleep, be positioned on their side or back. . . . This recommendation is made with the full recognition that the existing studies have methodologic limitations, and were conducted in countries with infant care practices and other Sudden Infant Death Syndrome risk factors that differ from those in the United States. . . . However, taken as a group the studies are convincing." The task force recommendation took into account not only the data relating sleeping position to the incidence of SIDS, but also the fact that there were no data "even strongly suggesting that sleeping in the lateral or supine position is harmful to healthy infants." Conceivably, the task force could have recommended that no action regarding sleeping position be taken until randomized trials had been conducted to address the issue. However, they viewed the data from the non-randomized studies to be compelling, enough so that it would be unethical to ask parents to allow the sleeping position of their child to be decided at random.

The hypothesis that sleeping position can influence an infant's risk of SIDS subsequently has received support from the experience of populations in which large changes have taken place in the proportion of infants who sleep prone. In England, for example, a "Back to Sleep" campaign was mounted beginning in December of 1991 in the wake of the studies mentioned above. This campaign was associated with a decline in prone sleeping: Based on two samples of newborns, the prevalence fell from 21% in mid-1991 to 4% in mid-1992 (Hiley and Morley, 1994). A striking change in mortality from SIDS accompanied the change in sleeping position: There were 912 SIDS deaths in England in 1991, but only 456 in 1992.

Critics of epidemiologic research have argued that epidemiologic studies can raise questions but cannot answer them. The studies of sleeping position and SIDS, the causal inferences drawn from them, and the benefits of the actions that were based on those inferences, would appear to be a good rebuttal to an argument of this sort.

EXERCISES

1. The following is excerpted from a letter to the editor of the *New England Journal of Medicine* (1998; 338:921):

> Although the link between sexual behavior, human papilloma virus (HPV) infection, and anogenital cancer is strong, there are clearly other factors of equal or greater importance, because many more people are infected with HPVs than have cancer. To view these malignant conditions as simply being caused by sexually transmitted infections is misleading. In the context of a multi-factorial disease, attributing cause to one recognized infectious step in the process has the potential to confuse clinicians and arouse undue fear in the general population. We would urge caution in the use of terms such as "cause," which can be over-interpreted. We believe public health is best served by the more difficult approach involving education about the multi-factorial nature of risk associated with disease.

(a) When seeking to infer whether or not HPV infection is a cause of anogenital cancer, is it desirable to consider whether:

   i. ". . . there are clearly other factors of equal or greater importance . . ."?
   ii. An inference of cause and effect may ". . . confuse clinicians and arouse undue fear in the general population"?

(b) Is inferring a causal relation between HPV and anogenital cancer inconsistent with "the multi-factorial nature of risk"?

2. The following appeared in the "News" section of the *Lancet* of March 27, 1999:

> Excessive breast self-examination may promote anxiety. A new study of women with a family history of breast cancer adds to evidence that excessive breast self-examination is counterproductive, because it increases anxiety and may make early detection of breast cancer more difficult.
>
> Researchers from the University of Wales College of Medicine, Cardiff, UK; and Sheffield University, UK, surveyed 833 women aged 17–77 years, from families with histories of breast cancer. 18% claimed to examine their breasts daily or weekly, 56% once or twice a month, and 26% rarely. General anxiety and cancer-specific anxiety were lowest among women who examined themselves least often, and highest among the hypervigilant women—differences that were strongly significant.

What is another plausible interpretation of these data, other than that "excessive" breast self-examination increases a woman's level of anxiety?

3. An Australian study (Orlowski et al., 1990) observed no association between a child's use of aspirin and the occurrence of Reye's syndrome. The authors noted that all prior studies of this issue had found a strong association. The following paraphrases the concluding sentences of their paper:

> A different burden of proof is required if one attempts to prove a hypothesis than if one wants to disprove the proposal. This is best understood with a simple analogy. If one observes 100 swans that are all white, one might propose that all swans are white. But only one black swan is needed to prove that all swans are not white. Our study is the black swan that proves that aspirin does not cause Reye's syndrome.

Assume the authors' own study is both large and flawless. Do you agree with their conclusion? If yes, why? If no, why not?

ANSWERS

1. *(a)* i. Ranking of causal factors serves no purpose here. The fact that other causes of anogenital cancer exist does not detract from an inference that HPV infection does so, too.

   ii. The assessment of a possible causal relation between an exposure, such as HPV infection, and cancer incidence is a separate task from communicating that inference to clinicians and to the population as a whole.

   (b) HPV infection is not sufficient to produce an anogenital cancer; other factors must be involved. But if it is judged that some persons could be spared developing a cancer by not acquiring an HPV infection, then it would be incorrect not to speak of HPV infection as a cause of cancer.

2. Another interpretation, arguably a more plausible one: Anxiety leads to "excessive" self-examination.

3. From this study, the only hypothesis that can be refuted is that *all* epidemiologic studies will find an association between aspirin and Reye's syndrome. It is true that an inference of cause and effect is strengthened by an association between exposure and disease having been observed consistently across studies. Nonetheless, we recognize that an agent with the capacity to cause disease may not be able to exert its deleterious influence if other necessary factors are not present. The fact that Reye's syndrome was unassociated with aspirin in the authors' study population—perhaps some additional, interacting factor (e.g., a flu epidemic) was absent in that population—does not preclude it from being a cause in another setting.

REFERENCES

AAP Task Force on Infant Positioning and SIDS. Positioning and SIDS. Pediatrics 1992; 89:1120–26.

Brinton LA, Gridley G, Persson I, Baron J, Bergqvist A. Cancer risk after a hospital discharge diagnosis of endometriosis. Am J Obstet Gynecol 1997; 176:572–79.

Carpenter KJ. The history of scurvy and vitamin C. Cambridge, UK: Cambridge University Press, 1986.

de Vicenzi I. A longitudinal study of human immunodeficiency virus transmission by heterosexual partners. European Study Group on Heterosexual Transmission of HIV. N Engl J Med 1994; 331:341–46.

Dwyer T, Ponsonby AL. The decline of SIDS: a success story for epidemiology. Epidemiology 1996; 7:323–25.

Dwyer T, Ponsonby AL, Newman NM, Gibbons LE. Prospective cohort study of prone sleeping position and sudden infant death syndrome. Lancet 1991; 337:1244–47.

Forsyth BW, Horwitz RI, Acampora D, Shapiro ED, Viscoli CM, Feinstein AR, et al. New epidemiologic evidence confirming that bias does not explain the aspirin/Reye's syndrome association. JAMA 1989; 261:2517–24.

Guntheroth WG, Spiers PS. Sleeping prone and the risk of sudden infant death syndrome. JAMA 1992; 267:2359–62.

Halpin TJ, Holtzhauer FJ, Campbell RJ, Hall LJ, Correa-Villasenor A, Lanese R, et al. Reye's syndrome and medication use. JAMA 1982; 248:687–91.

Hiley CMH, Morley CJ. Evaluation of government's campaign to reduce risk of cot death. BMJ 1994; 309:703–4.

Hill AB. The environment and disease: association or causation. Proc R Soc Med 1965; 58:295–300.

Hurwitz ES, Barrett MJ, Bregman D, Gunn WJ, Pinsky P, Schonberger LB, et al. Public Health Service study of Reye's syndrome and medications. Report of the main study. JAMA 1987; 257:1905–11.

Marks JS, Halpin TJ. Guillain-Barré syndrome in recipients of A/New Jersey influenza vaccine. JAMA 1980; 243:2490–94.

Orlowski JP, Campbell P, Goldstein S. Reye's syndrome: a case-control study of medication use and associated viruses in Australia. Cleve Clin J Med 1990; 57:323–29.

Qian GS, Ross RK, Yu MC, Yuan JM, Gao YT, Henderson BE, et al. A follow-up study of urinary markers of aflatoxin exposure and liver cancer risk in Shanghai, People's Republic of China. Cancer Epidemiol Biomarkers Prev 1994; 3:3–10.

Schumacher MC, Jick SS, Jick H, Feld AD. Cimetidine use and gastric cancer. Epidemiology 1990; 1:251–54.

Selby JV, Friedman GD, Quesenberry CP Jr, Weiss NS. A case-control study of screening sigmoidoscopy and mortality from colorectal cancer. N Engl J Med 1992; 326:653–57.

U S Public Health Service. Smoking and health. Report of the Advisory Committee to the Surgeon General of the Public Health Service. PHS Pub. No. 1103. Washington, D.C.: U.S. Department of Health, Education, and Welfare, 1964.

Veterans Administration Cooperative Study Group on Antihypertensive Agents. Effects of treatment on morbidity in hypertension. JAMA 1967; 202:116–22.

Wang LY, Hatch M, Chen CJ, Levin B, You SL, Lu SN, et al. Aflatoxin exposure and risk of hepatocellular carcinoma in Taiwan. Int J Cancer 1996; 67:620–25.

Weiss NS. Inferring causal relationships: elaboration of the criterion of "dose-response." Am J Epidemiol 1981; 113:487–90.

Weiss NS. Can the "specificity" of an association be rehabilitated as a basis for supporting a causal hypothesis? Epidemiology 2002; 13:6–8.

9

MEASURES OF EXCESS RISK

In Tasmania during 1988–1990, information was obtained from the parents of 2607 one-month-old infants regarding their baby's usual sleeping position (Dwyer et al., 1991). The cumulative incidence of crib death (sudden infant death syndrome) through one year of age in these children was compared between those who were usually put to sleep prone (on their stomach) or in another position (side or back). The results shown in Table 9–1 were obtained.

In order to estimate the occurrence of crib death in relation to sleeping position, the risk in one group can be divided by that in the other. Let us label, arbitrarily, infants who were usually put to sleep prone as "exposed" and the others "non-exposed." The cumulative incidence in the exposed (I_e) is $9/846 = 10.64$ per 1000. The cumulative incidence in the non-exposed (I_o) is $6/1761 = 3.41$ per 1000. The relative incidence, or *relative risk* (*RR*) is:

$$RR = \frac{I_e}{I_o} = \frac{10.64}{3.41} = 3.1$$

Alternatively, from studies of this sort, the observed number of exposed persons who develop the illness or injury under study can be divided by the number that would have been "expected"; that is, the number predicted to occur if exposed persons had the same risk as the non-exposed. This represents another way of calculating the relative risk. In this example, there were nine crib deaths that occurred among infants put to sleep in the prone position. The expected number, based on the risk in the other infants, is $6/1761 \times 846 = 2.88$. The ratio of observed-to-expected deaths, $9/2.88$, is 3.1, the same number that was obtained above when dividing I_e by I_o.

To begin to introduce other measures of altered risk, let's consider Table 9–2, which is the generic version of the data table we just produced in the example on crib death.

The *difference* in risk between exposed and non-exposed persons would be:

$$I_e - I_o = \frac{a}{a+b} - \frac{c}{c+d}$$

Table 9–1. Sleeping Position and Crib Death

USUAL SLEEPING POSITION	Crib Death?		TOTAL
	YES	NO	
Prone	9	837	846
Other	6	1755	1761
Total	15	2592	2607

Table 9–2. Layout of Data Relating a Dichotomous Exposure
Variable and a Dichotomous Disease Outcome

EXPOSURE	Disease		ALL PERSONS
	PRESENT	ABSENT	
Yes	a	b	$a + b$
No	c	d	$c + d$

$$I_e = \text{cumulative incidence in exposed} = \frac{a}{a + b}$$

$$I_o = \text{cumulative incidence in non-exposed} = \frac{c}{c + d}$$

$$I_t = \text{overall cumulative incidence} = \frac{a + c}{a + b + c + d}$$

In the example, the risk difference would be:

$$I_e - I_o = 10.64 \text{ per } 1000 - 3.41 \text{ per } 1000 = 7.23 \text{ per } 1000$$

If the association between exposure and disease is suspected to represent a causal one, then the term *attributable risk (AR)* can be used to describe the difference in risk. It corresponds to the added risk of disease due to the exposure. The *AR* also can be expressed as a percentage of the incidence in the exposed:

$$\frac{I_e - I_o}{I_e} \times 100\%$$

In the present example, the attributable risk percent (*AR%*) would be:

$$\frac{9/846 - 6/1761}{9/846} \times 100\% = 68.0\%$$

This value is an estimate of the percentage of crib death occurrence among prone-sleeping infants that is due to this sleeping position (assuming an inference has been made that the prone sleeping position is in fact a cause of crib death), and not to other causes of crib death all infants are subject to.

The $AR\%$ is commonly used to describe the results of prevention trials (for example, of a vaccine), where it is termed *efficacy*. In calculations done using the results of vaccine studies, unvaccinated persons constitute the "exposed" group, vaccinated persons the "non-exposed." For example, in a trial of polio vaccine from the 1950s, the cumulative incidence of polio in unvaccinated children during the several-month duration of the study was 57 per 100,000; the corresponding incidence in vaccinated children was 16 per 100,000. The vaccine efficacy was estimated as:

$$\frac{\text{Incidence (unvaccinated)} - \text{Incidence (vaccinated)}}{\text{Incidence (unvaccinated)}}$$

$$= \frac{57/100,000 - 16/100,000}{57/100,000} \times 100\% = 71.9\%$$

In a population in which there are both exposed and nonexposed individuals, the contribution to overall incidence of a given exposure (the *population attributable risk*, or *PAR*) is calculated as $I_t - I_o$, where $I_t = $ total incidence in the population. In the example on crib death, $I_t = 15/2607$. Thus, the *PAR* would be:

$$\frac{15}{2607} - \frac{6}{1761} = 2.35 \text{ per } 1000$$

If the association with sleeping position were causal, these data suggest that in Tasmania during the time of the study, 2.35 crib deaths per 1000 infants could be attributed to being put to sleep in the prone position.

Note that in some study designs; e.g., most case-control studies; it will not be possible to calculate I_t directly from the results obtained. In such instances, it may be possible to estimate I_t from information available apart from the study itself.

The *PAR* can also be expressed as a percentage of the total incidence (the *population attributable risk percent*), which in the present example would be:

$$\frac{15/2607 - 6/1761}{15/2607} \times 100\% = 40.8\%$$

That is, about 41% of the incidence of crib death in Tasmania would have been due to sleeping prone.

All of the above terms for expressing an altered *risk* have a counterpart when it is an altered *rate* that is being considered. So, there is a relative rate (or rate ratio), rate difference, attributable rate, attributable rate percent, population attributable rate, and population attributable rate percent. It is the unusual epidemiologist who rigorously distinguishes each of these, however, when writing or speaking, from the analogous term that pertains to "risk."

Table 9–3 lists the measures of excess risk, along with the factors that influence the size of each measure, and the purpose each one can be put to. As indicated in Chapter 8, the principal use of the *relative risk* is to guide inferences of cause and effect when an association is observed between an exposure and disease occurrence

Table 9–3. Application of Measures of Excess Risk in Epidemiology

MEASURE OF EXCESS RISK	ABBREVIATION	FORMULA	HELPS ANSWER THE QUESTION:
Relative risk	RR	I_e/I_o	Does exposure (E) cause disease (D)?
Risk difference (attributable risk to the exposed)	AR	$I_e - I_o$	(If E is believed to cause D) Among persons exposed to E, what amount of the incidence of D is E responsible for? Should anything be done to modify or eliminate E?
Attributable risk (%)	AR%	$\dfrac{RR - 1}{RR} \times 100\%$	(If E is believed to cause D) What proportion of the occurrence of disease in exposed individuals was due to the exposure?
Attributable risk to the population	PAR	$I_t - I_o$	(If E is believed to cause D) Should resources be allocated to controlling E or, instead, to exposures causing greater health problems in the population?
Attributable risk to the population (%)	PAR%	$\dfrac{I_t - I_o}{I_t} \times 100\%$	(If E is believed to cause D) What portion of D in the population is caused by E? Should resources allocated to combating D be directed toward etiologic research or control of known etiologies (e.g., E)?

I_e = incidence in exposed
I_o = incidence in non-exposed
I_t = incidence in all persons, exposed plus non-exposed

in epidemiologic studies. The *risk difference* quantifies the potential importance of this association in absolute terms: Over a given period of time, how many additional ill or injured persons would there be out of the total number who were exposed? For a relative risk of a given size, the risk difference associated with a given exposure will be larger for a commonly occurring illness than for a rare one. If the condition in question is common enough, even small relative risks can have a relatively large impact on disease occurrence. For example, consider the relationship between cigarette smoking and the incidence of two adverse outcomes among persons with type 2 diabetes: myocardial infarction (MI); and leg amputation or death due to peripheral arterial disease. Diabetics who smoke one pack of cigarettes per day double (approximately) their risk of an MI, but increase their risk of peripheral arterial disease by about a factor of 10 (Weiss, 1972). Both associations probably reflect the causal influence of smoking. The *attributable risk* (since we have drawn a causal inference, we are entitled to use this term instead of *risk difference*) related to smoking for each condition is shown in Table 9–4.

Smoking one pack of cigarettes per day makes a greater relative contribution to the incidence of peripheral arterial disease than to MI. Nonetheless, the absolute impact of smoking on the rate of MI—10 per 1000 person-years—actually exceeds that of peripheral vascular disease—4.5 per 1000 person-years—due to the much higher rate of MI in the absence of smoking.

For associations believed to be causal in nature, it is the *AR* (estimated collectively from all available studies) that is used to weigh the adverse and beneficial effects of the exposure on health outcomes. For example, observations in the 1970s of a fourfold increase in the rate of MI associated with current use of oral contraceptives (OCs) resulted in recommendations against such use for women in their mid-40s. The incidence among women in their mid-40s who did not use OCs was about 10 per million person-years, so the *AR* was about $(4 \times 10) - 10 = 30$ per million person-years. This contrasts with the absence of any such proscription for women under the age of 35, despite the fact that the *RR* for MI was the same in

Table 9–4. Cigarette Smoking in Relation to Vascular Complications in Persons with Type 2 Diabetes

CONDITION	Annual Incidence per 1000 Person-Years		*RR*	AR^a
	SMOKERS (I_e)	NONSMOKERS (I_o)		
Myocardial infarction	20	10	2	10
Peripheral arterial disease	5	0.5	10	4.5

^{a}Rate per 1000 person-years.

them as for a 45-year-old. In these younger women, whose annual rate of MI in the absence of OC use was only about 0.8 per million, the *AR* for MI associated with OC use was:

$$(4 \times 0.8) - (0.8) = 2.4 \text{ per million person-years.}$$

This figure seemed quite small relative to the health and other benefits that use of OCs was known to provide.

For some persons, the reciprocal of the attributable risk—the number of exposed persons or exposed person-time needed for one additional outcome event to occur—is easier to grasp than the attributable risk itself. So, one would say that among women in their mid-40s in the 1970s, the number of person-years of OC use necessary to produce one additional case of MI was 1/30 per million person-years = 33,333 person-years. The corresponding figure for women under the age of 35 was 1/2.4 per million person-years = 416,667 person-years. When applied in a clinical setting, this approach to considering the added risk or benefit of an intervention is referred to as the "number needed to treat."

Even in a person who has been exposed to an agent and who has developed the illness that the agent has the capacity to cause, the person's illness might have occurred through other means (unless the agent is a necessary cause of the disease). The *AR%* indicates what fraction of exposed individuals who developed a disease indeed did so because of the causal action(s) of that exposure. Among a group of diseased individuals who had received the exposure, almost never is there the equivalent of a fingerprint left behind by the causal exposure (in the form of a specific illness manifestation), so there is no way to discern which persons became ill specifically because of its effects. Thus, in any one such person, all that can be said is that the *AR%* for the group translates into his/her likelihood that the disease occurred as a result of his/her exposure to the agent in question. This notion of the likelihood of causation in an ill, exposed individual has application in civil litigation (Weiss, 1997)—though some question the validity of this sort of application (Greenland, 1999)—since in that setting a typical question is whether, more probably than not, a person's illness occurred because of her/his exposure to an agent. If it has been inferred that exposure to that agent has the capacity to cause the illness, then the *AR%* would appear to provide the relevant probability.

If it is believed that a given exposure can cause a given illness, it may be useful to calculate the *PAR*, which quantifies the contribution to the overall incidence of that illness in the population at large that can be attributed to the exposure. The information provided by the *PAR* can potentially be useful in allocating resources for prevention: a higher priority generally would be given to efforts to eliminate or modify exposures that are believed to produce a large burden of disease in the population (for example, cigarette smoking in most societies) than to exposures whose impact is smaller.

The *PAR%* is used to address a somewhat different question: What fraction of the population's incidence of a given disease can be accounted for by the presence of a particular causal agent? If that fraction is high, an argument can be made that directing resources towards modifying or eliminating the agent (or the factors it interacts with to allow it to produce the disease) might be a better investment than trying to identify other causal pathways leading to the same disease. It is likely that the campaigns mounted in many countries beginning in the mid-1990s to have parents place their infants in the supine position were stimulated by the high percentage (in addition to the high absolute rate) of crib-death occurrence that was estimated to be attributable to the prone sleeping position.

Sometimes we wish to estimate the reduction in a population's incidence of disease that might occur from the elimination of more than one of its causes. This cannot be accomplished simply by adding the *PAR%* calculated for each exposure alone: in a person with both exposures, the illness can only be prevented once. What must be done is to obtain a new *PAR%* associated with the presence of *either* the first or second exposure. For example, assume that among the 1755 infants in the Tasmanian study of crib death who usually were put to sleep on their back or side—the low-risk position—three events occurred in the 500 who had been passively exposed to cigarette smoke in their home (another risk factor for crib death). The *PAR%* for the two exposures, the prone sleeping position and exposure to passive smoking, would be estimated as shown in Table 9–5. From this calculation we would conclude that, if the causal actions of prone sleeping and passive smoking on the occurrence of crib death could be blocked or eliminated, the incidence of crib death in Tasmania would diminish by 58.7%.

Table 9–5. Calculation of *PAR%* for Two Exposures Associated with an Increased Risk of Crib Death

EXPOSURE STATUS	Crib Death?		TOTAL
	YES	NO	
Prone sleeping or passive smoking	$9 + 3 = 12$	$837 + 497 = 1334$	$846 + 500 = 1348$
Neither of the above	$6 - 3 = 3$	$1755 - 497 = 1258$	$1761 - 500 = 1261$
Total	15	2592	2607

$$PAR\% = \frac{15/2607 - 3/1261}{15/2607} \times 100\% = 58.7\%$$

As indicated in Table 9–3, the size of both the *PAR* and the *PAR%* is influenced by the frequency of the exposure: The more common a factor that predisposes to a given disease, the greater amount or percentage of that disease it will be responsible for. Thus, a *PAR* or *PAR%* estimated from a study in one population will not accurately characterize the same parameter in a second population if the prevalence of the exposure differs between the two.

Statistical significance is often calculated when a possible association between exposure and disease is investigated. It is not a measure of excess risk. Instead, it assesses the likelihood of observing an association at least as large as the one seen, if in truth no association were present in the population from which the study subjects were drawn. The size of the p-value that is generated in statistical hypothesis testing is heavily dependent on the size of the study population: the larger the number of subjects, the smaller the p value. The size of the study is to some extent arbitrary, so we ought not use the p value for any purpose other than evaluating the role of chance. Similarly, we would not use the *RR* for any purpose beyond that which it could achieve: guidance in an inference of possible cause and effect. And so on for the other measures in Table 9–3: each has a role in answering a particular question from among the several questions that can be posed concerning the influence of an exposure on disease occurrence.

ESTIMATING THE RELATIVE RISK WHEN INCIDENCE RATES CANNOT BE CALCULATED

Case-Control Studies

These studies compare antecedent exposures or characteristics of ill or injured persons (cases) with those of persons at risk of the illness or injury (see Chapter 15). Even though incidence rates are typically not obtained, either for exposed or for non-exposed persons, the data gathered often can be used to provide a good estimate of the relative risk. To understand how this can be done, consider a cohort study in which exposed and non-exposed persons are followed for a certain period of time. Table 9–6 summarizes their experience with regard to a particular disease.

The cumulative incidence of the disease in exposed and non-exposed persons over a given period of follow-up is $a/(a + b)$ and $c/(c + d)$, respectively. The relative risk (*RR*) is defined as:

$$\frac{a/(a + b)}{c/(c + d)}$$

Table 9–6. Data Layout for a Hypothetical
Cohort Study

| | Disease | | |
EXPOSED	YES	NO	TOTAL
Yes	a	b	$a+b$
No	c	d	$c+d$

Table 9–7. Hypothetical Results of a
Cohort Study

| | Disease | | |
EXPOSED	YES	NO	TOTAL
Yes	100	9,900	10,000
No	300	89,700	90,000

$$RR = \frac{100/10,000}{300/90,000} = 3.00$$

If the incidence of the disease is relatively low during the follow-up period in both exposed and non-exposed persons, then a will be small relative to b, and c will be small relative to d. Therefore

$$RR = \frac{a/(a+b)}{c/(c+d)} \approx \frac{a/b}{c/d} = \frac{a/c}{b/d}$$

The expression $\frac{a/c}{b/d}$ is the *odds ratio (OR)*: the numerator a/c is the odds of exposure in persons who develop the disease, and the denominator b/d is the odds of exposure in persons who remain well. It is important to note that the numerator of the odds ratio can be estimated from a sample of cases, while the denominator can be estimated from a sample of non-cases. Neither estimate is influenced by the proportion of cases among the subjects actually chosen for study.

In the hypothetical example shown in Table 9–7, assume that 100 of 10,000 persons exposed to a particular substance or organism developed a disease, in contrast with 300 of 90,000 non-exposed persons.

Table 9–8. Effect of Case-Control Sampling Within a
Hypothetical Cohort Study

| EXPOSED | Disease | |
	YES	NO
Yes	$100 \times 0.5 = 50$	$9,900 \times 0.01 = 99$
No	$300 \times 0.5 = 150$	$89,700 \times 0.01 = 897$

$$RR \approx OR = \frac{50/150}{99/897} = 3.02$$

If a case-control study including 50 per cent of cases but only 1 per cent of non-cases had been performed, the results shown in Table 9–8 would be expected.

When controls are chosen in this way—from persons who had not developed the disease by the end of the same time period during which other persons (the cases) had developed it—the less common the disease in both exposed and non-exposed persons during the period, the better the odds ratio will estimate the ratio of cumulative incidence (Zhang and Yu, 1998). In the previous example, only 1% and 0.33% of exposed and non-exposed persons, respectively, developed the illness, so the relative cumulative incidence and odds ratio were in close correspondence (3.00 versus 3.02). But it is also possible to choose controls from persons free of disease only until the corresponding cases have been diagnosed; a person can appear in the study first as a control and later as a case. If this approach is used, the odds ratio will be a valid estimate of the ratio of incidence rates (i.e., number of cases divided by the person-time at risk) irrespective of the disease frequency (Greenland and Thomas, 1982; Rodrigues and Kirkwood, 1990; Pearce, 1993).

Proportional Mortality (Morbidity) Studies

It may happen that in a particular setting you know the number of exposed individuals who have developed an illness or have died, but you have no means of enumerating either the total number of exposed persons or the person-time from which the illnesses or deaths occurred. Let us say you have available to you records of deaths among members of a particular labor union. While information on cause of death is present in the files—perhaps a death certificate had to be submitted to receive benefits—the union is not able to tell you the size of its membership over time, so the denominator needed to calculate a death rate for any given cause cannot be determined. Nonetheless, what *can* be calculated is the *proportional mortality*—the fraction of all deaths that are due to a particular cause of death. To assess whether this fraction is atypical, it can be compared to the corresponding fraction for demographically comparable persons who died in the geographic population in which the union members resided. So, for example, if five percent of deaths in union members were due to nonmalignant respiratory disease, but only two percent of deaths in the population at large were due to this cause, one could estimate the relative risk of death from respiratory disease associated with union membership as being $0.05/0.02 = 2.5$.

The potential limitations of the *proportional mortality ratio* calculated above are evident: Even if the rate of death from respiratory disease among union members were identical to that in the remainder of the population, the *proportion of* deaths from this cause would be elevated if the death rate from all other causes (combined) in union members were relatively low. Or that proportion would be depressed if the rate of death from other causes in union members were relatively high. Therefore, proportional mortality (or morbidity) ratios must be interpreted cautiously, since their magnitude takes into account more than the one thing we are using them to estimate; i.e., the ratio of the rate of death or illness between exposed and non-exposed persons. (For a more complete discussion of the uses and limitations of the proportional mortality ratio, see Chapter 3.)

ESTIMATING EXCESS RISK FROM RESULTS OF CASE-CONTROL STUDIES

Occasionally, a case-control study identifies a large odds ratio relating an exposure and a disease, and for this and other reasons a causal influence of the exposure may be suspected. The decision to limit or eliminate that exposure requires weighing its negative and positive consequences. This weighing must be done in absolute rather than in relative terms, since the same relative increase (or decrease) in risk is of far greater consequence for common than for rare outcomes. As we have seen, the absolute increase in the risk of disease believed to be due to a dichotomous exposure, the attributable risk $I_e - I_o$, can be obtained directly from studies that directly measure the incidence in exposed (I_e) and non-exposed persons (I_o). Since I_e can be expressed as the relative risk (RR) times I_o, the term $I_e - I_o$ can be rewritten as $(RR \cdot I_o) - I_o$, or as $I_o(RR - 1)$. Since the RR can be estimated from the results of a case-control study by means of the odds ratio, the only additional piece of information needed to estimate the AR is an estimate of I_o. For the population in which the study has been conducted, I_o can be estimated if:

1. The overall incidence (I) of the disease in that population is known or can be approximated; and
2. The frequency of exposure (p_e) in the controls selected for study reasonably reflects that of the population that gave rise to the cases.

Given (1) and (2) above,

$$I = I_e(p_e) + I_o(1 - p_e)$$
$$= I_o \cdot RR(p_e) + I_o(1 - p_e)$$
$$= I_o[p_e(RR - 1) + 1],$$

and so $I_o = \dfrac{I}{p_e(RR - 1) + 1}.$

Thus, $AR = I_o(RR - 1)$

$$= \frac{I(RR - 1)}{p_e(RR - 1) + \frac{RR-1}{RR-1}}$$

$$= \frac{I}{p_e + \frac{1}{RR-1}}$$

For example, consider a disease with an incidence rate of 10 per 100,000 person-years in a population in which five percent of persons have been exposed during a relevant period of time. The following table summarizes data from a hypothetical case-control study conducted in that population:

EXPOSED?	CASES	CONTROLS	OR
Yes	15%	5%	3.35
No	85%	95%	1

The AR that corresponds to the estimated 3.35-fold increase in risk is:

$$AR = \frac{I}{p_e + \frac{1}{RR-1}}$$

$$= \frac{10}{0.05 + \frac{1}{3.35-1}}$$

$$= 21.0 \text{ per } 100{,}000 \text{ person-years.}$$

From the results of case-control studies that suggest a causal relation, it is also possible to estimate the percentage of exposed persons with the disease who developed it because of their exposure, rather than through one or more causal pathways not involving the exposure. This measure, the attributable risk percent ($AR\%$) among exposed persons, was defined earlier as:

$$AR\% = \frac{I_e - I_o}{I_e} \times 100\%$$

The terms in the formula for the $AR\%$ can be rearranged as:

$$\frac{I_e - I_o}{I_e} = \frac{I_e}{I_e} - \frac{I_o}{I_e}$$

$$= 1 - \frac{1}{RR}$$

$$= \frac{RR}{RR} - \frac{1}{RR}$$

$$= \frac{RR - 1}{RR} \times 100\%$$

Therefore, estimates of the $AR\%$ can be obtained from case-control studies that can estimate the RR, by means of the odds ratio (see earlier in chapter), even if neither I_e nor I_o is known. So, in the hypothetical study that obtained an odds ratio of 3.35, the $AR\%$ could be estimated as:

$$\frac{3.35 - 1}{3.35} \times 100\% = 70.1\%$$

It is also possible to estimate the percentage of a disease's occurrence in the population as a whole that resulted from the actions of a given exposure. This measure, the population attributable risk percent ($PAR\%$), is simply the $AR\%$ multiplied by the proportion of cases in that population who were exposed (p_c):

$$PAR\% = AR\%(p_c)$$

$$= \frac{RR - 1}{RR} \times p_c \times 100\%$$

In the present example, the $PAR\% = 70.1\% \times 0.15 = 10.5\%$.

EXERCISES

1. You are the epidemiology consultant to a large local factory. Because of some suspicion by physicians who provide care to employees there, you conduct a study of the occurrence of a particular respiratory disease among the workers, and obtain the following results.

   - Incidence of respiratory disease among workers exposed to chemical A = 200 per 100,000 person-years.
   - Incidence of respiratory disease among workers not exposed to chemical A = 20 per 100,000 person-years.
   - Incidence in the general population in which the factory is situated = 21 per 100,000 person-years.

   Assume that no one who works outside of the factory is exposed to chemical A.

   (a) What are the relative rate (RR), attributable rate (AR), and the population attributable rate percent (PAR%) associated with occupational exposure to this chemical?
   (b) How can you account for the low PAR% in view of the high RR?
   (c) Based on the high RR and other available information, you believe that the association between occupational exposure to chemical A and the incidence of this respiratory disease to be a causal one.

       i. Among exposed workers who developed the respiratory disease, what fraction of them did so as a result of their employment?
       ii. In making your recommendations to management and labor as they consider the benefits and costs of extra protection for the workers, which measure of excess risk would you use? Why?

2. Consider a randomized trial in which the incidence of disease X has been monitored in persons who were and were not vaccinated against the disease. The incidence in the latter (unvaccinated) group was three times that of the former group.

   Is this information adequate to permit an estimate of the efficacy of vaccination against disease X? If yes, what is that estimate? If no, why not?

3. Approximately 12 percent of the deaths in children aged five through nine in the United States in 1987 were due to cancer. In contrast, approximately one-fourth of the deaths at ages 60 to 64 were due to this condition. Is it correct to say that the risk of death from cancer was approximately twice as great in the older age group? If not, why not?

4. Comment on the following (paraphrased from a letter to the editor of a medical journal):

> Prospective and retrospective studies conducted during the 1950s all concluded that cigarette smoking accounted for only about 20% of lung cancer incidence in women. Therefore, the steady rise in lung cancer in women since that time must have some other cause, and air pollution by carcinogens is the obvious answer. Enthusiasm for the cigarette theory should not be allowed to hold back the thorough investigation of every possible factor.

5. The following data are taken from a study by Braddon (1907) on the epidemiology of beri-beri in Singapore:

	HOSPITAL ADMISSIONS (ALL CAUSES) PER 1000 POPULATION IN 1900	NEW BERI-BERI CASES PER 1000 HOSPITAL ADMISSIONS IN 1900
Chinese	62	150
Europeans	310	1.4

Do these data support the hypothesis that the incidence of beri-beri was greater among Chinese than European residents of Singapore? If yes, to what degree? If no, why not?

6. The data shown in Table 9–9 were obtained in a study of smoking in relation to the incidence of bladder cancer (Cole et al., 1971). Among women, the relative risk of bladder cancer for each category of intensity or duration of smoking was the same as or slightly higher than the relative risk among men. However:

   (a) The population attributable rate percent among men was greater, 39% to 29%. How could this be?

   (b) The attributable rate among male smokers was more than double that among female smokers. Why?

Table 9–9. Incidence and Attributable Rate per 100,000 Person-years and Population Attributable Rate Percent

	MEN	WOMEN
Incidence in smokers	48.0	19.2
Incidence in non-smokers	25.4	9.6
Total incidence	41.8	13.5
Attributable rate in smokers	22.6	9.6
Population attributable rate	16.4	3.9
Population attributable rate percent	39%	29%

7. The data shown below come from a case-control study of cigarette smoking and lung cancer in British men, among the very first on this topic (Doll and Hill, 1950):

	Daily Cigarette Consumption				
	NONE OR < 5	5–14	15–24	25–49	50+
Men with lung cancer	26	208	196	174	45
Controls	65	242	201	118	23

(a) Estimate the risk of lung cancer to cigarette smokers in each category of daily consumption relative to the risk of men who never smoked or smoked less than five cigarettes per day.

(b) Estimate the proportion of lung cancer among British males in this age group that could have been prevented if no man had ever smoked more than four cigarettes per day during his lifetime.

(c) Assuming that the incidence of lung cancer among males in this age group is 80 per 100,000 per year, what is the incidence of lung cancer in smokers of more than four cigarettes per day attributable to their smoking?

ANSWERS

1. (a)

$$RR = 200/20$$
$$= 10$$

$$AR = 200 \text{ per } 100,000 - 20 \text{ per } 100,000$$
$$= 180 \text{ per } 100,000 \text{ person-years}$$

$$PAR\% = \frac{21 - 20}{21} \times 100\%$$
$$= 4.8\%$$

(b) The size of the PAR% depends on two things:

- the size of the relative risk; and
- the proportion of the population exposed.

The PAR% is low because occupational exposure to chemical A must be relatively uncommon in this population.

(c) i. $AR\% = \frac{200-20}{200} \times 100\% = 90\%$. Only 10% of exposed workers with the respiratory disease would have developed it without exposure to chemical A.

ii. Attributable rate—it alone describes the extra absolute risk to the workers themselves. In deciding whether exposure to chemical A should continue or not continue, the AR for respiratory disease would be weighed along with the other risks and benefits related to this exposure.

2. Vaccine efficacy can be calculated as follows:

$$\text{Vaccine efficacy} = \frac{I_{unvacc} - I_{vacc}}{I_{unvacc}}$$

$$= \frac{I_{unvacc}}{I_{unvacc}} - \frac{I_{vacc}}{I_{unvacc}}$$

$$= 1 - \frac{1}{3}$$

$$= 66.7\%.$$

3. It is not correct to conclude that the risk of death from cancer is twice as great in the older age group. The statement compares the proportional mortality for deaths due to cancer in the 5–9 year age group with that for the group 60–64 years of age. Differences in the occurrence of the denominator event, rate of death from other causes, can also influence the size of the proportionate mortality. Since the rate from "other" causes of death is far higher in the older than the younger age group, the true risk of death from cancer at ages 60–64 years is far more than twice that at ages 5–9 years. To illustrate this, consider the following table that presents approximate death rates for persons in these two age groups:

	Annual Death Rate per 100,000		CANCER DEATHS ÷
AGE (YEARS)	CANCER	ALL CAUSES	TOTAL DEATHS
5–9	6	50	.12
60–64	750	3000	.25

Although the percentage of deaths from cancer at ages 60–64 is about twice that at age 5–9 (.25 vs. .12), the ratio of annual cancer mortality *rates* is far larger: 750 per 100,000 vs. 6 per 100,000, or 125.

4. The figure of 20% is the population attributable risk percent. This measure depends on the size of the relative risk as well as the proportion of the population

exposed. If smoking among women had become more frequent over time, it could have led to both an increase in the overall incidence of lung cancer and an increase in the *PAR%* due to smoking.

5. Incidence of beri-beri in 1901:

$$\text{Chinese:} \quad 62/1000 \times 150/1000 = 9.3/1000$$
$$\text{Europeans:} \quad 310/1000 \times 1.4/1000 = 0.43/1000$$

Relative incidence:

$$\text{Based on cases per 1000 admissions:} \quad 150/1.4 = 107.1$$
$$\text{Based on incidence:} \quad 9.3/.43 = 21.6$$

The incidence of beri-beri among Chinese residents of Singapore was 21.6 times that of Europeans. The ratio based on cases per hospital admissions is inflated, due to the relatively low incidence of hospitalization for other reasons among Chinese.

6. *(a)* The prevalence of smoking among men in this population must be higher than that among women.

   (b) Among nonsmokers, the incidence of bladder cancer in men (25.4 per 100,000 person-years) is greater than in women (9.6). The identical *RR* associated with smoking will therefore produce a larger added rate in men than in women.

7. *(a)*

	Daily Cigarette Consumption				
	NONE OR < 5	5–14	15–24	25–49	50+
Odds ratio[a]	1.0	2.15	2.44	3.69	4.89

[a] Approximates the relative risk.

(b)
$$PAR\% = \frac{RR - 1}{RR} \times (\text{proportion of cases exposed}) \times 100\%$$

$$RR = OR = \frac{623/26}{65/584} = 2.67$$

Of the 649 men with lung cancer, 623 had smoked $\geq$ 5 cigarettes per day, so:

$$PAR\% = \frac{2.67 - 1}{2.67} \times \frac{623}{649} \times 100\% = 60\%$$

(c) The question asks for the added incidence of lung cancer among men who smoked $\geq$ 5 cigarettes per day, i.e., the attributable rate.

$$AR = \frac{I}{P_e + \frac{1}{RR - 1}}$$

$$= \frac{80}{\frac{584}{649} + \frac{1}{2.67 - 1}}$$

$$= 53.4 \text{ per } 100,000 \text{ per year}$$

REFERENCES

Braddon WL. The cause and prevention of beri-beri. London: Rebman Ltd., 1907.

Cole P, Monson RR, Haning H, Friedell GH. Smoking and cancer of the lower urinary tract. N Engl J Med 1971; 284:129–34.

Doll R, Hill AB. Smoking and carcinoma of the lung. BMJ 1950; 2:739–48.

Dwyer T, Ponsonby AL, Newman NM, Gibbons LE. Prospective cohort study of prone sleeping position and sudden infant death syndrome. Lancet 1991; 337:1244–47.

Greenland S. Relation of probability of causation to relative risk and doubling dose: a methodologic error that has become a social problem. Am J Public Health 1999; 89:1166–69.

Greenland S, Thomas DC. On the need for the rare disease assumption in case-control studies. Am J Epidemiol 1982; 116:547–53.

Pearce N. What does the odds ratio estimate in a case-control study? Int J Epidemiol 1993; 22:1189–92.

Rodrigues L, Kirkwood BR. Case-control designs in the study of common diseases: updates on the demise of the rare disease assumption and the choice of sampling scheme for controls. Int J Epidemiol 1990; 19:205–13.

Weiss NS. Cigarette smoking and arteriosclerosis obliterans: an epidemiologic approach. Am J Epidemiol 1972; 95:17–25.

Weiss NS. "General concepts of epidemiology." In: Faigman D, Kaye D, Saks M, Sanders J (eds.). Modern scientific evidence: the law and science of expert testimony. St. Paul, Minn.: West, 2002.

Zhang J, Yu KF. What's the relative risk? A method for correcting the odds ratio in cohort studies of common outcomes. JAMA 1998; 280:1690–91.

10

MEASUREMENT ERROR

In epidemiology, victories are few and at this point a whole field may be on the verge of propagating pathological science, which means they cannot get good enough resolution to identify the effects they're studying. Epidemiologists may be seeing and reporting that there are canals on Mars because they're looking at Mars through Galileo's telescope. And that's the nature of the field and all the statistical wizardry in the world isn't going to change that.

G. Taubes

Although it is likely that few epidemiologists would share Taubes's pessimistic outlook, most would agree that improving the resolution of their measurement tools will allow them to more accurately describe the relationship between exposures and diseases they are studying. This chapter addresses the sources, assessment, and consequences of measurement error. It also gives examples of exposure–disease relationships that, figuratively, were as large as Mars itself, not just its "canals," and could readily be detected by epidemiologic tools whose accuracy was similar to that of Galileo's telescope.

SOURCES OF MEASUREMENT ERROR

Mismeasurement of *exposure* status or level is present to at least some degree in nearly every epidemiologic study, since nearly every means of ascertaining the presence or level of exposure is imperfect. Interviews or questionnaires can obtain erroneous information: a subject may have been misinformed about his or her exposure status, or may even intentionally misrepresent it. The methods used to make direct measurements on study subjects (e.g., blood pressure by means of a cuff), or on samples taken from them, often err. For characteristics that vary over time within an individual, such as blood pressure, the problem is compounded if (as is often the case) an opportunity exists to make measurements on each subject on only a single occasion, since the value obtained on that occasion may not correspond to the person's longer-term average value. Records that might contain information on past exposures or on correlates of these—such as employment, medical, or vital records—not only have the potential limitations given above, they may be incomplete or not faithfully transcribed.

Error in measurement of health *outcomes* can occur in epidemiologic studies as well. For example:

- Current diagnostic technology may not be applied to all persons who might meet the criteria for being a "case": for example, the prevalence of gallstone disease or endometriosis would be substantially underestimated if reliance were placed exclusively on a positive result from a particular diagnostic test, since so many people with these conditions are asymptomatic and are not given the test.
- The available diagnostic technology may be limited in its ability to discriminate sub-groups within a larger group of ill persons who have experienced a similar pathophysiologic process. For example, among all persons with arthritis there will be some in whom it will be uncertain whether or not they have a particular type; e.g., rheumatoid arthritis.
- Even when the appropriate diagnostic tests have been used in the care of a particular individual, the results of those tests may not be available to those conducting the epidemiologic study in which that individual is a subject. For example, in a large study of the efficacy of pneumococcal vaccine that relied exclusively on computerized data available on Medicaid recipients, the investigators (Gable et al., 1990) compared the incidence of pneumonia between persons who had and had not been vaccinated. Though they would have preferred to study pneumococcal pneumonia per se, the computerized records could only specify the broader outcome, pneumonia, irrespective of its microbiological etiology. This likely led to a substantial degree of misclassification in this study, since typically pneumococcal pneumonia constitutes less than a third of all pneumonia.

ASSESSING MEASUREMENT ERROR

As used here, the term *measure* refers broadly to almost any way of capturing data on a certain characteristic of study subjects. The underlying characteristic itself can be anything: disease status, exposure status, a potential confounder or effect modifier, and so on. The data-gathering method may be by self-administered questionnaire, personal interview, physical examination, laboratory test, extraction of information from medical records, direct observation of behavior, or other approaches.

Regardless of the characteristic or data-collection method, there is a *true* value of the characteristic for each study subject. For example, each study subject has a certain true body weight at a certain time. The true value for each subject is often unknown; only the measured value may be available, such as body weight as self-reported to a telephone interviewer. Any discrepancy between the true value and the measured value is measurement error.

As we shall see, the consequences of measurement error depend on how much of it is present, so ways of quantifying it are needed. Quantitative indices of measurement error can be useful when choosing among different measures of the same characteristic during the study-design phase, for detecting data quality problems during staff training and data collection, and for gauging how large a role measurement error may have played in determining study results during data analysis. This section offers a brief introduction to indices of measurement error, a topic that has been studied extensively. Good sources for more information include Armstrong et al. (1992); Fleiss (1986, 1980); and Thomas et al. (1993).

To begin with, two properties are desirable in any measurement:

- *Reliability.* A good measurement should yield the same value if applied repeatedly under circumstances in which the underlying characteristic is believed to remain the same.
- *Validity.* A good measurement method should yield the *correct* value. (Being consistent is not good enough if the results are consistently wrong.)

Reliability and validity apply broadly to any kind of measurement, but the approach to quantifying them depends on the *scale* of measurement. Those of most interest to epidemiologists include:

1. *Continuous.* The measure can in principle take on any numeric value, including fractional values, over a defined range. For example, body weight can be almost any positive real number, depending on the units in which it is expressed. For practical reasons, continuous measures are recorded to a fixed number of digits of precision, but this choice is arbitrary and not an intrinsic property of the measure.
2. *Categorical*
   (a) *Ordinal.* Three or more discrete values are possible, which fall into a natural sequence according to how much of the characteristic being measured is present. For example, disease severity can be mild, moderate, or severe.
   (b) *Nominal.* Two or more discrete values are possible, but there is no particular ordering among them. For example, marital status can be currently married, never married, divorced, separated, or widowed.

Sometimes only two values are possible, and the nominal scale is referred to as *binary*. For example, a certain disease can be either present or absent; gender can be either male or female.

Measurement error on a categorical measure is commonly termed *misclassification*.

The above list of measurement scales is itself ordered from "fine" to "coarse." A relatively fine measurement can often be converted to a coarser one by grouping values together. For example, age can be converted from a continuous variable to an ordinal one by assigning each person to one of several age groups based on the original age value. Marital status can be converted from a nominal variable to a binary one (currently married or not, say). "Degrading" the scale of measurement in this way may be done for convenience in data analysis or presentation, although information is often lost in the process.

Reliability

As noted earlier, *reliability* concerns agreement among repeated measurements. Reliability is also termed *reproducibility*. Adjectives are sometimes applied to it to indicate how the repeated measurements are related. For example, *intra-observer* reliability refers to agreement among measurements made by the same observer, while *inter-observer* reliability refers to agreement among measurements taken by different observers. *Test-retest* reliability refers to agreement among measurements on the same subjects at different times. But overall, similar approaches to quantifying reliability are used in all these situations.

Concordance (percent agreement)

Concordance applies to categorical measures. Suppose that a certain categorical measurement is obtained twice under similar circumstances on each of several study subjects. Concordance is simply the proportion of all tested subjects for whom both measurements are the same. Expressed as a percentage, this quantity is also termed the *percent agreement*. Either way, it is easy to calculate and to grasp, which probably explains why it continues to appear in the literature.

Unfortunately, concordance has a serious limitation: it fails to account for agreement that chance alone could produce. For example, say that the measurement of interest is binary, and that two independent measurements are made on every study subject. Each result is either positive or negative. The results can be organized as in Table 10–1: a, b, c, and d are the number of subjects with each combination of results, and N is the total number of people tested. The observed concordance is $(a + d)/N$.

Table 10–1. Data Layout for Reliability Assessment
on a Binary Measure

| | Measurement No. 2 | | |
MEASUREMENT NO. 1	+	−	TOTAL
+	a	b	$a + b$
−	c	d	$c + d$
Total	$a + c$	$b + d$	N

Table 10–2. Expected Results If Two Observers Each Assign
a Positive Result to a Random 10% of Study Subjects

| | Observer No. 2 | |
OBSERVER NO. 1	+	−
+	1	9
−	9	81

Now suppose that the underlying characteristic being measured is truly present in 10% of people. Suspecting this, two lazy data collectors could simply record "+" for a random 10% of tested subjects and "−" for the rest, without ever doing any real observations. The expected results would be as shown in Table 10–2. The lazy observers would have recorded the same result for 82% of subjects. This might naïvely be interpreted as an impressive degree of concordance, but in truth it merely reflects agreement by chance.

Because of this problem, concordance alone is of rather limited value as an index of reliability. It is used, however, in calculation of a better index, *kappa*.

Kappa

Widely used as a measure of reliability for categorical measures *kappa* (κ) is designed to correct for chance agreement (Cohen, 1960; Fleiss, 1980). It is defined as

$$\kappa = \frac{P_o - P_e}{1 - P_e} \tag{10.1}$$

where P_o is the observed concordance, and P_e is the concordance expected by chance. P_e is based only on the row and column totals—that is, on the distribution of results for each observer (or measurement occasion) considered separately. For

Table 10–3. Guidelines for Interpretation of Kappa

KAPPA	INTERPRETATION
>.80	Almost perfect
.61–.80	Substantial
.41–.60	Moderate
.21–.40	Fair
.00–.20	Slight
<.00	Poor

[*Source:* Landis and Koch (1977).]

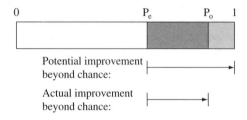

Figure 10–1. Graphical Interpretation of Kappa.

a binary variable, using the notation of Table 10–1,

$$P_o = \frac{a + d}{N}$$

$$P_e = \left[\frac{(a + b)(a + c)}{N} + \frac{(b + d)(c + d)}{N} \right] \bigg/ N$$

(Those familiar with the χ^2 test may recognize the two terms within the brackets in the formula for P_e. They are expressions for the expected number of study subjects in the a and d cells, respectively, if the row and column factors are independent. P_o and P_e are thus similar, one being based on observed cell frequencies and the other on expected cell frequencies.)

Figure 10–1 sketches the idea behind kappa. As with any proportion, concordance can range from 0 to 1. P_e is the concordance expected by chance, so $1 - P_e$ can be thought of as the amount of "room for improvement" between P_e and perfect agreement. Kappa represents the amount by which the observed concordance (P_o) exceeds that expected by chance (P_e), expressed as a proportion of the potential improvement beyond chance.

Kappa normally falls between 0 and 1, but it can become negative if $P_o < P_e$, indicating that agreement is even worse than chance alone could produce. Landis and Koch (1977) offered the guidelines in Table 10–3 for interpretation of kappa.

Example: Wright and colleagues (2000) studied genital-tract human papillomavirus (HPV) testing as a possible screening test for cervical cancer. Among other things, they examined the agreement between test results on swabs obtained by clinicians with test results on swabs obtained by screenees themselves. For 1415 women, both kinds of specimens were obtained. The results were:

	Self-collected		
CLINICIAN-COLLECTED	+	−	TOTAL
+	170	132	302
−	128	985	1113
Total	298	1117	1415

The observed concordance was $(170 + 985)/1415 = .816$, but chance alone would lead to

$$\left(\frac{302 \times 298}{1415} + \frac{1113 \times 1117}{1415}\right)\bigg/ 1415 = .666$$

concordance. Kappa was $(.816 - .666)/(1 - .666) = 0.45$, representing only moderate agreement beyond chance.

More complex variants of kappa have been developed to quantify reliability for categorical variables with more than two levels, as described in Appendix 10A.

The value of kappa depends in part on the true prevalence of the characteristic being measured. Thompson and Walter (1988) described the mathematical basis for this relationship, showing that kappa declines as prevalence approaches 0 or 1. This property should be kept in mind when comparing kappas among populations in which the prevalence of the characteristic under study differs substantially.

Kappa can be useful in interpretation of study results, especially when there is concern that an observed association may be seriously attenuated by errors in measurements of disease or exposure. Thompson (1990) derived a mathematical relation between kappa, sensitivity, and specificity (see below), and the amount of bias in an observed odds ratio, under certain assumptions. As kappa approaches zero, attenuation of the odds ratio becomes severe, and a true exposure–disease association may go undetected due to measurement error.

Intraclass correlation coefficient

For continuous measures, reliability can be quantified using the *intraclass correlation coefficient (ICC)*, which is based on the analysis of variance (Snedecor and Cochran, 1980). There are several forms of the *ICC*, each corresponding to a different analysis of variance model. These models differ according to whether the replicate observations on each subject are considered interchangeable; and if not, which statistical model best captures the sources of variation likely to affect an observed value (Armstrong et al., 1992; Fleiss, 1986).

The simplest situation is when two independent observations of the same characteristic have been made on each study subject, and those two observations are considered interchangeable. For example, suppose that in a study of dietary sodium intake, urine specimens have been obtained from each of 50 people. To determine the reliability of the urinary sodium assay, two separate aliquots of urine are extracted from each person's original specimen, and the assay is run on all 100 resulting aliquots. For any particular person, it would not matter which aliquot is labelled #1 and which #2—they are interchangeable.

Even for this simple situation, the computing formula for the *ICC* is complex, so it is not given here but is available elsewhere (Armstrong et al., 1992; Fleiss, 1986; Rosner, 1995). Nowadays the calculations would usually be done by computer using standard statistical software. But the underlying idea is straightforward. In the urinary-sodium example, the total variance among the 100 observations can be partitioned statistically into two components, *between*-person variance (B) and *within*-person variance (W), such that total variance $= B + W$. The intraclass correlation coefficient is

$$ICC = \frac{B}{B + W}$$

In other words, it is the fraction of the total variance that is due to between-person variation. The $ICC = 1$ if all of the variation is between people—that is, if the two urinary sodium measurements for each person agree exactly. The $ICC = 0$ if $B = 0$, which occurs if the means for all 50 people are no more variable than if the 100 urine samples had simply been allocated at random into 50 pairs.

The value of the *ICC* can be interpreted using the same descriptors as for kappa, as shown in Table 10–3. Confidence limits for it can be obtained using methods described by Fleiss (1986) and Rosner (1995). A discussion of other epidemiologic research situations in which the replicate observations for each person would *not* be considered interchangeable can be found in Armstrong et al. (1992).

Validity

Validity concerns whether a measurement reflects the truth. To evaluate the validity of a measure, each study subject's true status on the characteristic of interest must generally be known. This need is usually met by a different *criterion measure* whose validity is already established or can be safely assumed, often called a *gold standard*.

In epidemiology, the true characteristic of interest is often binary, such as presence or absence of a certain disease condition or exposure. For example, the gold standard for determining whether Alzheimer's disease is present or absent might be microscopic examination of brain tissue by a competent neuropathologist. But applying a gold standard test to everyone may be too risky, invasive, time-consuming, or costly, which motivates a search for more feasible alternative measures.

Sensitivity and specificity

Suppose that the characteristic of interest is the presence or absence of a certain disease condition, and that a gold standard test for true disease status has been applied to a set of study subjects. Some subjects prove to have the condition; others prove not to have it. Now imagine that a new test for the condition yields a binary result, positive or negative, and is applied to the same people. The correspondence between the new test result and the gold standard result can be summarized as in Table 10–4, where

a = number of *true positives*
b = number of *false positives*
c = number of *false negatives*
d = number of *true negatives*

Table 10–4. Data Layout for Assessing
the Validity of a Binary Test

TEST RESULT	Condition Present?	
	+	−
+	a	b
−	c	d
Total	$a + c$	$b + d$

Sensitivity $= a/(a + c)$
Specificity $= d/(b + d)$

Two key aspects of the test's validity are defined as follows:

- *Sensitivity.* When the condition is truly present, how often does the test detect it? Here there are $a + c$ true cases, and the test yields a positive result on a of them. Its estimated *sensitivity* is defined as $a/(a + c)$.
- *Specificity.* When the condition is truly absent, how often does the test give a negative result? There are $b + d$ true non-cases, and the test is negative on d of them. Its estimated *specificity* is defined as $d/(b + d)$.

Sensitivity and specificity are proportions that can range from 0 to 1. Confidence limits for them can be obtained as described in appendix 4A. They can also be interpreted as conditional probabilities: if T_+ and T_- denote positive and negative test results, respectively, and C_+ and C_- denote presence or absence of the underlying condition, then

$$\text{Sensitivity} = \Pr(T_+ \mid C_+)$$

$$\text{Specificity} = \Pr(T_- \mid C_-)$$

High sensitivity and high specificity are both desirable, but neither can be considered in isolation. For example, a patently worthless test that always yields a positive result, regardless of the person's true status, would have excellent sensitivity (1.0), but terrible specificity (0.0). In practice, almost every test is imperfect, with sensitivity and specificity falling somewhere between 0 and 1.

Example: Catanzaro and colleagues (2000) sought to evaluate a new rapid diagnostic test for active pulmonary tuberculosis (TB), called the Extended *Mycobacterium tuberculosis* Direct test (E-MTD), designed to detect genetic material from the TB bacillus. This test was applied to 338 patients being evaluated for possible TB at seven clinical sites. Each patient also received an extensive clinical work-up including medical history, physical examination, sputum cultures, X-rays, and other tests, which were later used to determine whether active TB was truly present or absent according to a standardized protocol. Of the 72 patients who were determined to have active TB, 60 had a positive E-MTD test, for an estimated sensitivity of $60/72 = 0.833$. Of the 266 patients who were determined to be free of TB, 259 had a negative E-MTD test, for an estimated specificity of $259/266 = .974$.

Sensitivity and specificity are useful for comparing the performance of competing tests. For example, in the study of TB, microscopic examination of sputum smears for acid-fast bacilli (AFB) was also carried out for all patients and was found to have sensitivity = .597 and specificity = .917, both lower than for the E-MTD test. Accordingly, the E-MTD test was more accurate overall: regardless of whether the person tested did or did not have active TB, the E-MTD test was more likely to give a correct result than was the AFB test.

Sensitivity and specificity are often treated as fixed properties of a test or measure. As can be seen from their computing formulas (Table 10–4), sensitivity depends only on how the test performs among those *with* the characteristic (such as a disease), and specificity depends only on how it performs among those *without* the characteristic. Thus neither property depends directly on the prevalence of the characteristic itself.

But in reality, for many tests, sensitivity and specificity do appear to vary from one setting or target population to another (Brenner and Gefeller, 1997; Ransohoff and Feinstein, 1978). For example, among the patients with possible TB studied by Catanzaro, et al., the sensitivity of the AFB test was found to be $5/12 = .42$ among patients in whom the initial clinical suspicion of TB was low, but it was $33/40 = .83$ among patients in whom the initial suspicion of TB was high. Perhaps TB bacilli may be more abundant and thus easier to detect in the sputum of patients with more advanced, clinically apparent disease. In general, sensitivity and specificity estimates are best interpreted to reflect how the test performs when applied in a certain way in a certain target population.

Closely related concepts of test performance are the *predictive value* and the *likelihood ratio* associated with a certain test result. Because these measures are closely related to screening for disease, discussion of them is deferred to Chapter 18.

Receiver operating characteristic (ROC) curves

In epidemiology, the underlying characteristic of interest is often binary, but a test or measure for it may yield a result on an ordinal or continuous scale. How can the validity of such a result be evaluated? Consider an example:

Example: Buchsbaum and colleagues (1991) sought to determine the degree to which responses to a four-item questionnaire called the CAGE could be used to divide medical outpatients into those with and without an alcohol abuse or dependence disorder. Each CAGE question could be answered "yes" or "no," and each was worded so that a response of "yes" suggested an alcohol problem—for example: "Have you ever felt you should cut down on your drinking?" The CAGE score was defined as how many questions a person answered with "yes," and it could range from 0 to 4.

Table 10–5. CAGE Questionnaire Scores in Patients With
and Without True Alcohol Abuse or Dependence

	True Alcohol Abuse or Dependence	
CAGE SCORE	PRESENT	ABSENT
4	56	1
3	74	10
2	86	34
1	45	54
0	33	428
Total	294	527

[*Source:* Buchsbaum et al. (1991).]

The gold standard was a much more elaborate, structured interview—the alcohol module of the Diagnostic Interview Schedule—which had been previously validated as a measure of alcohol use or dependence according to widely accepted psychiatric criteria.

The results are shown in Table 10–5. CAGE scores among patients with alcohol abuse or dependence were generally higher than among patients without such a condition, but the two distributions of CAGE scores overlapped.

One way to assess the performance of such a test in relation to a binary gold standard is to select a *cutoff* value that can be used to split the numerical test results into two ranges. Results falling above the cutoff are considered positive, while those falling below it are considered negative. Sensitivity and specificity can then be calculated as before, using that cutoff.

For example, in the CAGE data, suppose that a cutoff value between 1 and 2 is chosen, so that CAGE scores of 2, 3, or 4 are classified as positive and scores of 0 or 1 as negative. The sensitivity of the CAGE score would then be $(56 + 74 + 86)/294 = .735$, and its specificity would be $(54 + 428)/527 = .915$.

The resulting sensitivity and specificity clearly depend on the particular cutoff value selected. Moving the cutoff value higher or lower on such a test involves trading off sensitivity against specificity. For the CAGE data, as shown in Table 10–6, sensitivity can take on any of six unique values, depending on where the cutoff falls in relation to each of the five possible CAGE scores, and likewise for specificity.

A *receiver operating characteristic* (ROC) plot shows sensitivity versus specificity for *all possible* cutoff values (Zweig and Campbell, 1993). ROC curves

Table 10–6. Sensitivity and Specificity of CAGE Questionnaire Score at Six
Possible Cutoff Values

| CAGE SCORE | True Alcohol Abuse or Dependence | | CUTOFF LOCATION | SENSITIVITY | SPECIFICITY |
	PRESENT	ABSENT			
			←	0.000	1.000
4	56	1			
			←	0.190	0.998
3	74	10			
			←	0.442	0.979
2	86	34			
			←	0.735	0.915
1	45	54			
			←	0.888	0.812
0	33	428			
			←	1.000	0.000
Total	294	527			

were originally developed to describe and compare the accuracy of radar receivers, which explains their odd name. By convention, sensitivity on the vertical axis is plotted against 1− specificity on the horizontal axis. Three ROC curves are shown in Figure 10–2:

- The thick middle curve shows the trade-off between sensitivity and specificity actually obtained for the CAGE score at all possible cutoff values. It is a graphical summary of the rightmost two columns in Table 10–6.
- The diagonal line labelled "uninformative test" shows, for illustration, an ROC curve for a hypothetical test that is unable to discriminate at all between positives and negatives on the gold standard. Every gain in sensitivity due to changing the cutoff value results in an equal-sized loss of specificity, and vice versa.
- The right-angled curve labeled "perfect test" shows an ROC curve for a different hypothetical test at the other extreme, which is able to discriminate perfectly between positives and negatives on the gold standard if the right cutoff value is chosen. Its ROC curve first hugs the vertical axis, showing that gains in sensitivity due to changing the cutoff value involve no loss of specificity. The curve eventually reaches the upper left corner of the plot, where sensitivity and specificity both equal 1.0. Whatever cutoff value

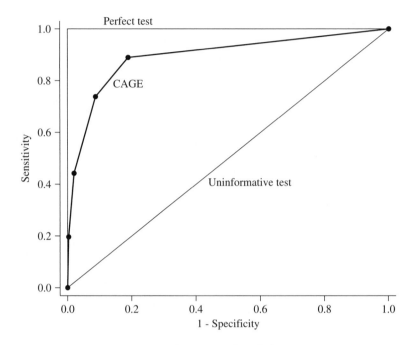

Figure 10–2. A Receiver Operating Characteristic (ROC) Plot.

corresponds to that point is the optimal value at which to divide test results into positive and negative, because then agreement with the gold standard will be perfect. (Multiple cutoff values over a certain range may satisfy this condition.) From the upper-left point, the ROC curve continues horizontally to the upper right corner.

In general, the more accurate a test is, the farther toward the upper left its curve falls in an ROC plot. This rule can be used to discern at a glance which of two tests is more accurate when both ROC curves are shown on the same plot. The rule applies even if the two tests yield results in entirely different units on totally different scales. Methods are available to determine whether the ROC curves for two tests applied to the same persons differ more than chance alone could easily explain (Hanley and McNeil, 1983).

The *area under the curve* (abbreviated *AUC*) is sometimes used as a single summary measure of test accuracy. For an uninformative test, $AUC = 0.5$; for a perfect test, $AUC = 1.0$. For the CAGE score's ROC curve in Figure 10–2, $AUC = 0.89$. Hanley and McNeil (1982) described computational methods for estimating *AUC* and its confidence limits.

Sometimes no suitable gold standard is available for the underlying characteristic of interest. Fairly complex statistical methods have been proposed to permit sensitivity and specificity to be estimated indirectly in this situation (Hui and Zhou, 1998). These methods generally require that several imperfect tests be applied to the same study subjects, and they often require making untestable assumptions about independence of measurement error across tests. Other related methods have been proposed when a gold standard test exists but can be applied only when an imperfect test has yielded a positive result (Walter, 1999).

If both the gold standard and the measure being evaluated are continuous, the Pearson product–moment correlation can be used to quantify validity (Armstrong et al., 1992). If both are ordinal, the Spearman rank correlation can be used. Computing formulas for both types of correlation can be found in Rosner (1995).

CONSEQUENCES OF MEASUREMENT ERROR

The impact of measurement error on the results of a given epidemiologic study depends in part on the way the error has arisen. If differential (selective) mismeasurement of exposure status has occurred—that is, when the ascertainment of exposure has been influenced by the presence or absence of disease—then the results can be biased positively or negatively. If, for example, ill persons are better able to recall a prior exposure than well persons who were chosen as a basis for comparison—perhaps the illness has prompted a heightened awareness of events that occurred prior to the onset of that illness—then a positive association between that exposure and illness will be observed in an interview-based case-control study even if none truly is present.

As another example of differential measurement error, the weight of persons after they have been diagnosed with type II diabetes may not reflect their weight during the period of time when the diabetes was developing. Because of the effects of dietary modification, it is often lower. A comparison of weight in persons with type II diabetes (of more than a very short duration) and non-diabetic controls, in order to assess the possible etiologic role of being overweight, could underestimate the size of the true association, since in the controls a corresponding stimulus to weight reduction would not generally have been present.

Similarly, differential misclassification of disease status can give rise to a falsely high or a falsely low estimate of the risk associated with a given exposure. Studies that are most susceptible to this type of bias are those of conditions whose recognition can be influenced by knowledge of exposure status.

Example: To some extent, Reye's syndrome is a disease of exclusion: there is no pattern of test results that is unequivocally indicative of the presence of this disease. For a number of years before any formal epidemiologic studies of Reye's syndrome were done, there was a widespread suspicion that taking aspirin might predispose children to this disease. As a consequence, investigators of the relationship of Reye's syndrome to prior aspirin use had to design their studies to deal with the possibility that some physicians might have incorporated a child's prior use of aspirin as one criterion for diagnosing him or her as having Reye's syndrome. Specifically (Hurwitz et al., 1987), they included only clinically serious cases (in whom it was believed this potential bias was less likely to operate); defined the disease using standardized criteria across collaborating institutions; and had the records of all cases reviewed by an expert panel whose members were ignorant of the child's prior use of medications.

Had steps not been taken to minimize it, the differential misclassification of outcome in this instance (differential because the likelihood of diagnosing the disease differed depending on exposure status) could have led to a falsely large estimate of the size of the association.

Nondifferential (nonselective) error in measurement of *exposure* is present when errors in assessing a subject's exposure status are similar in frequency and degree between ill and well persons. Nondifferential misclassification of *outcome* is present when errors in assessing a subject's illness or injury status are similar whether that subject has been exposed or not. The presence of nondifferential mismeasurement of exposure, which is ubiquitous in epidemiologic studies, generally leads to an attenuation of the estimated size of a true association between exposure and disease (Thomas, 1995). As an illustration of this point, consider the following hypothetical example:

Example: Assume that in a case-control study in which a dichotomous exposure was measured perfectly, the following results would be obtained:

EXPOSURE	CASES	CONTROLS	ODDS RATIO
Yes	150	75	
			$\dfrac{150}{150} \div \dfrac{75}{225} = 3.0$
No	150	225	
	300	300	

However, if one-third of exposed persons were misclassified as being non-exposed, both among cases and controls, the results would instead look like this:

EXPOSURE	CASES	CONTROLS	ODDS RATIO
Yes	150 − 50*	75 − 25*	
			$\dfrac{100}{200} \div \dfrac{50}{250} = 2.5$
No	150 + 50	225 + 25	
	300	300	

*$150 \times 1/3 = 50, 75 \times 1/3 = 25$

The observed odds ratio is now closer to the null value of 1.0.

The bias towards the null would increase further if some truly non-exposed persons were to be incorrectly classified as having been exposed. Assume this occurs in 20% of truly non-exposed persons, both among cases and controls:

EXPOSURE	CASES	CONTROLS	ODDS RATIO
Yes	150 − 50 + 30	75 − 25 + 45	
			$\dfrac{130}{170} \div \dfrac{95}{205} = 1.65$
No	150 + 50 − 30*	225 + 25 − 45	
	300	300	

*$150 \times .2 = 30, 225 \times .2 = 45$

This result is even closer to the null, and differs enough from the true odds ratio that the interpretation of the results of the study could well be influenced.

To what extent will a true association be attenuated by the presence of non-differential misclassification of exposure? The larger the degree of misclassification, the greater the attenuation. For a dichotomous exposure, misclassification can be thought of as having two components:

1. Some persons with the exposure are falsely labeled as having been non-exposed; that is, the measure being used to assess exposure status has less than 100% *sensitivity;* and

2. Persons without the exposure are falsely labeled as exposed; that is, there is less than 100% *specificity* of the measure. While either a low sensitivity or a low specificity of the means by which exposure is identified will lead to bias toward the null result, the degree of bias depends on the frequency of exposure in the population from which the study subjects were sampled.

Example: Let's say that we are comparing the one-year cumulative incidence of a certain illness in persons who do or do not consume food A. Assume there is no error in ascertaining the presence of the illness, which occurs at a rate 10 times higher in consumers of A than the annual incidence of 10 per 10,000 persons who do not eat A. If one in 11 persons in the study population ate food A, the results of a study with perfect ascertainment of A consumption would look like this:

The truth:

CONSUMPTION OF FOOD A	Illness			RELATIVE RISK
	YES	NO	TOTAL	
Yes	10	990	1000	
				10
No	10	9990	10,000	

If eating A had been correctly ascertained in only 80% of A consumers (sensitivity = 80%), both in ill and well persons, but all non-eaters of A were correctly classified as such (specificity = 100%), the results would appear as follows:

Exposure status ascertained with 80%
sensitivity and 100% specificity:

CONSUMPTION OF FOOD A	Illness			RELATIVE RISK
	YES	NO	TOTAL	
Yes	10(.8) = 8	990(.8) = 792	800	
				8.5
No	10 + 2 = 12	9990 + 198 = 10,188	10,200	

On the other hand, had all A eaters been correctly classified (100% sensitivity), but 20% of A non-eaters had been misclassified as A eaters (80% specificity), the results would instead look like this:

Exposure status ascertained with 100%
sensitivity and 80% specificity:

CONSUMPTION OF FOOD A	Illness		TOTAL	RELATIVE RISK
	YES	NO		
Yes	$10 + 2 = 12$	$990 + 1998 = 2988$	3000	4.0
No	$10(.8) = 8$	$9990(.8) = 7992$	8000	

In this instance, because a relatively small proportion (one of 11) of the population ate food A, the absolute number of misclassified persons was much higher when there was less-than-perfect specificity than where there was less-than-perfect sensitivity. Though the true relative risk of 10 was underestimated in both scenarios where nondifferential misclassification of exposure was present, the degree of underestimation was particularly great in the presence of less-than-100% specificity. If food A had been consumed by the majority of persons, rather than the minority, then the degree of underestimation of the relative risk would be influenced more by the sensitivity of ascertainment than by the specificity, since even a small relative impairment of sensitivity would lead to a relatively larger number of misclassified persons. This topic has been discussed in greater detail elsewhere (Flegal et al., 1986).

The foregoing discussion applies entirely to studies that ascertain exposure status for individual subjects within a population. In ecological studies, in which the possible effect of an exposure is estimated by correlating disease rates across groups with differences in their exposure prevalence, nondifferential misclassification of the latter can actually lead to an inflated estimate of the influence of exposure on disease risk (Brenner et al., 1992). An example is given in Chapter 12.

In cohort studies, if ascertainment of *disease status* is incomplete, but is comparably incomplete for exposed and non-exposed persons, then the *ratio* of observed disease incidence between the exposed and the non-exposed (i.e., the relative risk), will be the same as if this type of misclassification had not been present. (In case control studies this will be true for the odds ratio as well, except when the disease in question occurs with extremely high frequency in the study population.) In contrast, to the extent that persons without a disease are falsely labeled as having it, the observed relative risk will be closer to the null than the true value.

Example: Let's return to the example of illness in relation to consumption of food A, this time assuming that it is illness status and not exposure status that is subject to misclassification. Again, in the absence of any misclassification the data would look like this:

The truth:

| CONSUMPTION | Illness | | | RELATIVE |
OF FOOD A	YES	NO	TOTAL	RISK
Yes	10	990	1000	
				10
No	10	9990	10,000	

If 10 percent of persons who became ill were not recognized as such (sensitivity = 90%), the following numbers would result:

Illness status ascertained with 90%
sensitivity and 100% specificity:

| CONSUMPTION | Illness | | | RELATIVE |
OF FOOD A	YES	NO	TOTAL	RISK
Yes	10(0.9) = 9	990 + 1 = 991	1000	
				10
No	10(.9) = 9	9990 + 1 = 9991	10,000	

The under-ascertainment of cases has no influence on the denominator of the cumulative incidence in exposed and nonexposed persons, and, since the numerators remain the same *relative* to one another, there is no impact on the size of the relative risk.

In contrast, if specificity in ascertaining illness is less than 100%, the influence on the relative risk can be substantial. Consider the situation in which just one percent of well persons were inadvertently believed to have developed the illness:

Illness status ascertained with 100%
sensitivity and 99% specificity:

CONSUMPTION OF FOOD A	Illness			RELATIVE RISK
	YES	NO	TOTAL	
Yes	$10 + 10 = 20$	$990(.99) = 980$	1000	
				1.82
No	$10 + 100 = 110$	$9990(.99) = 9890$	10,000	

The observed relative risk in the presence of less-than-perfect specificity is reduced considerably towards the null value of 1.0, from 10.0 to 1.82.

The minimization of measurement error is, of course, the objective of every epidemiologic study. Whether for exposure or disease, we would like our tools to be reliable—obtaining the same value or result each time we make a measurement—and to be valid—obtaining the true value or result. The means of enhancing reliability and validity depends on just what tool is being used, the setting in which the study is done, and on other factors. This topic is beyond the scope of the present book; an introduction to it can be found in Armstrong et al. (1992).

Largely because of our inability to accurately measure certain exposures, a number of etiologic questions of great interest have not been satisfactorily addressed in epidemiologic studies. To this day we are unsure of the role of certain types of air and water pollution on health, or of the long-term consequences of certain dietary or occupational exposures, primarily because it is not possible to quantify with great reliability and validity how much study participants have been exposed to these agents. Nonetheless, we should not lose sight of the possibility that a potential association we wish to investigate may be so strong that misclassification, sometimes even a substantial degree of it, will not wholly obscure that association.

Example: In order to explore the possibility that anal intercourse could in some way predispose to the subsequent occurrence of anal cancer, Daling et al. (1982) conducted a case-control study. Men diagnosed with anal cancer in western Washington State during 1974–1979 were compared to controls (men with other cancers) for a history of syphilis, as determined from records of the Washington State Health Department. These investigators knew that for a number of years prior to the time of the study, the majority of men in Washington with a new diagnosis of syphilis reported a history of recent sexual contact with another man. They found eight of 47 men with anal cancer (17.0%) also were listed in health department records as having syphilis, in contrast to only 1–2% of men with the other forms of cancer studied.

Daling et al. pursued this lead by comparing the distribution of marital status between men with anal cancer and controls. They reasoned that men who engaged in receptive anal intercourse would be less likely to be married to a woman than would other men. Because marital status is ascertained routinely by cancer registries in the US, they were able to use data from US registries outside of Washington State as well. The results again supported their hypothesis: 24.4% of men with anal cancer had never been married, in contrast to about eight percent of men with colon or rectal cancer (controls). No corresponding difference in the distribution of marital status was present between women with anal cancer and control women.

These registry-based studies were rife with misclassification. In the second study, for example, it is likely that only the minority of never-married men had had anal intercourse, the actual exposure of interest. But the strong association observed using the misclassified exposure status quickly led to an interview-based case-control study (Daling et al., 1987), which observed an even stronger one: 25.9% of men with anal cancer versus only 1.6% of controls stated they had previously engaged in anal intercourse.

Example: In Britain, procedures to inactivate live virus in blood products were initiated in 1985. Screening of blood products for hepatitis B virus began there earlier, in 1972. Thus, while hemophiliacs (in whom receipt of blood products is nearly universal) treated in Britain beginning in 1972–1985 would be expected to have become infected with hepatitis C virus (because this infection was probably present in an appreciable proportion of blood samples that were donated), few of them should have been infected with hepatitis B virus.

In an effort to learn of long-term consequences of infection with hepatitis C virus, the mortality from liver cancer and other liver disease was documented among hemophiliacs treated in Britain during 1972–1985 (Darby et al., 1997). Five deaths from liver cancer occurred among members of this cohort, with only 0.90 expected based on mortality rates in demographically similar men. The corresponding numbers for other liver disease: 51 deaths observed, versus 3.05 expected.

The investigators did not assess the presence of hepatitis C infection in a single study subject, and so it is not known if there were some hemophiliacs who escaped infection with this virus. Also, in the general British male population that served as the basis for comparison, there were certainly a small number of non-hemophiliac men who were infected with hepatitis C. Yet the presence of what must be a *very* strong association between hepatitis C infection and fatal liver disease, combined with the relatively modest level of exposure misclassification, permitted the study to contribute to our knowledge of some deleterious consequences of hepatitis C infection.

APPENDIX 10A

Variants of Kappa for Categorical Variables with Three or More Categories

Kappa can also be used to quantify the reliability of nominal measures that can take any of, say, h unordered values. The data for two replicate measurements can be arranged as in Table 10–7, which contains one cell for each possible combination of values. The n's represent the number of subjects in each cell, r's are row totals, and c's are column totals.

The observed concordance is

$$P_o = \frac{\sum_{i=1}^{h} n_{ii}}{N}$$

The concordance expected by chance is

$$P_e = \frac{\sum_{i=1}^{h} r_i \cdot c_i / N}{N} \tag{10.2}$$

and kappa is calculated as before (equation 10–1).

Table 10–7. Data Layout for Reliability Assessment on a Categorical Measure with 3+ Possible Values

FIRST MEASUREMENT	Second Measurement				
	VALUE 1	VALUE 2	...	VALUE h	TOTAL
Value 1	n_{11}	n_{12}	...	n_{1h}	r_1
Value 2	n_{21}	n_{22}	...	n_{2h}	r_2
$\vdots$	$\vdots$	$\vdots$	...	$\vdots$	$\vdots$
Value h	n_{h1}	n_{h2}	...	n_{hh}	r_h
Total	c_1	c_2	...	c_h	N

The resulting value of kappa depends in part on h, the number of categories, which in turn may reflect a choice made by investigators on how finely or coarsely study subjects are grouped (Maclure and Willett, 1987). Other things being equal, kappa decreases as h increases. For example, kappa measuring agreement between two different sources of information on race is likely to be greater if race is categorized as "white / black / other" than if race is categorized as as "white / black / Native American / Chinese / Japanese / Hawaiian / Pacific Islander / other."

Weighted kappa is a variant of kappa that can be used for ordinal measures. The data layout shown in Table 10–7 still applies, as long as the values defining the rows and columns are arranged in their proper order—e.g., from mild to severe. As before, perfect agreement occurs when all observations fall on the main diagonal from upper left to bottom right. But among the off-diagonal cells, the severity of disagreement depends on how far off the main diagonal a cell lies. Cells that lie just adjacent to the main diagonal, such as the n_{12} and n_{21} cells, contain observations for which the discrepancy between the two measurements was relatively mild— just one category. In contrast, cells farthest from the main diagonal, such as the n_{1h} and n_{h1} cells, contain observations for which the two measurements fell toward opposite ends of the scale, representing serious disagreements.

Weighted kappa is designed to give "full credit" when the two observations for a study subject agree exactly, and "partial credit" if they disagree, depending on how far apart the two measurements are. Various weighting schemes can be used, but a common choice is to give the cell in row i and column j a weight of

$$w_{ij} = 1 - \frac{(i - j)^2}{(h - 1)^2} \tag{10.3}$$

For example, if $h = 4$, then weights of 1, .89, .55, and 0 apply to cells representing discrepancies of 0, 1, 2, and 3 categories, respectively. The weighted concordance observed is then

$$P_o = \frac{\sum_{i=1}^{h} \sum_{j=1}^{h} w_{ij} \cdot n_{ij}}{N}$$

The weighted concordance expected by chance is

$$P_e = \frac{\sum_{i=1}^{h} \sum_{j=1}^{h} w_{ij} \cdot r_i \cdot c_j / N}{N}$$

and kappa is again calculated from equation 10.1. Using the weights above, weighted kappa converges to the intraclass correlation coefficient as N increases (Fleiss, 1980). Brenner and Kliebsch (1996) showed that the value of weighted kappa tends to increase with h, which should be borne in mind when comparing measures of the same characteristic but with different numbers of categories.

Weighted kappa and other methods of reliability assessment for ordinal data are also reviewed by Nelson and Pepe (2000).

Fleiss (1980) gives formulas for the approximate standard error of kappa and weighted kappa, which can be used to obtain confidence limits for them. He also describes extensions of kappa to more than two measurements per study subject.

EXERCISES

1. As part of a randomized trial of alternative strategies for treatment of low-grade abnormalities on cervical cytology, Stoler and Schiffman (2001) collected a cervical cytology specimen on each of 4948 women referred to the trial. Monolayer cytology preparations were evaluated independently by two highly trained pathologists. Each pathologist then assigned each specimen to one of four categories:

   - Negative
   - ASCUS—atypical squamous cells of undetermined significance
   - LSIL—low-grade squamous intraepithelial lesion
   - ≥HSIL—high-grade squamous intraepithelial lesion, or more advanced disease

   The results are shown in Table 10–8. How would you summarize quantitatively the reproducibility of the pathologists' interpretations?
2. Tobacco smoking is a common exposure in epidemiologic studies. In a sample of hospital outpatients, Jarvis and colleagues (1987) compared several methods for ascertaining smoking status, including self-report and biochemical markers in breath, saliva, blood, and urine.

Table 10–8. Independent Interpretations of Cervical Cytology Specimens on 4948 Women in the ASCUS-LSIL Triage Study

FIRST PATHOLOGIST'S INTERPRETATION	Second Pathologist's Interpretation				
	NEGATIVE	ASCUS	LSIL	≥HSIL	TOTAL
Negative	1325	322	52	8	1707
ASCUS	568	633	245	27	1473
LSIL	57	292	908	78	1335
≥HSIL	14	98	117	204	433
Total	1964	1345	1322	317	4948

[*Source:* Adapted from Stoler and Schiffman (2001).]

Table 10–9. Sensitivity and Specificity of Four Biochemical
Markers for Smoking

BIOCHEMICAL TEST	SENSITIVITY	SPECIFICITY
Breath carbon monoxide	.90	.89
Plasma nicotine	.88	.99
Plasma cotinine	.96	1.00
Plasma thiocyanate	.84	.91

[*Source:* Adapted from Jarvis et al. (1987).]

(a) Initially, self-reported smoking status was used as the gold standard against which several biochemical tests were evaluated. Of 211 patients studied, 90 reported being current smokers. The plasma cotinine test, which measures a metabolite of nicotine, was reported to have sensitivity = .94 and specificity = .81 at a cutoff of 13.7 ng/ml.

Other studies and later analyses in the Jarvis study suggested that self-report may not be a good gold standard because some current smokers deny that they smoke. The plasma cotinine test itself is thought to be more accurate overall. Suppose you are interested in estimating the sensitivity and specificity of *self-report* when *plasma cotinine* is used as the gold standard, using the same cutoff value. Can you do so from the data given?

(b) In later analyses, the investigators used a "composite" gold standard instead. Any patient who reported being a smoker *or* who had a positive plasma cotinine test was classified as a true smoker; otherwise, he or she was classified as a true nonsmoker. Relative to this gold standard, the sensitivity and specificity of several biochemical markers were reported as shown in Table 10–9. What concern might you have in concluding from these data that plasma cotinine was the most sensitive and specific test for current smoking?

3. As part of the Collaborative Perinatal Project (a prospective study of pregnancy, labor, and child development conducted in the United States from 1959 to 1966), serum samples were obtained from approximately 42,000 women at the beginning of their pregnancy. Serum samples from the 591 women who subsequently experienced a spontaneous abortion during that pregnancy, and a matched sample of 2558 controls, were assayed for levels of paraxanthine (a metabolite of caffeine). The results are summarized in Figure 10–3, based on Klebanoff et al. (1999).

The half-life of paraxanthine in serum is approximately five hours. Therefore, serum paraxanthine is a marker only of short-term caffeine intake, so

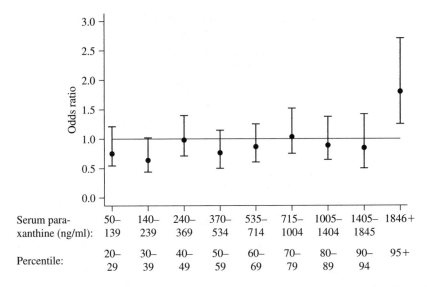

Figure 10-3. Odds Ratio for Spontaneous Abortion in Relation to Serum Paraxanthine (based on Klebanoff et al., 1999).

the values obtained on the samples of these subjects may not mirror those present when the events leading to the spontaneous abortion took place. Had the "relevant" levels of serum paraxanthine been possible to obtain—e.g., long-term levels, or levels closer to the time when the pathology leading to this spontaneous abortion occurred—would you anticipate the odds ratio associated with a value of more than 1845 ng/ml to be greater than, the same as, or less than the odds ratio of 1.9 observed in this study? Why?

4. Assume you have conducted two case-control studies of the efficacy of seatbelt use against the incidence of a skeletal fracture among persons involved in an automobile crash. The studies were done a number of years apart, 1975 and 1990, and the prevalence of seatbelt use was greater in the more recent of the two. The "cases" in each study were persons who sustained a fracture in a car crash. "Controls" were persons in crashes that were identical to those in which the cases were involved (in terms of such characteristics as vehicle speed, vehicle type), who did not sustain a fracture, and who were similar to the cases in terms of demographic and other characteristics that influence the likelihood of fracture.

   Assume that in each of the two studies, in which 1000 cases and 1000 controls had been enrolled, the "correct" data (i.e., those that would have been obtained had there been no misclassification) were as shown in Table 10–10.

   (a) What would be the odds ratio for each of the two years relating use of seatbelts to fracture risk in the absence of any misclassification?

Table 10–10. True Association Between Seat
Belt Use and Case-Control Status, by Year

Correct Data, 1975		
SEAT BELT USE	CASES	CONTROLS
Yes	50	100
No	950	900
Correct Data, 1990		
SEAT BELT USE	CASES	CONTROLS
Yes	322	500
No	678	500

(b) What would the two odds ratios be if 10% of both cases and controls who were unbelted reported, incorrectly, having worn a seatbelt at the time of the crash (i.e., 90% specificity of the ascertainment modality)?

(c) What would these odds ratios be if misclassification arose exclusively from the ascertainment modality being only 90% sensitive, i.e., if 10% of the cases and controls who truly had worn a belt were labeled as unbelted?

When misclassification of exposure status is present, why do the odds ratios obtained in the study conducted in 1975 differ from the corresponding odds ratios obtained in 1990?

ANSWERS

1. One approach is to treat the pathologists' interpretation as a four-category nominal scale. The concordance between pathologists was $(1325 + 633 + 908 + 204)/4948 = .620$, implying that the they agreed with each other's interpretations 62% of the time.

   Because some of this agreement could be due to chance, however, kappa would also be appropriate. The concordance expected by chance, obtained using equation 10.2, was .296. Kappa can be calculated as $(.620 - .296)/(1 - .296) = .461$, indicating a moderate level of agreement.

   Another reasonable approach is to treat the four-category scale of interpretations as being ordered as to degree of abnormality, from none to highly abnormal. This view of the data lends itself to using weighted kappa. Using the weighting scheme described in equation 10.3, weighted kappa can be calculated as .704. It is higher than the four-category (unweighted) kappa because it gives

partial credit for relatively small discrepancies of one or two categories, which
were common here.

2. *(a)* Yes. We know that .94 × 90 = 85 of the self-reported smokers had a
positive plasma cotinine test. We also know that .81 × (211 − 90) = 98
of the self-reported *non*-smokers had a negative plasma cotinine test. Thus
we can construct the following table:

PLASMA COTININE	Self-reported Smoking +	−	TOTAL
+	85	23	118
−	5	98	103
Total	90	121	211

If we now treat plasma cotinine as the gold standard, the sensitivity of
self-report is 85/118 = 0.72, and its specificity is 98/103 = .95.

(b) Because the plasma cotinine test result itself was used as part of the composite gold standard, plasma cotinine is not being evaluated against an
independent criterion measure. In particular, a false positive result was
logically impossible, because any patient with a positive plasma cotinine
test had already been classified as a true smoker. Thus the specificity of
1.00 for plasma cotinine was an automatic consequence of how the gold
standard was defined, not an empirical finding.

3. If the "relevant" serum levels were correctly classified, one would expect that the
resulting *OR* would be greater than 1.9. The use of the non-differentially misclassified value of serum paraxanthine for each subject is expected to produce
a result spuriously close to the null.

4. The true odds ratio relating seatbelt use to skeletal fracture is 2.11 in each year
(Table 10–11). If the method of ascertaining seatbelt use were 90% *specific*, the
odds ratio (*OR*) observed in the earlier study would be more biased (towards the
null) by nondifferential misclassification than the *OR* in the later study, since
the absolute number of misclassified individuals would be greater in the earlier
study. The impact of less-than-perfect specificity of the criterion for exposure
leads to a larger number of misclassified subjects when the exposure frequency
is low (e.g., seatbelt use in 1975) than when it is high (e.g., in 1990). When
the *sensitivity* is 90%, the observed odds ratios are relatively close to the true
value of 2.11. Nonetheless, the 1990 analysis is more biased than that for 1975,
since the absolute number of individuals misclassified regarding seatbelt use
was greater than in 1990.

Table 10–11. Seat Belt Use in Relation to Case-Control Status Under Misclassification

YEAR	SEAT BELTS	Truth		Misclassified Exposure Status: Sensitivity of Interview = 100% Specificity of Interview = 90%		Misclassified Exposure Status: Sensitivity of Interview = 90% Specificity of Interview = 100%	
		CASES	CONTROLS	CASES	CONTROLS	CASES	CONTROLS
1975	No	950	900	$950 - 95 = 855$	$900 - 90 = 810$	$950 + 5 = 955$	$900 + 10 = 910$
	Yes	50	100	$50 + 95 = 145$	$100 + 90 = 190$	$50 - 5 = 45$	$100 - 10 = 90$
		$\text{O.R.} = \dfrac{950/50}{900/100} = 2.11$		$\text{O.R.} = \dfrac{855/145}{810/190} = 1.38$		$\text{O.R.} = \dfrac{955/45}{910/90} = 2.10$	
1990	No	678	500	$678 - 68 = 610$	$500 - 50 = 450$	$678 + 32 = 710$	$500 + 50 = 550$
	Yes	322	500	$322 + 68 = 390$	$500 + 50 = 550$	$322 - 32 = 290$	$500 - 50 = 450$
		$\text{O.R.} = \dfrac{678/322}{500/500} = 2.11$		$\text{O.R.} = \dfrac{610/390}{450/550} = 1.91$		$\text{O.R.} = \dfrac{710/290}{550/450} = 2.00$	

Moral: The impact of misclassification of exposure status depends not only on the relative degree of misclassification, but on the relative size of the part of the study population that is misclassified.

REFERENCES

Armstrong BK, White E, Saracci R. Principles of exposure measurement in epidemiology. New York: Oxford, 1992.

Brenner H, Gefeller O. Variation of sensitivity, specificity, likelihood ratios, and predictive values with disease prevalence. Stat Med 1997; 16:981–91.

Brenner H, Greenland S, Savitz DA. The effects of nondifferential confounder misclassification in ecologic studies. Epidemiology 1992; 3:456–69.

Brenner H, Kliebsch U. Dependence of weighted kappa coefficients on the number of categories. Epidemiology 1996; 7:199–202.

Buchsbaum DG, Buchanan RG, Centor RM, Schnoll SH, Lawton MJ. Screening for alcohol abuse using CAGE scores and likelihood ratios. Ann Intern Med 1991; 115:774–77.

Catanzaro A, Perry S, Clarridge JE, Dunbar S, Goodnight-White S, LoBue PA, et al. The role of clinical suspicion in evaluating a new diagnostic test for active tuberculosis. Results of a multicenter prospective trial. JAMA 2000; 283:639–45.

Cohen J. A coefficient of agreement for nominal scales. Educ Psychol Meas 1960; 20:37–46.

Daling JR, Weiss NS, Hislop TG, Maden C, Coates RJ, Sherman KJ, et al. Sexual practices, sexually transmitted diseases, and the incidence of anal cancer. N Engl J Med 1987; 317:973–77.

Daling JR, Weiss NS, Klopfenstein LL, Cochran LE, Chow WH, Daifuku R. Correlates of homosexual behavior and the incidence of anal cancer. JAMA 1982; 247:1988–90.

Darby SC, Ewart DW, Giangrande PL, Spooner RJ, Rizza CR, Dusheiko GM, et al. Mortality from liver cancer and liver disease in haemophilic men and boys in UK given blood products contaminated with hepatitis C. Lancet 1997; 350:1425–31.

Flegal KM, Brownie C, Haas JD. The effects of exposure misclassification on estimates of relative risk. Am J Epidemiol 1986; 123:736–51.

Fleiss JL. Statistical methods for rates and proportions (2nd ed.). New York: John Wiley and Sons, 1980.

Fleiss JL. The design and analysis of clinical experiments. New York: Wiley and Sons, 1986.

Gable CB, Holzer SS, Engelhart L, Friedman RB, Smeltz F, Schroeder D, et al. Pneumococcal vaccine. Efficacy and associated cost savings. JAMA 1990; 264:2910–15.

Hanley JA, McNeil BJ. The meaning and use of the area under a receiver operating characteristic (ROC) curve. Radiology 1982; 143:29–36.

Hanley JA, McNeil BJ. A method of comparing the areas under receiver operating characteristic curves derived from the same cases. Radiology 1983; 148:839–43.

Hui SL, Zhou XH. Evaulation of diagnostic tests without gold standards. Stat Meth Med Res 1998; 7:354–70.

Hurwitz ES, Barrett MJ, Bregman D, Gunn WJ, Pinsky P, Schonberger LB, et al. Public Health Service study of Reye's syndrome and medications. Report of the main study. JAMA 1987; 257:1905–11.

Jarvis MJ, Tunstall-Pedoe H, Feyerabend C, Vesey C, Saloojee Y. Comparison of tests used to distinguish smokers from nonsmokers. Am J Public Health 1987; 77:1435–38.

Klebanoff MA, Levine RJ, DerSimonian R, Clemens JD, Wilkins DG. Maternal serum paraxanthine, a caffeine metabolite, and the risk of spontaneous abortion. N Engl J Med 1999; 341:1639–44.

Landis JR, Koch GG. The measurement of observer agreement for categorical data. Biometrics 1977; 33:159–74.

Maclure M, Willett WC. Misinterpretation and misuse of the kappa statistic. Am J Epidemiol 1987; 126:161–69.

Nelson JC, Pepe MS. Statistical description of interrater variability in ordinal ratings. Stat Meth Med Res 2000; 9:475–96.

Ransohoff DF, Feinstein AR. Problems of spectrum and bias in evaluating the efficacy of diagnostic tests. N Engl J Med 1978; 299:926–30.

Rosner B. Fundamentals of biostatistics (4th edition). New York: Duxbury Press, 1995.

Snedecor G, Cochran WG. Statistical methods (6th ed.). Iowa City, Iowa: Iowa State University Press, 1980.

Stoler MH, Schiffman M. Interobserver reproducibility of cervical cytologic and histologic interpretations. Realistic estimates from the ASCUS-LSIL Triage Study. JAMA 2001; 285:1500–5.

Taubes G. Epidemiology Monitor 1996; 17:1–14.

Thomas D, Stram D, Dwyer J. Exposure measurement error: influence on exposure–disease relationships and methods of correction. Annu Rev Public Health 1993; 14:69–93.

Thomas DC. Re: "When will nondifferential misclassification of an exposure preserve the direction of a trend?" Am J Epidemiol 1995; 142:782–83.

Thompson WD. Kappa and attenuation of the odds ratio. Epidemiology 1990; 1:357–69.

Thompson WD, Walter SD. Variance and dissent. A reappraisal of the kappa coefficient. J Clin Epidemiol 1988; 41:949–58.

Walter SD. Estimation of test sensitivity and specificity when disease confirmation is limited to positive results. Epidemiology 1999; 10:67–72.

Wright TC Jr, Denny L, Kuhn L, Pollack A, Lorincz A. HPV DNA testing of self-collected vaginal samples compared with cytologic screening to detect cervical cancer. JAMA 2000; 283:81–86.

Zweig MH, Campbell G. Receiver-operating characteristic (ROC) plots: a fundamental evaluation tool in clinical medicine. Clin Chem 1993; 39:561–77.

11

CONFOUNDING AND ITS CONTROL

Confounding occurs in epidemiologic research when the measured association between an exposure and disease occurrence is distorted by an imbalance between exposed and non-exposed persons with regard to one or more other risk factors for the disease. An example of likely confounding is the association between low blood levels of beta-carotene and an increased incidence of several types of cancer observed in a number of cohort and case-control studies. Persons randomized to receive supplements of beta-carotene do not have a lower incidence of these cancers than persons randomized to receive a placebo (Alpha-Tocopherol, Beta Carotene Cancer Prevention Study Group, 1994; Omenn et al., 1996), so it is likely that the association present in the non-randomized studies is due to confounding. Perhaps one or more nutrients contained in the same foods in which beta-carotene is found protect against the development of the cancers in question, rather than beta-carotene itself.

RATE ADJUSTMENT

Rationale and Mechanics

To see in a quantitative way how confounding operates, as well as one of the ways confounding can be dealt with, consider the following hypothetical example. Let us say you have obtained mortality rates for a one-year period for two communities: Community A, located in the developed world, and Community B, located in the developing world. You would like to compare these rates. Characteristic of many communities in the developing world at present, Community B has a younger population than Community A. Reviewing the data shown in Table 11–1, you observe that within each of the three age groups for which data are available, the mortality rates in Community B are exactly double those of Community A.

The rates for persons of all ages combined were obtained by simply dividing the total number of deaths in each community by the size of the total

Table 11–1. Mortality Rates in Two Hypothetical Communities

AGE	Community A			Community B		
	NO. OF DEATHS	MID-YEAR POPULATION	RATE[a]	NO. OF DEATHS	MID-YEAR POPULATION	RATE[a]
Young	1	1000	1	10	5000	2
Middle	15	3000	5	40	4000	10
Old	50	5000	10	20	1000	20
Total	66	9000	7.3	70	10,000	7.0

[a]Deaths per 1000 person-years.

population: $66/9{,}000 = 7.3$ per 1000 person-years in Community A, and $70/10{,}000 = 7.0$ per 1000 person-years in Community B. In this example, a comparison of rates obtained in this way—termed "crude" rates—provides what at first glance may be surprising: the overall mortality rate in Community B is not twice that of Community A, as it is for individuals within each of the three age categories. In fact, it is less than that of Community A (7.0 versus 7.3 per 1000 person-years)! The explanation for the disparity between comparisons of crude and age-specific rates lies in:

- The relationship of age to mortality rates—in both communities these rates rise sharply with increasing age; and
- The difference in the age distribution of the two communities—on average, persons in A are older than those in B.

The crude rates permit the differences in mortality by age to be mixed in with (confound) the community-related differences in mortality. Community A, with its relatively higher proportion of older (and therefore higher-risk) persons is "penalized" in the comparison to Community B, so much so that the truly lower mortality rate present in residents of Community A at any given age is not only obscured when considering persons of all ages combined, it is reversed.

Armed with the data in the above table, however, it is possible by means of adjustment—also called standardization—to nullify the confounding effect of age. One approach to adjustment involves calculating what would have been the overall mortality rates in A and B if they had had the same age composition. It proceeds as follows:

1. Pick a reference population distribution. One way (of many) to do this is to combine the two populations:

$$\text{Young} = 1000 + 5000 = 6000$$

$$\text{Middle} = 3000 + 4000 = 7000$$

$$\text{Old} = 5000 + 1000 = 6000$$

2. Apply age-specific rates for each population under study to the reference population, and add up the expected deaths across the age categories. In this instance, one obtains the number of deaths that would be expected if the community's age-specific rates had operated on the reference population's size and age distribution.

	Community A				Community B	
RATE[a]	REFERENCE POPULATION	EXPECTED DEATHS	RATE[a]		REFERENCE POPULATION	EXPECTED DEATHS
1 ×	6000 =	6	2	×	6000 =	12
5 ×	7000 =	35	10	×	7000 =	70
10 ×	6000 =	60	20	×	6000 =	120
	19,000	101			19,000	202

[a]Deaths per 1000 person-years.

3. Divide the number of expected deaths in each group by the reference population:

Community A: $101/19,000 = 5.3$ per 1000 person-years

Community B: $202/19,000 = 10.6$ per 1000 person-years

In the above calculation, the age disparity between the two communities has been eliminated. The overall rates, now termed *age-adjusted* or *age-standardized rates,* are in the ratio of 2:1, exactly the ratio seen in the comparison of age-specific rates of the communities.

As was noted in Chapter 4, the crude rate in each community is a weighted average of the age-specific rates in that community. But because their age distributions differ, the weights for the age-specific rates also differ. In Community A, the rates for older people get relatively more weight because older people comprise a larger proportion of Community A's population. In Community B, the rates for younger people get more weight. It is also possible to think of the adjustment process as the application of a standard set of "weights" to the category-specific rates in the exposure groups to be compared. In the present example, using as before the combined mid-year populations of the two communities to derive the standard weights, the following would be obtained:

AGE GROUP	STANDARD WEIGHTS
Young	$\dfrac{1000 + 5000}{19,000} = 0.316$
Middle	$\dfrac{3000 + 4000}{19,000} = 0.368$
Old	$\dfrac{5000 + 1000}{19,000} = 0.316$
	$\overline{1.000}$

Applying this set of weights to the age-specific rates observed in each community would produce the same pair of adjusted rates as before:

Community A				Community B			
RATE[a]		WEIGHT		RATE[a]		WEIGHT	
1	×	0.316	= 0.316	2	×	0.316	= 0.632
5	×	0.368	= 1.84	10	×	0.368	= 3.68
10	×	0.316	= 3.16	20	×	0.316	= 6.32
			5.3[a]				10.6[a]

[a] Deaths per 1000 person-years.

Choice of a Standard Population

The decision to use the combined mid-year populations of Community A and Community B was an arbitrary one. What would the results of rate adjustment have looked like had another age distribution been used? Here are two other sets of "weights" based on the respective age distributions of Community A and Community B.

	Standard Population	
AGE	COMMUNITY A	COMMUNITY B
Young	1000/9,000 = 0.111	5000/10,000 = 0.50
Middle	3000/9,000 = 0.333	4000/10,000 = 0.40
Old	5000/9,000 = 0.555	1000/10,000 = 0.10

The age-adjusted rates can be calculated using these weights instead:

	Standard Population	
ADJUSTED RATE[a] IN:	COMMUNITY A	COMMUNITY B
Community A	7.33	3.5
Community B	14.65	7.0
Ratio (B/A)	2.0	2.0
Difference (B − A)	7.33	3.5

[a] Deaths per 1000 person-years.

The size of the adjusted rate in each community varies depending on the standard population chosen. Using the age distribution of A as the standard produces high absolute rates (14.65 and 7.33 per 1000 person-years) because of the relatively great weight (0.555) given to the rates in older persons. Conversely, since the choice of B's age distribution as a standard assigns a weight of only 0.10 to the rates in older persons, the absolute rates in this case are smaller (7.0 and 3.5 per 1000 person-years). Because the ratio of the rates is exactly 2.0 in each age category, however, the *ratio* of the age-adjusted rates is 2.0 no matter what age distribution is chosen to assign the weights.

In this example, because the difference in rates between the two communities is not constant across age categories, the size of the difference between the adjusted rates will be influenced by the choice of the standard:

- 7.33 per 1000 person-years if the age distribution of A is the standard;
- 3.5 per 1000 person-years if that of B is the standard.

There are situations in which it is desirable to compare lifetime cumulative incidence or lifetime cumulative mortality across populations with different age structures. In these situations, it is also necessary to incorporate adjustment for age to avoid introducing confounding. One approach (Day, 1976) simply involves adding age-specific rates across equal-size age strata to produce (for all but very common illnesses or causes of death) a good approximation of the cumulative incidence of (or mortality from) that condition through a given age, one that is standardized to a uniform age distribution. Another approach provides a "standardized lifetime risk" (Sasieni and Adams, 1999) by weighting the age-specific rates in a given population by the proportion of a standard population that survives until the end of each particular age interval.

Presentation of Results as Observed and Expected Number of Cases

Sometimes, data such as those collected to describe mortality rates in Community A and Community B are summarized by indicating the observed number of deaths that occurred in B, and then comparing that number to the one expected, had the age-specific rates in the comparison population, A, been present in a population of the same size and age distribution as B. In this instance the observed number of deaths is 70. The expected number, adjusted for age, is:

MID-YEAR POPULATION OF B	RATE IN A (PER 1000 PERSON-YEARS)	EXPECTED NUMBER OF DEATHS IN B
5000	1	5
4000	5	20
1000	10	10
		35

The ratio of the observed expected number of deaths, called the *standardized mortality ratio* (SMR), is $70/35 = 2.0$. Note that this calculation of the SMR is very similar to the calculation performed above of the adjusted rate using the age distribution of Community B as the standard population. To make the calculations identical, all that is needed is to divide the observed and expected numbers—70 and 35—by the size of the denominator—10,000 person-years—to arrive at the rates obtained earlier, 7.0 per 1000 person-years in B and 3.5 per 1000 person-years in A.

ADJUSTMENT OF RELATIVE RISKS AND ODDS RATIOS

If it is believed that the measure of interest (e.g., relative risk, risk difference) truly varies from stratum to stratum, it is not useful to obtain a summary estimate of this measure across strata, crude or standardized. Instead, the results should be presented for the individual strata separately. The observation of inter-stratum variation in the measure of interest does not necessarily mean there truly *is* variation, of course, since chance can be an explanation for this as well. (A discussion of the bases for regarding observed inter-stratum variability in the size of an exposure–disease association as reflecting genuine effect modification appears in Chapter 17.) If despite the presence of variation there is no reason to believe that it is due to more than chance, it is reasonable to summarize across strata and, if necessary, adjust for the variable(s) that define the strata. But now, the choice of weights to be attached to the strata can make a difference in the estimate of the overall size of the association: If large weights are attached to the strata where the association is relatively large, the estimate will be greater than if small weights are chosen. What is a fair way to go about assigning stratum-specific weights in this circumstance?

The standardized mortality (or morbidity) ratio, SMR, is often used as the adjusted relative risk in occupational cohort studies, or in any cohort study in which the rates are to be compared between a relatively small exposed population and a much larger one (e.g., a national population). In calculating the SMR, the weights attached to the stratum-specific rates derive from the distribution of the confounding variable(s) in the exposed group. So in the above example, thinking of residents of Community B as the "exposed" persons, it was their age distribution that served as the standard. This approach has the virtue of attaching the greatest weights to the strata that are numerically the largest in the exposed group. It avoids the possibility of having an externally derived set of weights inadvertently giving relatively great emphasis to a stratum with very few observations.

But in other cohort studies, and in virtually all case-control studies, the weights that provide the most statistically stable estimate will be obtained from all persons included in the study, both exposed and non-exposed. Specifically, the weight attached to each stratum should be in proportion to the inverse of its variance. A computationally easy method of approaching this was proposed by Mantel and Haenszel (1959) for case-control studies, and this method has been adapted for cohort studies as well. (For a discussion of other approaches to standardizing relative risks, see Rothman and Greenland, 1998, pp. 265–72.)

To illustrate how this method works, let's consider the data shown in Table 11–2 from three hypothetical studies of the incidence of coronary heart disease (CHD) in women of reproductive age in relation to current use of high-potency oral contraceptives (OCs). One is a study of a closed cohort of women in which we seek to estimate the cumulative incidence of CHD in OC users relative to that in nonusers. The second deals with person-time data and seeks to estimate the relative incidence rates. The third is a case-control study in which the odds ratio is to be calculated as an estimate of the relative risk. In each study there is the same confounding factor—physical activity—for which adjustment has to be made.

Table 11–2. Data Layout in Three Hypothetical Studies of CHD Incidence in Relation to OC Use, by Physical Activity Status

A. Example

PHYSICAL ACTIVITY	Cumulative Incidence Study		Study with Person-Time Data		Case-Control Study		
	CHD CASES	NO. OF WOMEN	CHD CASES	NO. OF PERSON-YEARS	CHD CASES	CONTROLS	TOTAL
Sedentary							
OC users	6	29,000	6	29,000	6	29	
OC nonusers	3	44,000	3	44,000	3	44	
		73,000		73,000	9	73	82
Active							
OC users	7	57,000	7	57,000	7	57	
OC nonusers	1	33,000	1	33,000	1	33	
		90,000		90,000	8	90	98

B. General Case

POTENTIAL CONFOUNDER		NO. OF PERSONS		PERSON-TIME		CONTROLS	TOTAL
	CASES	PERSONS	CASES	TIME	CASES		
Stratum i							
Exposed	a_i	N_{i1}	a_i	T_{i1}	a_i	c_i	
Nonexposed	b_i	N_{i0}	b_i	T_{i0}	b_i	d_i	
		N_i		T_i	$a_i + b_i$	$c_i + d_i$	N_i

In the "General case" panel of Table 11–2, in the ith stratum:

a_i = No. of exposed cases
b_i = No. of nonexposed cases
N_{i1} = No. of exposed persons
N_{i0} = No. of nonexposed persons
N_i = Total no. of persons
T_{i1} = Amount of person-time among the exposed
T_{i0} = Amount of person-time among the nonexposed
T_i = Total person-time
c_i = No. of exposed controls
d_i = No. of nonexposed controls

The adjusted relative risk, adjusted relative rate, and adjusted relative odds are calculated as follows:

Cumulative incidence study:

$$\text{Adjusted relative risk} = \frac{\sum_i a_i \cdot N_{i0}/N_i}{\sum_i b_i \cdot N_{i1}/N_i}$$

$$= \frac{6 \cdot 44{,}000/73{,}000 + 7 \cdot 33{,}000/90{,}000}{3 \cdot 29{,}000/73{,}000 + 1 \cdot 57{,}000/90{,}000}$$

$$= 3.39$$

Study with person-time data:

$$\text{Adjusted rate ratio} = \frac{\sum_i a_i \cdot T_{i0}/T_i}{\sum_i b_i \cdot T_{i1}/T_i}$$

$$= \frac{6 \cdot 44{,}000/73{,}000 + 7 \cdot 33{,}000/90{,}000}{3 \cdot 29{,}000/73{,}000 + 1 \cdot 57{,}000/90{,}000}$$

$$= 3.39$$

Case-control study:

$$\text{Adjusted odds ratio} = \frac{\sum_i a_i \cdot d_i/N_i}{\sum_i b_i \cdot c_i/N_i}$$

$$= \frac{6 \cdot 44/82 + 7 \cdot 33/98}{3 \cdot 29/82 + 1 \cdot 57/98}$$

$$= 3.39$$

MULTIVARIATE METHODS

Often more than one variable will have the potential to distort a given association, so it is necessary to be able to deal with each of them to arrive at an unconfounded estimate of the ratio of, or difference between, the rates. If the number of confounding variables is not too large, and there are not too many levels of confounding variables, the approach of stratification that has been employed in this chapter until now can continue to work well. So, for example, if mortality rates in communities A and B were to be adjusted not only for age but for sex as well, the data would be assembled in six strata—three age groups for men, three for women. Or the relative risk of CHD associated with OC use could be examined within categories of both physical activity and another confounding factor, such as parity. If there were three levels of physical activity and three for parity (e.g., 0, 1–2, >3), the adjustment would be performed within a total of nine strata.

While stratification as a means of controlling confounding is easy to describe and to use, in some circumstances it has noteworthy limitations:

- Stratifying simultaneously on many potential confounding factors can be problematic. Many known or suspected risk factors for a disease may already have been identified before research on a possible new cause begins. The incidence of coronary heart disease, for example, is known to be elevated in association with advancing age, male gender, hypertension, diabetes, high cholesterol, smoking, sedentary lifestyle, family history of heart disease, and several other factors. For research on a possible new exposure, all of these known risk factors become potential confounders.

  When the study sample is stratified by multiple potential confounders at once, however, some observations may end up being lost from the analysis altogether. This happens (1) when all study subjects in a certain stratum are exposed to the new risk factor under study, or when none are exposed; or (2) when all subjects in a certain stratum are disease cases, or when none are cases. These kinds of non-informative strata become more and more common as the number of strata increases. They are, in effect, ignored by the Mantel-Haenszel-style analysis methods described in Table 11–2, because these strata contribute zero to sums in both the numerator and denominator.

- All potential confounders (and exposures) must be analyzed as categorical variables. Confounding factors that are naturally measured as continuous variables must nonetheless be converted into categorical form in order to stratify by them. Age, for example, must be divided into a set of age groups in order to carry out age adjustment. When making this conversion, it is tempting to form just a few broad categories in order to keep the number of strata low. But using coarse strata opens the door to *residual confounding,* meaning that confounding may still be present within the broad categories.

Multivariate analysis provides statistical tools for dealing with confounding that are much less subject to these limitations. This section introduces some basic theory behind multivariate analysis and illustrates its use with two examples. More extensive coverage can be found in Holford (2002); Breslow and Day (1980, 1987); Selvin (2001, 1996); Clayton and Hills (1993).

Theory

Multivariate analysis in epidemiology is based on the idea that a person's disease risk can depend on multiple characteristics about him or her. One such characteristic is often an exposure of main interest. Other characteristics (*covariates*) may include factors that can confound or modify the effect of the exposure and that may be risk factors for disease in their own right. Conceptually,

$$\text{Disease risk} = f(\text{Characteristic \#1, Characteristic \#2, \ldots})$$

where $f(\ )$ is a function that specifies just *how* information on these various characteristics is translated into a risk level. In the three hypothetical studies shown in Table 11–2, for example, a woman's risk of developing coronary heart disease is investigated as a function of two characteristics: her use of oral contraceptives and her level of physical activity.

Understanding the function $f(\ )$ is clearly at the heart of the matter. The possibilities are infinite, and obviously the investigator cannot consider them all. In epidemiologic research, candidates are usually limited to functional forms known as *generalized linear models* (McCullagh and Nelder, 1989). These models are mathematically convenient and flexible enough to permit a good fit of the model to empirical observations in many contexts.

To understand what is meant by "generalized linear models," remember from basic geometry that if y and x are linearly related, their relationship can be expressed as

$$y = a + bx$$

where a and b are two constants: a is the intercept, and b is the slope. Once values of a and b are known, then for any value of x, the corresponding value of y can be calculated.

To adapt this framework for epidemiologic research, think of y as a *response* variable representing, in some form, disease risk or disease frequency. For example, y might be the probability or odds of disease in a certain person, or the hazard rate of disease in a certain person at a certain point in time, or the number of disease cases in a certain amount of person-time. The particular form of multivariate analysis used depends on specifically what y represents, which depends in turn on the study design. Several forms of multivariate analysis of importance in epidemiology are described below.

Meanwhile, the right side of the equation involves not just one x but multiple x-variables. Each represents a different characteristic that may be related to disease occurrence, such as age, gender, or exposure to a certain risk factor. The x-variables are often termed *predictors*. An x-variable may be a continuous variable, such as age. Or it may be an *indicator* variable (sometimes called a "dummy" variable) that can take on either of two values, usually 1 or 0, reflecting the presence or absence of a certain characteristic, such as male gender. Sometimes a single characteristic is represented in the statistical model by a set of two or more x-variables, particularly when the original characteristic is a categorical factor with several possible values (such as race or marital status).

Ultimately, instead of $a + bx$, the right side of the statistical model incorporates what is termed a *linear combination* of the x-variables:

$$a + b_1 x_1 + b_2 x_2 + \cdots + b_k x_k \qquad (11.1)$$

The form of this expression is what makes the model a linear one. It specifies a certain way information on the x-variables is combined. In particular, each x-variable is multiplied by its own slope coefficient (b), which thus governs how large a contribution the term involving that x-variable makes toward the overall sum. These b-coefficients (and a) are estimated from the data and are treated as constant across all study subjects, while the values of the x-variables vary among subjects.

Some of the most important results of multivariate analysis are estimates of the b-coefficients. The statistical methods for obtaining these estimates— usually maximum likelihood estimation—are beyond the scope of this book (see McCullagh and Nelder, 1989; Breslow and Day, 1980, 1987). In broad terms, values of the b-coefficients are selected to maximize agreement between the pattern of disease occurrence actually observed and what the statistical model would predict. All standard computer programs for epidemiologic analysis produce point estimates and confidence limits (or standard errors) for the b-coefficients. It is the epidemiologist's job to interpret and apply this information properly. To that end, three properties of the b-coefficient estimates should be noted:

- Each b-coefficient estimate reflects the size of the corresponding x-variable's contribution to disease risk *after accounting for the contributions of all of the other x-variables.* In other words, a b-coefficient represents the "incremental" association between a certain x-variable and disease risk, after adjusting statistically for the effects of the other x-variables.

  As shown below, the estimated b-coefficient for a key exposure variable can be converted easily into an adjusted estimate of the magnitude of the exposure's association with disease, such as an adjusted relative risk. The task of evaluating confounding via multivariate analysis then involves comparing the relative risk estimates for an exposure across two or more statistical models. A model that includes the exposure as the only x-variable yields a "crude" or "unadjusted" relative risk estimate for the exposure. A model that includes the exposure and other x-variables as covariates yields a relative risk estimate for exposure, adjusted for those other x-variables. The extent of confounding can then be gauged by comparing relative risk estimates with and without adjustment for the suspected confounder(s), in much the same way that one compares relative risks before and after rate standardization.

- The estimated size of a b-coefficient reflects the amount by which a *one-unit* increase in the corresponding x changes the sum. As a special case, if x is an indicator variable, coded as 1 when a certain characteristic is present and as 0 when it is absent, then the size of b reflects the amount of change in the sum in relation to presence of that characteristic. This property also applies to an adjusted relative risk estimate derived from b, which thus reflects the factor by which risk is multiplied in association with a one-unit increase in x.

- If the estimated value of a b-coefficient is zero or nearly zero, this finding implies that the corresponding x evidently contributes little toward predicting disease risk after accounting for the effects of other x-variables in the model. This is because if $b = 0$, then $bx = 0$, and the term involving x makes no net contribution to the sum. It might just as well be omitted from the statistical model altogether. Such a result may signal an opportunity to simplify the statistical model by omitting a relatively unimportant x-variable.

These features apply to all of the most commonly used forms of multivariate analysis in epidemiology, because all can be formulated as having a linear combination of x-variables on the right side of a prediction equation. But beyond this point they diverge according to what appears on the left side of the equation.

- **Logistic regression** is commonly used for case-control studies, for cohort studies of relatively rare diseases that yield cumulative incidence data without censoring, and for studies of prevalence. The log odds of disease risk appears on the left:

$$\ln \left[\frac{\text{Pr(disease)}}{1 - \text{Pr(disease)}} \right] = a + b_1 x_1 + b_2 x_2 + \cdots + b_k x_k \qquad (11.2)$$

  The log odds is also called the *logit,* from which the adjective *logistic* is derived. Two nice features of logistic regression help explain its popularity. First, after the b-coefficients have been estimated, $\exp(b_i)$ can be interpreted as an estimate of the *adjusted odds ratio* for x_i. Because the odds ratio is a good estimate of relative risk whenever the disease is rare, logistic regression can be used to obtain adjusted relative risk estimates for rare diseases in the context of several standard epidemiologic study designs, including cohort studies, case-control studies, and even randomized trials.
  Second, equation (11.2) can be rearranged as:

$$\text{Pr(disease)} = \frac{\exp(a + b_1 x_1 + b_2 x_2 + \cdots + b_k x_k)}{1 + \exp(a + b_1 x_1 + b_2 x_2 + \cdots + b_k x_k)} \qquad (11.3)$$

  to obtain a *predicted probability of disease* in a person with specified values of the x-variables. Regardless of the values of the x-variables, the b-coefficients, and a, equation (11.3) always yields a predicted value for Pr(disease) that lies between 0 and 1, as expected of any quantity that is to be interpreted as a probability. (Note, however, that if [11.3] is used with estimates derived from case-control study data, Pr[disease] refers only to the probability of being a case *within the study,* not the probability of disease in the source population from which cases and controls were derived.) A variant of logistic regression, called *conditional logistic regression,* is used for matched case-control studies (Breslow et al., 1978).
  Logistic regression is actually just one member of a larger family of *binomial regression* methods for binary outcomes, such as disease status. Other members of this family use $\ln[Pr(\text{disease})]$ or simply Pr(disease) on the left side of the prediction equation. When applied to cumulative incidence data, these techniques permit estimating *adjusted relative risks* or *adjusted attributable risks,* respectively, from the b-coefficients, rather than adjusted odds ratios. But both techniques have the disadvantage of

sometimes yielding predicted values of Pr(disease) that fall outside the range 0–1, which are awkward to try to interpret as probabilities.

- **Poisson regression** is commonly used for studies that yield incidence rate data. The left side of the prediction equation is the logarithm of the incidence rate:

$$\ln\left(\frac{\text{No. of cases}}{\text{Person-time}}\right) = a + b_1 x_1 + b_2 x_2 + \cdots + b_k x_k$$

Once the b-coefficients have been estimated, $\exp(b_i)$ is interpretable as an estimate of the adjusted incidence rate ratio (rate ratio) for x_i.

- **Cox proportional-hazards regression** is a form of survival analysis used for cohort studies or randomized trials that involve censored data, or when the values of x-variables can change over time in study subjects. The left side of the prediction equation is the logarithm of a ratio of hazard rates:

$$\ln\left[\frac{h(t)}{h_0(t)}\right] = b_1 x_1 + b_2 x_2 + \cdots + b_k x_k$$

Here $h(t)$ represents the hazard of disease in a certain person at a certain time t, to which the specified values of the x-variables pertain. The quantity $h_0(t)$ is a reference or "baseline" hazard at time t in a person for whom all of the x-variables equal zero. Once the b-coefficients have been estimated, $\exp(b_i)$ is interpretable as an estimate of the *adjusted hazard ratio* for x_i.

For each of these techniques, the quantity on the left side of the equation should be regarded as a *predicted* or *expected* quantity. Input to a model-fitting computer program typically consists of a set of *observed* values of disease status, x-variables, and other method-specific data such as person-time at risk or time of disease onset. The model-fitting program then finds estimates of a and the b-coefficients that maximize agreement between observed disease occurrence and what the model predicts.

Example 1: Oral Contraceptives, Physical Activity, and Coronary Heart Disease (Revisited)

Table 11–2 showed data from three hypothetical studies of coronary heart disease (CHD) in women, each study using a different design. Oral contraceptive (OC) use was the exposure of main interest, while physical activity level was a confounding factor. Let us see how multivariate analysis could be applied for each type of study.

Cumulative incidence study

After data collection, each of the 163,000 study women would have values on three binary variables:

$$CHD = 1 \text{ if a case}$$

$$= 0 \text{ if not a case}$$

$$OC \text{ use: } x_1 = 1 \text{ if an OC user}$$

$$= 0 \text{ if an OC non-user}$$

$$Physical \text{ activity: } x_2 = 1 \text{ if active}$$

$$= 0 \text{ if sedentary}$$

The raw data could be represented as the data matrix in Table 11–3, wherein women are listed arbitrarily according to a study ID number ranging from 1 to 163,000. A total of 17 women (the cases) would have CHD = 1, while 86,000 women (the OC users) would have $x_1 = 1$, and 98,000 women (those who were physically active) would have $x_2 = 1$.

In this instance, there are only eight possible combinations of values on CHD, OC use, and physical activity. Hence the essential data can be represented more compactly by listing each of the eight combinations as one row and adding to each row the value of a fourth variable, N, which is a *frequency weight*—i.e., how many study women had that combination of values. This data layout is shown in Table 11–4.

Table 11–5 shows selected results of fitting two logistic regression models to these data. The constant term a in each model appears in the coefficient column and the intercept row. This is usually a byproduct of model-fitting and is of little

Table 11–3. Raw Data Matrix for Cumulative Study of Coronary Heart Disease in Women (Based on Table 11–2)

ID NUMBER	CHD	OC USE (x_1)	PHYSICAL ACTIVITY (x_2)
1	1	0	0
2	1	1	0
3	0	1	1
4	1	1	0
⋮	⋮	⋮	⋮
163,000	0	0	0

Table 11–4. Compact Data Layout for Cumulative Incidence Study
of Coronary Heart Disease in Women

CHD	OC USE (x_1)	PHYSICAL ACTIVITY (x_2)	N
1	1	0	6
1	0	0	3
1	1	1	7
1	0	1	1
0	1	0	28,994
0	0	0	43,997
0	1	1	56,993
0	0	1	32,999

Table 11–5. Logistic Regression Analysis Results for Cumulative Incidence Study
of CHD in Women

	Coefficient			Odds Ratio	
MODEL TERM	POINT ESTIMATE	STANDARD ERROR	p	POINT ESTIMATE	(95% CONFIDENCE INTERVAL)
Model no. 1					
(Intercept)	−9.865	.500	...	...	...
x_1 (OC use)	1.068	.572	.062	2.91	(.95–8.93)
Model no. 2					
(Intercept)	−9.657	.521	...	...	...
x_1 (OC use)	1.204	.583	.039	3.33	(1.06–10.45)
x_2 (Phys. act.)	−.579	.495	.243	.56	(.21–1.48)

substantive interest, although it is used when calculating predicted probabilities of disease.

Each odds ratio estimate was calculated from the b-coefficient in its row as $OR = \exp(b)$, and 95% confidence limits were computed as $\exp[b \pm 1.96 \cdot s.e.(b)]$. Most computer programs produce these automatically, or as an option.

In Model no. 1, x_1 (OC use) was the only x-variable. Hence the odds ratio, 2.91, reflects the "unadjusted" effect of OC use on CHD risk. It exactly equals the odds ratio that can be computed from the simple 2×2 table formed by cross-classifying case/control status by OC use, ignoring physical activity.

In Model no. 2, both x_1 and x_2 were included. The odds ratio for OC use, 3.33, reflects the effect of OC use on CHD risk, adjusted for physical activity.

Note that it agrees closely with the $OR = 3.39$ obtained earlier from the Mantel-Haenszel analysis of the same data. The small discrepancy results from differences in the method of statistical estimation, which weight the experience of active and sedentary women slightly differently.

As a byproduct, Model no. 2 also yields $OR = 0.56$ for physical activity. This odds ratio is adjusted for the effects of OC use. Note that its 95% confidence limits include the null value of 1.0, even though physical activity does modestly confound the effect of OC use: compare the odds ratios for OC use between Models no. 1 and no. 2, which differ by about 15%. Thus, although physical activity has no "statistically significant" association with CHD risk in Model #2, it merits inclusion because of the study's primary focus on obtaining as unconfounded an estimate as possible for the effect of OC use.

A slight disadvantage of using logistic regression here is that it yields odds ratios rather than true relative risks. In this instance, however, fitting relative-risk models yields almost identical numerical results, as might be expected in view of the rarity of CHD in the population from which these data were derived.

Incidence rate study

For the second hypothetical study of CHD in women, yielding incidence rate data, the data layout is as shown in Table 11–6. Each row represents a different combination of OC use and physical activity. Poisson regression was used for multivariate analysis.

In this case, fitting two Poisson regression models to the data yields numerical results almost exactly the same as those in Table 11–5, so they are not shown again. The only change needed is to relabel "Odds ratio" as "Incidence rate ratio."

Case-control study

For the hypothetical case-control study of CHD in women, the data layout is just like that for the cumulative incidence study (Table 11–4), except that values for N in the last four rows become 29, 44, 57, and 33, respectively. This

Table 11–6. Data Layout for Incidence Rate Study of Coronary Heart Disease in Women

CHD CASES	PERSON-YEARS	OC USE	PHYSICAL ACTIVITY
6	29,000	1	0
3	44,000	0	0
7	57,000	1	1
1	33,000	0	1

Table 11–7. Logistic Regression Analysis Results for Case-Control Study of Coronary Heart Disease in Women

MODEL TERM	Coefficient			Odds Ratio	
	POINT ESTIMATE	STANDARD ERROR	p	POINT ESTIMATE	(95% CONFIDENCE INTERVAL)
Model no. 1					
(Intercept)	−2.958	.513	. . .	. . .	. . .
x_1 (OC use)	1.068	.593	.072	2.91	(.91–9.30)
Model no. 2					
(Intercept)	−2.749	.537	. . .	. . .	. . .
x_1 (OC use)	1.207	.609	.047	3.34	(1.01–11.02)
x_2 (Phys. act.)	−.584	.530	.270	.56	(.20–1.57)

reflects the fact that only a small fraction of potentially eligible non-cases would actually be studied. After this change, logistic regression was applied in the same manner as for the cumulative incidence study, yielding the results shown in Table 11–7.

The interpretation of these results is closely similar to that of the other two study designs. In comparison with the cumulative incidence study results, which were also obtained from logistic regression, the confidence limits are wider around the odds ratio estimates for OC use and physical activity in Table 11–7 because of the smaller number of non-cases studied. But the increase in width is small in light of the nearly 1000-fold difference in the total number of women studied— an illustration of how efficient the case-control design can be for study of rare diseases.

Example 2: Low Birth Weight, Maternal Coffee Consumption, and Cigarette Smoking

This example illustrates how a continuous x-variable can be handled in multivariate analysis.

In 1980, based on animal studies, the U.S. Food and Drug Administration recommended that pregnant women avoid foods and beverages containing caffeine. To determine whether drinking coffee during pregnancy was associated with low infant birth weight in humans, Linn and colleagues (1982) studied 12,205 mother-baby pairs in the Boston area within one to two days after delivery. Mothers were asked about coffee intake and cigarette smoking during pregnancy, among other topics. A summary of the results is shown in Table 11–8.

Table 11-8. Frequency of Low Infant Birth Weight in Relation to Mother's Smoking
and Coffee Intake During Pregnancy

| | Currently Smoke Cigarettes? | | | | | |
| COFFEE INTAKE | NO | | YES | | TOTAL | |
(CUPS PER DAY)	N	% LBW[a]	N	% LBW	N	% LBW
0	5460	6.1	1457	11.8	6917	7.3
1	1950	7.2	552	10.9	2502	8.0
2	1057	7.7	463	11.5	1520	8.8
3	396	6.1	278	10.8	674	8.0
4-6	228	4.8	263	14.1	491	9.8
7+	25	4.0	76	17.1	101	13.9
Total	9,116	6.5	3,089	11.8	12,205	7.8

[a] % of infants weighing <2500 grams at birth.
[*Source:* Linn et al. (1982).]

To prepare these data for analysis, a raw-data matrix resembling that shown in Table 11-4 was constructed. The four input variables were LBW (0 = no, 1 = yes); SMOKING (1 = current smoker, 0 = not a current smoker); COFFEE (coded as 0, 1, 2, 3, 5, or 8 cups/day); and N, a frequency-weight variable specifying how many mothers had each unique combination of data values. LBW was the response variable, COFFEE the key exposure, and SMOKING a potential confounder.

Table 11-9 shows results from a sequence of four logistic regression models fitted to these data. As before, each row of results within a given model corresponds to a different x-variable, and the "(Intercept)" row shows the constant term (a) and its standard error. The four models form a progression and are discussed in order.

Ignoring smoking for the moment, in Model no. 1, each of the six categories of daily coffee intake was treated as a separate exposure level. One level (0 cups/day) was selected as a *reference* level to which others were compared. Five indicator variables were then created, one for each higher level of coffee intake. For example, $x_1 = 1$ for mothers who drank exactly one cup of coffee daily, while $x_1 = 0$ for all other mothers, and similarly for $x_2 \ldots x_5$. All five indicator variables were then included in the model. The column of five odds ratios for Model no. 1 shows how the odds of having a low-birth-weight baby varied in relation to daily coffee intake, always relative to mothers who drank no coffee. There is a strong suggestion of increasing odds with increasing coffee intake, but it is not a perfectly regular trend. For example, the observed odds ratio for mothers who drank three cups per day was actually lower than that for mothers who drank two cups per day.

Table 11–9. Logistic Regression Analysis Results for Study of Coffee, Smoking and Low Birth Weight

MODEL TERM	Coefficient			Odds Ratio	
	POINT ESTIMATE	STD. ERROR	p	POINT ESTIMATE	(95% CONFIDENCE INTERVAL)
Model no. 1					
(Intercept)	−2.537	.046	...	...	...
x_1 (1 cup)	.094	.087	.280	1.098	(.926–1.303)
x_2 (2 cups)	.201	.102	.048	1.222	(1.002–1.492)
x_3 (3 cups)	.096	.149	.518	1.101	(.821–1.475)
x_4 (4–6 cups)	.315	.159	.047	1.370	(1.003–1.870)
x_5 (7+ cups)	.710	.292	.015	2.035	(1.149–3.603)
Model no. 2					
(Intercept)	−2.531	.042	...	...	...
COFFEE	.071	.022	.001	1.073	(1.028–1.120)
Model no. 3					
(Intercept)	−2.667	.043	...	...	...
SMOKING	.657	.070	<.001	1.929	(1.682–2.213)
Model no. 4					
(Intercept)	−2.687	.046	...	...	...
COFFEE	.028	.023	.213	1.028	(.984–1.075)
SMOKING	.638	.072	<.001	1.893	(1.645–2.180)

Model no. 2 treated daily coffee intake as a continuous variable, including the original COFFEE variable as the only predictor. The resulting odds ratio implies that each one-cup increase in daily coffee intake was associated with a 1.073-fold increase in the odds of having a low-birth-weight baby. This increase would be compounded with additional cups, so the estimated odds ratio for mothers who drank, say, three cups per day would be $1.073 \times 1.073 \times 1.073 = 1.236$, relative to women who drank no coffee.

Model no. 3 examined the effect of SMOKING, already coded as an indicator variable, considered by itself. The odds ratio estimate implies a 93% increase in odds of low infant birth weight among smoking mothers, relative to non-smoking mothers.

Model no. 4 includes both COFFEE and SMOKING, providing a chance to determine the extent to which each confounds the effect of the other. Comparing the unadjusted odds ratio for COFFEE in Model no. 2 with the SMOKING-adjusted odds ratio for COFFEE in Model no. 4, it appears that most of the original association with coffee intake disappeared after adjusting for smoking status. Both 1.073

(from Model no. 2) and 1.028 (from Model no. 4) are so close to 1.0 that they look at first glance like weak associations. But remember that each represents the odds ratio for a *one-cup* increase in daily coffee intake, which is a fairly small exposure increment. Viewed differently, the original 7.3% increase in odds with each added cup is reduced to a 2.8% increase after controlling for smoking. Moreover, the confidence limits around 1.028 in Model no. 4 indicate that the remaining weak association with coffee intake could easily be explained by chance.

Comparing the odds ratios for SMOKING between Models no. 3 and no. 4, it appears that coffee intake confounded the association between smoking status and low birth weight to only a minor degree.

Propensity Scores

The applications of multivariate analysis discussed above all involve modeling the outcome variable, usually disease status or disease frequency, as a function of exposure and other covariates. In some studies, a useful alternative approach to controlling for multiple potential confounders simultaneously involves using a *propensity score* (Rosenbaum and Rubin, 1983; Rubin, 1997; D'Agostino, 1998). In brief, the analyst first models the *exposure* variable as a function of the potential confounders, using logistic regression or a related method. This model is used to calculate an expected probability ("propensity") of exposure for each study subject. The main analysis then involves examining the exposure-outcome association while controlling for the propensity score by stratification, matching, or covariate adjustment. This approach can be attractive when multiple outcome variables are to be studied in relation to a single key exposure, because the same propensity score can be used for analysis of several different outcome variables. In addition, if outcome events are rare but exposure is common (within the study), then a multivariate model for exposure may be able to accommodate more important potential confounders than a model for outcome because of the limited number of outcome events. These circumstances often occur in quasi-experiments and cohort studies.

Concluding Comments on Multivariate Analysis

In broad terms, multivariate analysis methods are like power tools: one can do bigger, more complicated jobs with them than would otherwise be possible, but they can also wreak havoc if used improperly. One danger is that the user has a relatively detached perspective on the data. The analyst cannot always detect from a computer-generated table of regression coefficients that sample sizes in a critical subgroup were exceedingly small, or that an implausible data value is the real explanation for some striking finding. Experienced analysts use multivariate analysis in tandem with simpler methods, such as descriptive statistics and crosstabulations, to stay in close touch with the data. Multivariate methods also rely on assumptions about the form of the data that need to be be kept in mind and that can often be checked.

Most future epidemiologists will want to study multivariate analysis in more depth than can be covered in this brief introduction. Nonetheless, the discussion here may motivate such further study by showing why and how these methods can be used to facilitate epidemiologic research.

UNDER WHAT CONDITIONS WILL CONFOUNDING BE PRESENT?

Earlier it was shown that the comparison of mortality rates in hypothetical communities A and B was confounded by age, since death rates increased with increasing age and the two communities had different age distributions. Only a variable that in some way is related both to exposure and to disease has the potential to act as a confounder. But whether it actually confounds also depends on the nature of these relationships.

Relationship of Potential Confounding Variable to Exposure Status or Level

A characteristic or experience that occurs only as a consequence of a given exposure cannot distort the relationship of that exposure to disease occurrence, so it generally is not treated as a confounding variable. For example, bronchial epithelial changes occur in response to long-term cigarette smoking. Their presence increases the risk of bronchial cancer, but statistical control for these changes (if they could be measured) would not be appropriate when seeking to measure a possible association between cigarette smoking and bronchial cancer. To be a confounding factor, a variable would have to give rise to cigarette smoking or be associated with a characteristic that did—in addition to being related on its own to the incidence of bronchial cancer. Adjustment for a consequence of exposure can only serve to blunt the measured exposure–disease association.

There *are* circumstances in which adjustment is made for a consequence of exposure, but these arise only when there is interest in examining the possibility of an exposure–disease association *beyond* that arising from that specific consequence. For example, most epidemiologic studies seeking to assess whether use of OCs during the teenage years alters a woman's later risk of breast cancer have adjusted for the age at which she gives birth to her first child. They have done so

despite the fact that age-at-first-birth does not meet the usual criteria for a confounder. While late age-at-first-birth tends to predict an elevated risk of breast
cancer, use of OCs during the teenage years tends to delay a first pregnancy and
childbirth, not vice versa. Nonetheless, since these studies are interested in answering the question "Does teenage use of OCs affect breast cancer risk *beyond its
ability to delay a first pregnancy?*" an adjustment for this consequence of exposure
is warranted.

Temporal sequence aside, how does one judge whether a potential confounder
is associated with exposure? Should one simply look at the data that have been
gathered, or consider information external to the study? If, in the underlying population the study participants have been drawn from, there truly is no association
between the exposure and the potential confounding variable, that variable will
not be a true confounder. So, if a variable is not credibly related to exposure (e.g.,
day of the week of birth and cigarette smoking), one would not consider it a confounder. Any association that might be present in the data should be interpreted
as having occurred by chance and should be ignored. Since there are very few
variables, however, whose lack of association with exposure can be claimed with
confidence a priori, we tend to examine the data that have been gathered to guide
this judgment. That examination should not involve an assessment of the role of
chance as a possible explanation for any association observed between exposure
and potential confounder. A large *p*-value may say as much about the small size of
the sample as about the true absence of a relationship in the underlying population
that sample had been drawn from.

Relationship of Potential Confounding Variable to Outcome

No matter how strongly a variable is related to exposure status, if it is not also
related to the occurrence of the disease in question, it cannot be a confounder. The
nature of that relationship to disease may take one of several forms:

1. The potential confounding variable can be an actual cause of the disease.
   For example, an imbalance in cigarette smoking behavior between persons
   employed in a certain industry and a comparison group would distort the
   assessment of the association between employment in that industry and
   the occurrence of lung cancer.
2. The potential confounder can be associated with a cause of the disease that,
   in the context of the study, cannot be measured. A study of a possibly altered incidence of prostate cancer among white and black men who worked
   in the above industry would wish to deal with potential confounding by
   race, given the higher risk of this disease in black men. What would no
   doubt be ascertained in such a study would be racial phenotype, based on

some combination of skin pigment, hair characteristics, etc. *Un*measured in the study would be the characteristics of black men—genetic or environmental ones—that actually predispose to prostate cancer. The racial phenotype, which is not a cause of prostate cancer in and of itself, would be used as a surrogate for the genuine cause(s).

3. A variable can be a confounder if it is related to the *recognition* of the outcome in question, even if it has no relationship to the actual occurrence of that outcome. An example of such a variable might be cervical screening, when assessing a potential association between use of OCs and the development of preneoplastic lesions of the uterine cervix. Since these lesions are asymptomatic and are detected only by means of cervical screening, and OC users generally have a higher frequency of screening than do nonusers, a comparison of the occurrence of cervical preneoplastic lesions between users and nonusers of OCs would be confounded unless efforts were made to "force" (in the design or analysis) the level of screening to be similar between the two groups of women.

STRATEGIES FOR CONTROLLING CONFOUNDING

Confounding can be dealt with not only in the analysis of data gathered in an epidemiologic study, but in the design of those studies. As discussed in Chapter 13, addressing a possible association by means of a *randomized trial* generally achieves good control of confounding since, except in very small trials, the distribution of other factors that influence disease occurrence will be approximately balanced between persons assigned to the intervention and control arms of the study. In non-randomized studies, a commonly used approach to controlling confounding is *restriction* of the study population to a segment that is homogeneous with respect to a particular risk factor for disease. For example, nearly all studies of occupational factors in relationship to the incidence of breast cancer are restricted to women. The inclusion of men in such studies would: *(a)* lead to confounding (unless other measures to control confounding were employed), since men have a much lower incidence of breast cancer than women and the patterns of employment differ between sexes; and *(b)* not add appreciably to the power of the study to detect an association.

In cohort studies, control of confounding can be achieved by *matching* non-exposed subjects to exposed ones for the presence or level of a variable that is related to disease occurrence. For example, in their cohort study of the possible influence of induced abortion on the occurrence of adverse outcomes in a subsequent pregnancy, Daling and Emanuel (1975) matched one pregnant woman who had no history of induced abortion to each pregnant woman who did have such a history for age, number of prior pregnancies, and a history of prior stillbirth or miscarriage. Thus, the comparison of the two groups for the occurrence of fetal or neonatal deaths, prematurity, or congenital malformations in that pregnancy was not distorted by any dissimilarity between them with regard to the matching characteristics.

In case-control studies, controls can be matched to cases for the presence or level of characteristics (other than the exposure of interest) that predict the occurrence of that illness. The primary purpose of matching in this situation, however, is not control of confounding—if the matching variable is related to the exposure in question, it will be necessary to account for it in the analysis in any case if a valid result is to be obtained (see Chapter 15). Rather, the purpose is an increase in study efficiency. For example, if a case-control study of occupational influences on breast cancer did not restrict its subjects to women, almost surely that study would match controls to cases on the basis of sex. Failure to do so would generate a control group of roughly equal numbers of men and women. This would result in an analysis in which one stratum—that of men—contained a very high ratio of controls to cases, and therefore a study whose power to address the hypothesis would be substantially less than had it attempted to have the ratio of women to men be similar for cases and controls.

Some studies employ multiple strategies to isolate the possible effect of the exposure of interest from other factors related to the disease with which it is correlated.

Example: In a study conducted in two urban areas of Brazil, Victora et al. (1987) compared infants who died of diarrhea or respiratory disease with other infants in terms of breast feeding and other types of dietary intake (as ascertained through interviews with parents) during a period of time prior to the onset of the cases' illnesses. Because a number of correlates of breast-feeding practices are themselves related to infant mortality, the authors gave considerable attention to control of possible confounding. First, they *restricted* their study population to singletons of birth weight greater than 1500 grams who had not been hospitalized for more than two weeks beginning at birth. Prior to the start of the study, it was anticipated that infants excluded by these criteria would be relatively less likely to have been breast-fed through the first year of life and also at increased risk of death from diarrhea or respiratory disease. Also, it was expected that there would be so few of them—especially among exclusive breast-feeders—that statistical adjustment might not have been feasible. Later, in the analysis of their data, the authors adjusted for a number of additional characteristics, including interval from preceding birth, maternal education, father's occupation, and neighborhood of residence. (For purposes of efficiency, they had already chosen control infants from the same neighborhoods as the cases.) They also adjusted for one of the characteristics used to restrict their sample—birth weight—in categories of 500 grams beginning at 1500 grams.

Because of the care with which confounding was addressed in this study, the strong association of mortality with *not* breast-feeding that was observed could be interpreted with some confidence as reflecting a genuine protective effect of nursing during the first year of life.

RESIDUAL CONFOUNDING

An effort to control for a variable's confounding influence will be incomplete to the extent that:

- The variable has not been measured accurately, or
- The variable has not been categorized or modeled in such a way as to fully capture the nature of its relationship to disease and/or exposure.

Nondifferential mismeasurement of a confounder will lead to an estimate of the size of the exposure–disease association that is falsely close to the unadjusted (crude) estimate. In the extreme case, in which the means of measuring the confounding variable is completely inaccurate, the "adjusted" and crude estimates will be identical.

Example: To explore the possibility that sexually transmitted infections other than human papillomavirus (HPV) can predispose to cervical cancer, two case-control studies were conducted by investigators at the National Cancer Institute to examine whether a woman's risk of this disease was related to the number of sexual partners she had had. Each study controlled for the presence of cervical HPV DNA, but they used different methods. The first, conducted in 1986–1987, employed Southern blot DNA hybridization, whereas the second (conducted in 1989–1990) used PCR, a more sensitive technique that only then had become available for epidemiologic studies. Evidence of the enhanced ability of the second study to accurately assess HPV status was the much higher odds ratio it obtained for the HPV–cancer association—20.1—than the corresponding odds ratio obtained in the first study—3.7.

Table 11–10 (from Schiffman and Schatzkin, 1994) describes the association between the number of sexual partners and cervical cancer in each study, both with and without adjustment for HPV status.

Table 11–10. Effect of Adjustment for HPV Infection on the Association Between
Lifetime Number of Sexual Partners and the Risk of Cervical Intraepithelial Neoplasia

LIFETIME NO. OF SEXUAL PARTNERS	CASES	CONTROLS	CRUDE ODDS RATIO (95% CONF. INT.)		ADJUSTED ODDS RATIO[a] (95% CONF. INT.)	
Study 1 (1986–1987)						
1	25	69	1.0		1.0	
2	47	61	2.1	(1.2–3.9)	2.2	(1.2–4.0)
3–4	71	79	2.1	(1.2–3.7)	2.0	(1.1–3.6)
5–9	48	89	2.5	(1.4–4.3)	2.4	(1.3–4.3)
10+	48	89	1.5	(0.8–2.7)	1.5	(0.8–2.8)
Study 2 (1989–1990)						
1	40	113	1.0		1.0	
2	34	58	1.7	(0.9–2.9)	1.0	(0.5–1.9)
3–5	127	116	3.1	(2.0–4.8)	1.1	(0.6–1.9)
6–9	116	70	4.7	(2.9–7.5)	1.5	(0.9–2.7)
10+	116	74	4.4	(2.8–7.0)	1.6	(0.9–2.8)

[a] Adjusted for HPV DNA detection.
[*Source:* Schiffman and Schatzkin (1994).]

Adjustment for HPV infection had a large impact on the elevated odds ratios associated with increasing numbers of sexual partners in the second study, but almost no impact at all in the first study. Misclassification of HPV status in the first study appears to have substantially decreased the ability to adjust for that variable.

If even an accurately measured confounding variable is not categorized appropriately, adjustment will not remove all of its confounding influence. For example, in a study of degree of baldness in relation to the incidence of prostate cancer (perhaps to obtain clues regarding hormonal or genetic influences on this disease), adjustment for age in two groups—perhaps less than 60 years and 60 or greater—would almost certainly lead to the presence of residual confounding. Within each broad category of age, both the degree of baldness and the incidence of prostate cancer rises. Finer stratification on age—perhaps in five-year groups, or using multivariate methods that allow age to be modeled as a continuous variable—would be needed to remove most or all of the confounding.

If a method that requires categorization of a confounder is to be used, how narrow must one make the categories of the confounding variable? The answer to this question depends on the particulars of the relationship between the confounder and the exposure and disease, respectively. In the hypothetical study of baldness and prostate cancer, it may be necessary to control for race. If the incidence of prostate cancer is similar between Chinese, Japanese, and Filipino men, for example, it would be possible to combine them in a single stratum for analysis (in addition to strata for white and for black men) with no introduction of confounding by race. But there are other instances (e.g., age as a potential confounder of the association between baldness and prostate cancer) in which it is necessary to create relatively fine strata of the confounding variable to prevent its strong relationship to both exposure and disease from distorting the association.

EXERCISES

1. The data below came from the Surveillance, Epidemiology, and End Results Program, 1990, in which nine geographic areas of the U.S. were monitored for cancer incidence:

AGE (YEARS)	White Males		Black Males	
	NO. OF BLADDER CANCER CASES, 1990	NO. OF MALES IN SURVEY AREAS, 1990	NO. OF BLADDER CANCER CASES, 1990	NO. OF MALES IN SURVEY AREAS, 1990
0–54	319	7,574,000	20	1,088,000
55–59	253	388,000	10	37,000
60–64	370	382,000	16	34,000
65–69	524	346,000	27	30,000
70–74	550	265,000	20	21,000
75–84	817	288,000	27	21,000

(a) What are the crude incidence rates for bladder cancer for white males and for black males? What is the ratio of these two rates?

(b) What are the age-adjusted incidence rates for bladder cancer for white males and for black males (use the white male population as a standard)? Now, what is the incidence in white males relative to that in black males? Why is it lower than when using crude rates?

2. Below are the results of a (hypothetical) cohort study of use of hair coloring products in relation to mortality from prostate cancer:

AGE (YEARS)	Use of Hair Coloring		Non-Use of Hair Coloring	
	DEATHS	MAN-YEARS	DEATHS	MAN-YEARS
50–59	0	1,502	1	10,485
55–59	2	1,978	5	21,930
60–64	1	431	22	11,641

Adjusting for age, what is the ratio of the mortality rates from prostate cancer between users and nonusers of hair coloring products? What is the corresponding crude mortality rate ratio? Why do the two differ from each other?

3. The data in the following table describe the median serum creatinine levels obtained 2–5 years prior to diagnosis in persons who developed kidney cancer, and during the corresponding period of time in controls.

	Cases		Controls	
	NO. OF SUBJECTS	MEDIAN SERUM CREATININE[a]	NO. OF SUBJECTS	MEDIAN SERUM CREATININE[a]
Men & women combined	180	1.1	435	1.0
Men	114	1.2	173	1.2
Women	66	0.9	262	0.9

[a] mg per dl

The median serum creatinine level was the same for male cases and controls, and also for female cases and controls. It was not the same, however, for cases and controls of the two sexes combined. Why?

4. Screening for elevated blood glucose is recommended during the 24th–28th week of pregnancy to identify women with gestational diabetes mellitus (GDM), since untreated GDM predisposes to (among other things) respiratory distress syndrome (RDS) in the infant. You are an epidemiologist at a large health maintenance organization in which nearly every pregnant female member is screened for blood glucose levels. You would like to do a case-control study of RDS to determine whether, among women with glucose levels below the threshold for a diagnosis of GDM, the risk of RDS rises with increasingly high levels of blood glucose. If you find, for example, that infants of pregnant women just below the presently accepted threshold of blood glucose are at increased risk, an argument could be made for redefining the definition of GDM.

Controls for the study will be sampled from members of the organization who delivered a baby without RDS. You are aware that RDS is primarily a condition that affects premature babies. In this study, under what circumstances, if any, would you recommend matching controls to cases on the basis of gestational age at the time of delivery? Explain your recommendation. (Assume that, because of the widespread use of prenatal ultrasound in this health maintenance organization, accurate information on gestational age is available on all pregnancies.)

5. The following is paraphrased from an article published some years ago: "Among persons 25–64 years of age, the annual mortality rate in 1970 from coronary heart disease among edentulous men was 347.6 per 100,000 person-years compared to a rate of 215.1 per 100,000 person-years among men who had at least some teeth left. These data support the hypothesis that under-nutrition and/or lack of mastication play a role in the genesis of coronary heart disease." Despite the age restriction employed by the authors, it is likely that the comparison made is confounded by age. How can this be? Does the presence of confounding by age exaggerate or minimize whatever true difference may be present?

6. Shapiro et al. (2000) examined the association between cigar smoking and death from tobacco-related cancers in a prospective cohort study. The authors chose to restrict their analysis to the men in the total cohort who had never regularly smoked cigarettes, and so conceded that their results "may not be generalizable to cigar smokers who have previously smoked cigarettes." Nonetheless, there are at least two arguments in support of the authors' decision to exclude men who had smoked cigarettes. First, if the absolute impact of cigar smoking risk were the same in smokers and nonsmokers of cigarettes, the relative impact would be greater in the latter (who, relative to cigarette smokers, are at lower risk of cancer). What is a second argument?

7. Using data obtained in a prospective cohort study, let us say you observe that the incidence of cancer among persons in the upper fourth of the distribution of serum beta carotene is 60% that of persons in the lower three-fourths. In that study, the intake of a particular vegetable, V, was ascertained. But the instrument used to ascertain V did so in only a cursory way. Because V contains nutrients other than beta carotene that might reduce cancer risk, you would like to adjust for intake of V when assessing the association between beta carotene levels and cancer. When you do this, the RR associated with being in the upper fourth of the serum beta carotene distribution is now 0.8 instead of 0.6.

   If V intake could have been measured more accurately, and thus confounding by V more completely controlled, would you expect the adjusted RR associated with high serum beta carotene levels to have been:

   (a) Less than 0.8
   (b) 0.8
   (c) Greater than 0.8
   Why?

ANSWERS

1. (a) Crude incidence, 1990:

   White males   2,833/9,243,000 = 0.307 per 1000 person-years

   Black males   120/1,229,000 = 0.0976 per 1000 person-years

   $$\text{Relative incidence} = \frac{0.307}{0.0976} = 3.14.$$

(b)

AGE (YEARS)	AGE-SPECIFIC INCIDENCE PER 1000 PERSON-YEARS, 1990, BLACK MALES (1)	1990 WHITE MALE POPULATION (THOUSANDS) (2)	(1) × (2)
0–54	.0184	7,574	139.48
55–59	.270	388	104.86
60–64	.471	382	179.76
65–69	.900	346	311.40
70–74	.952	265	252.38
75–84	1.29	288	370.29
			1358.18

Incidence of bladder cancer in black males, adjusted to the age distribution of white males = 1358.18/9,243,000 = 0.147 per 1000 person-years.

Ratio of adjusted rates = 0.307/0.147 = 2.09.

The age-adjusted incidence of bladder cancer in black males is higher than the crude incidence, because it is based on a population distribution—that of white males—which is older than that of the black males themselves. Note, for example, that males in the youngest category, 0–54 years, constitute only 7,574,000/9,243,000 = 81.9% of the total in whites, as opposed to 1,086,000/1,229,000 = 88.4% of the total in blacks. Therefore, the ratio of age-adjusted rates will be lower than the ratio of the crude rates (2.09 versus 3.14).

2. Crude mortality rate ratio $= \dfrac{3/3911}{28/44,056} = 1.21.$

Age-adjusted mortality rate ratio (see Table 11–2)

$$= \frac{0 \cdot 10,485/11,987 + 2 \cdot 21,930/23,908 + 1 \cdot 11,641/12,072}{1 \cdot 1,502/11,987 + 5 \cdot 1,978/23,908 + 22 \cdot 431/12,072}$$

$$= 2.11.$$

The crude rate ratio was spuriously low because age was a confounding factor:

- Men who used a hair coloring product were younger, on average, than other men, as indicated by the different distributions of person-years across the three age groups; and
- Mortality rates from prostate cancer were seen to increase with increasing age.

Adjustment nullified the mortality advantage of the hair coloring group that resulted from their younger age, leading to an adjusted rate ratio that was higher than the crude one.

3. Confounding by gender. Men have higher creatinine levels than women, and the proportion of cases who are men is greater than the proportion of controls.

4. Even if it were believed that glucose levels were associated with gestational age at delivery, it would not be appropriate to match on this variable (or to otherwise adjust for it in the analysis). In this study of women without GDM, you are seeking to estimate the association between elevated glucose levels and RDS through whatever means those elevated levels may be acting, including a predisposition to premature delivery. (Only if a different hypothesis were being investigated—the relationship of blood glucose to RDS among infants delivered at a given gestational age—should matching on this variable be considered.)

5. Within the 25–64-year age stratum, there is probably a strong relationship between increasing age and both being edentulous and mortality from coronary heart disease. Since edentulous men are older, on average, than other men, in the absence of further adjustment for age their mortality rate from coronary heart disease will be falsely high relative to that in other men.

6. There may be errors in ascertaining cigarette-smoking history, or information may not have been sought about the part of the history which is of greatest etiologic relevance. Either of these would allow for the possibility of residual confounding when trying to adjust for differences in cigarette smoking between men who do and do not smoke cigars.

7. The correct answer is c. Incomplete adjustment for the confounding variable, intake of V, will result in an adjusted relative risk that is spuriously close to the crude relative risk. Therefore, since incomplete adjustment led to an increase in the relative risk of cancer associated with high levels of serum beta carotene—from an unadjusted relative risk of 0.6 to 0.8—more complete adjustment would be expected to lead to a relative risk that would be higher still.

REFERENCES

Alpha-Tocopherol, Beta Carotene Cancer Prevention Study Group. The effect of vitamin E and beta carotene on the incidence of lung cancer and other cancers in male smokers. N Engl J Med 1994; 330:1029–35.

Breslow NE, Day NE. Statistical methods in cancer research. Volume I: The analysis of case-control studies. Lyon, France: International Agency for Research on Cancer, 1980.

Breslow NE, Day NE. Statistical methods in cancer research. Volume II: The analysis of cohort studies. Lyon, France: International Agency for Research on Cancer, 1987.

Breslow NE, Day NE, Halvorsen KT, Prentice RL, Sabai C. Estimation of multiple relative risk functions in matched case-control studies. Am J Epidemiol 1978; 108:299–307.

Clayton D, Hills M. Statistical models in epidemiology. New York: Oxford University Press, 1993.

D'Agostino J R B. Propensity score methods for bias reduction in the comparison of a treatment to a non-randomized control group. Stat Med 1998; 17:2265–81.

Daling JR, Emanuel I. Induced abortion and subsequent outcome of pregnancy. Lancet 1975; 2:170–78.

Day NE. "A new measure of age-standardized incidence, the cumulative rate." In: Doll R, Payne P, Waterhouse J (eds.). Cancer incidence in five continents, Vol. 3. Geneva, Switzerland: International Union Against Cancer, 1976.

Holford TR. Multivariate methods in epidemiology. New York: Oxford University Press, 2002.

Linn S, Schoenbaum SC, Monson RR, Rosner B, Stubblefield PG, Ryan KJ. No association between coffee consumption and adverse outcomes of pregnancy. N Engl J Med 1982; 306:141–45.

Mantel N, Haenszel W. Statistical aspects of the analysis of data from retrospective studies of disease. J Natl Cancer Inst 1959; 22:719–48.

McCullagh P, Nelder JA. Generalized linear models. London: Chapman and Hall, 1989.

Omenn GS, Goodman GE, Thornquist MD, Balmes J, Cullen MR, Glass A, et al. Effects of a combination of beta carotene and vitamin A on lung cancer and cardiovascular disease. N Engl J Med 1996; 334:1150–55.

Rosenbaum PR, Rubin DB. The central role of the propensity score in observational studies for causal effects. Biometrics 1983; 70:41–55.

Rothman KJ, Greenland S. Modern epidemiology (2nd ed.). Philadelphia: Lippincott-Raven, 1998.

Rubin DB. Estimating causal effects from large data sets using propensity scores. Ann Intern Med 1997; 127:757–63.

Sasieni PD, Adams J. Standardized lifetime risk. Am J Epidemiol 1999; 149:869–75.

Schiffman MH, Schatzkin A. Test reliability is critically important to molecular epidemiology: an example from studies of human papillomavirus infection and cervical neoplasia. Cancer Res 1994; 54 Suppl:1944s–47s.

Selvin S. Statistical analysis of epidemiologic data (2nd ed.). New York: Oxford University Press, 1996.

Selvin S. Epidemiologic analysis: a case-oriented approach. New York: Oxford University Press, 2001.

Shapiro JA, Jacobs EJ, Thun MJ. Cigar smoking in men and risk of death from tobacco-related cancers. J Natl Cancer Inst 2000; 92:333–37.

Victora CG, Smith PG, Vaughan JP, Nobre LC, Lombardi C, Teixeira AM, et al. Evidence for protection by breast-feeding against infant deaths from infectious diseases in Brazil. Lancet 1987; 2:319–22.

12

ECOLOGICAL STUDIES

> No man is an island, entire of itself; every man is a piece of the continent, a part
> of the main.
>
> John Donne

Most U.S. citizens are legally entitled to own a gun for personal protection, but
whether it is to a person's advantage to do so has long been a matter of debate
(Cummings and Weiss, 1998; Kleck and Gertz, 1995). Some argue that keeping a
gun in the home can deter criminals and allow potential victims to defend themselves. Others argue that brandishing a gun may provoke gunfire from an intruder,
and that easy access to a gun in the home may escalate a domestic conflict into
firearm violence.

In 1993, Killias reported on a study that sought to clarify the relationship
between gun ownership and the risk of homicide or suicide (Killias, 1993). A random sample of households in 14 nations had participated in an international crime
survey, which yielded country-specific estimates of the proportion of households
with a gun. This information was then combined with death rates due to homicide
in each country. (Data from Northern Ireland were excluded because deaths from
explosions during civil strife there could not be separated from firearm deaths.)

Table 12–1 shows the results for homicides by any mechanism. The prevalence
of gun ownership was found to have a significant positive correlation with the
homicide rate. The prevalence of gun ownership was also positively correlated
with the death rates for gun-related homicides, for all suicides, and for gun-related
suicides, and with the proportions of homicides and of suicides due to guns. The
article concluded that "the correlations detected in this study suggest that the
presence of a gun in the home increases the likelihood of homicide or suicide."

The Killias study is an example of an *ecological* study. Ecological studies
examine exposure–disease associations *among* groups of people. In other words,
they seek to determine how the frequency of exposure in each of several groups is
related to the frequency of disease in that group.

Ecological studies are commonly undertaken for one of two reasons. First,
only aggregate information on exposure in each group may be available to the
investigator, even though exposure status does actually vary among individuals

Table 12–1. Proportion of Households with a Gun, Death Rate from Homicide, and Approximate 1990 Population in 13 Countries

COUNTRY	PERCENT OF HOUSEHOLDS WITH A GUN	HOMICIDE RATE[a]	APPROX. 1990 POPULATION[b]
Australia	19.6	19.5	16.7
Belgium	16.6	18.5	9.9
Canada	29.1	26.0	27.1
England and Wales	4.7	6.7	47.1
Finland	23.2	29.6	4.9
France	22.6	12.5	55.4
Netherlands	1.9	11.8	14.7
Norway	32.0	12.1	4.2
Scotland	4.7	16.3	5.1
Spain	13.1	13.7	40.5
Switzerland	27.2	11.7	6.2
United States	48.0	75.9	248.0
West Germany	8.9	12.1	60.7

[a] Homicides per million person-years.
[b] In millions.
[*Source:* Killias (1993); World Almanac (1990).]

within each group. For example, in the Killias study, only information about the prevalence of gun ownership was available for each country, not the gun-ownership status of each individual within each country. Hence there was no way to determine from the data available whether a particular homicide victim in one of the study countries was any more or less likely to own a gun than were other individuals in that country. Each of the 13 countries became a single unit of observation. In these circumstances, exposure–disease associations at the population level are commonly studied as a proxy for exposure–disease associations at the individual level. As we shall see, there are several potential pitfalls involved in making this inference across levels.

Second, the exposure of interest may actually vary only at the population level, not among individuals within the study populations. For example, legal penalties for drinking and driving vary among states, but everyone within a state is subject to the same state law. In these circumstances, exposure–disease associations must necessarily be examined at the aggregate level because there is no variation in exposure within a group.

In principle, the aggregate populations in ecological studies can be of any size, including households, classrooms, workplaces, communities, geographic regions, or entire nations. Most often they are geopolitically defined populations for which the necessary data are routinely collected, inasmuch as most ecological studies use existing data.

Helpful reviews of the uses of ecological studies and the special methodological issues that arise in them have been published by Morgenstern (1982; 1995; 1998), Walter (1991a; 1991b), and Susser (1994a; 1994b).

Ecological studies are really a class of study designs, not a single design. Whether aggregate populations or individuals are the units of study is one dimension on which study designs can be distinguished from each other. In other respects, ecological designs can be classified in much the same way as studies of individuals (see Chapter 5). For example:

- *Group-randomized trials.* Community intervention trials involve assigning entire communities at random to intervention or control conditions. They are the ecological counterparts to randomized trials of individuals. For example, the COMMIT study randomized 11 pairs of communities to either a community-wide antismoking campaign or no intervention (COMMIT Research Group, 1995a,b). After the campaign had been implemented, smoking prevalence was compared between the paired intervention and control communities.
- *Ecological cohort studies.* Disease rates can be compared between a set of exposed populations and a set of non-exposed control populations, even if the investigator had no control over which populations were exposed. For example, Jablon and colleagues (1991) compared cancer incidence and mortality rates in 107 counties that contained or were near a nuclear facility with rates in 292 matched control counties from the same regions.
- *Cross-sectional ecological studies.* Two or more characteristics that pertain to the same point in time or time period can be compared among several study populations, as in Killias's cross-national study of gun ownership and homicide rates.
- *Longitudinal ecological studies.* Studies of changes in disease rates over time in entire populations correspond to longitudinal studies of individuals. For example, Villaveces and colleagues (2000) compared homicide rates in Cali and Bogotá, Colombia, during periods with and without a citywide ban on carrying guns.

LEVELS OF MEASUREMENT

Populations are made up of individuals—a statement that highlights two levels of aggregation at which characteristics relevant to disease occurrence can be measured. *Individual-level* measures are familiar, such as a person's age, gender, gun-ownership status, and so on. Individual-level measurements, however, are often unavailable in an ecological study.

Population-level measures can be divided into two kinds:

- An *aggregate* measure simply summarizes the distribution of an individual-level factor that may vary within a population—in other words, it is a statistic derived from individual-level data. For example, mean age, median age, and proportion of persons aged 65 years or older are all different ways to distill the age distribution of population members into a single population-level number. Aggregate measures have also been termed *derived* or *contextual* variables (Susser, 1994a; Von Korff et al., 1992; Diez-Roux, 1998).

  Note that an aggregate measure of an individual characteristic can take on new meaning at the population level by describing a feature of the environment people live in. Returning to the issue of gun ownership and homicide, a person's risk of becoming a homicide victim may be influenced not only by whether he or she owns a gun, but also by the general availability of firearms in the community, as reflected by the population prevalence of gun ownership. Hence both individual gun ownership and population prevalence of gun ownership, which are the same characteristic measured at two different levels, could affect a person's homicide risk by different means.

- An *intrinsically population-level* measure (termed an *integral* measure by some authors [Pickett and Pearl, 2001; Susser, 1994a; Selvin and Hagstrom, 1963]) characterizes an entire population as a unit. For example, a city's size, its population density, and whether it has a law requiring registration of handguns are all intrinsically city-level characteristics. Each of them automatically applies to all members of a population, so there is no individual-level variation on such a factor within the population. One important class of intrinsically population-level measures is the presence of policies or programs that apply to all members of a population and that may affect disease risk.

More generally, populations may be divided up at several possible levels of aggregation, and hence of measurement—census tract, city, state, and nation are examples—which may be nested within each other to form a hierarchy of levels. *Multi-level modeling,* discussed later, is an analytic approach that can deal with data at multiple levels of aggregation. For present purposes, however, two levels are enough to introduce the main methodological issues in ecological studies, including special problems that arise when only aggregate-level data are available. Hence the rest of this chapter concerns just two levels, which are sometimes termed the *macro* and *micro* levels.

STUDYING EFFECTS OF INDIVIDUAL-LEVEL EXPOSURES

As noted earlier, one of the main uses of ecological studies in epidemiology has been to study the relationship between an individual-level exposure and individual-level disease risk, having the association between exposure prevalence and disease frequency at the population level serve as a proxy for the individual-level association of real interest. A close look at the author's conclusion in the Killias study shows that it fits this description. The analysis involved examining only cross-national associations between the prevalence of gun ownership and death rates, but the conclusion inferred an association at the individual level.

Historically noteworthy examples of ecological studies that sought to identify individual-level associations include:

- Smoking and lung cancer. Lung cancer mortality rates were found to be higher in countries where per capita tobacco sales were higher, which was used to support the inference that smoking causes lung cancer (Advisory Committee to the Surgeon General, 1964).
- Poverty and pellagra. Goldberger and colleagues (1920) found pellagra to be more common in South Carolina cotton mill villages where a higher proportion of men had per capita incomes below $6 or $8 per month. As summarized in Chapter 7, they went on to show that this association held at the individual level and appeared to be explained by income-related differences in diet.
- Fluoride in drinking water and dental caries. Dean (1938) observed that the prevalence of dental caries was lower among children in several midwestern communities that had relatively high fluoride content in their drinking water.

Advantages

One of the chief attractions of using ecological studies to examine individual-level associations is that pre-existing population-level data may be readily available. If so, an ecological study can be completed relatively quickly and at low cost.

A second advantage can arise when exposure frequency varies substantially *between* populations but not very much *within* populations. This situation is sketched in Figure 12–1, in which the exposure and outcome variables are assumed to be continuous for illustration. By construction, the true relation between exposure and outcome is positive and linear, with random error around a common regression line. Each rectangle encloses the individual-level observations from one of three hypothetical communities. Exposure varies only over a fairly narrow range within each community, but the mean exposure level varies considerably among

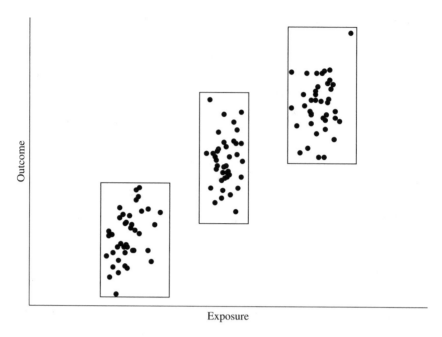

Figure 12–1. Example Showing Substantial Between-Population Variation in Exposure, But Little Within-Population Variation.

the communities. As a result, the underlying linear relation between exposure and outcome is easy to detect if data from all three communities are considered (Pearson's $r = .90$), but less evident within each community ($r = .42, .04,$ and $.20$, respectively).

For example, Rose noted that studying the relationship between water hardness and mortality from cardiovascular disease using traditional case-control methods within British regions would have been futile: nearly everyone obtained most of their water from public water supplies, resulting in relatively uniform exposure to hard or soft water within a region. Among regions, however, water hardness varied widely and permitted detection of an inverse association (Rose, 1985). Similarly, relatively large geographical and cultural differences in dietary fat intake may make it easier to detect associations between dietary fat and the incidence of breast cancer in ecological studies than in individual-level studies within geographical regions (Goodwin and Boyd, 1987).

A third advantage can become important if the exposure is subject to a high degree of measurement error or short-term biological variation at the individual level (Piantadosi et al., 1988; Susser, 1994a,b). If so, then aggregation of individual measurements to the population level can reduce the effects of such errors, enabling detection of associations that might otherwise be missed (Prentice and Sheppard, 1995).

Example: The association between dietary salt intake and blood pressure has appeared stronger in between-population studies than in within-population studies (Law et al., 1991; Frost et al., 1991). Daily salt intake has often been measured using 24-hour urinary sodium excretion. Liu and colleagues (1979) found sodium excretion to be highly variable from day to day in the same person, with *intra*-individual variance that was 3.2 times greater than *inter*-individual variance. Frost and colleagues (1991) used this result to show that this high intra-individual variability "diluted" the slope of the regression relation between sodium intake and blood pressure within a population to between 1/4 and 1/2 of its true value. Between-population studies were less affected by intra-individual variance because they aggregated measurements over many individuals. Once these sources of variation were accounted for statistically, the findings of between-population and within-population studies could be reconciled.

Estimating Attributable Risk and Relative Risk

The results of ecological studies are sometimes reported simply in terms of correlation coefficients, which at least reflect the direction and strength of the group-level association between exposure prevalence and disease rate. For the Killias study data in Table 12–1, the Pearson correlation between prevalence of gun ownership and homicide rate among countries is +.73, and the Spearman rank correlation is +.47, both suggesting moderately strong positive associations.

For epidemiologic purposes, however, relative risk and attributable risk are more informative measures of association and are easier to compare with results from other kinds of studies. Point estimates of relative risk and attributable risk can be obtained from ecological data using a generalization of a method described by Morgenstern (1982, 1995):

1. Apply regression analysis to the group-level data, modeling disease rate as a function of exposure prevalence. Several forms of regression can be used for this purpose, as described below.
2. Use the fitted regression model to predict the disease rate for a population in which everyone is exposed. Call that rate R_1. Similarly, predict the rate for a population in which nobody is exposed, and call that rate R_0.
3. Estimate relative risk as R_1/R_0 and attributable risk as $R_1 - R_0$.

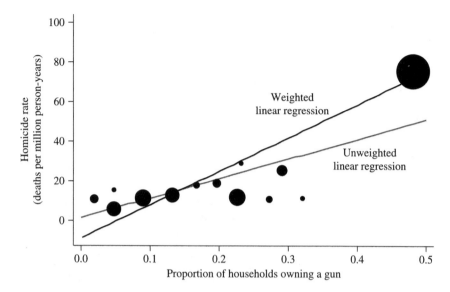

Figure 12-2. Two Linear Regression Analyses of Ecological Data from Table 12-1.

Although we will later note several pitfalls in inferring individual-level associations from ecological data, the data from the Killias study shown in Table 12–1 can be used to illustrate the calculations and some problems that can arise.

Figure 12–2 shows a scatterplot of homicide rate against prevalence of gun ownership. The area of each country's plotted circle is proportional to its population. The thinner regression line was fitted by linear least-squares regression, which gives each country equal weight.

A theoretically preferable analysis would give greater weight to data from larger countries, for which homicide rates were based on larger populations and thus are subject to less sampling error (Piantadosi et al., 1988; Walter, 1991b). The thicker regression line in Figure 12–2 was fitted by weighted least-squares regression. The data for each country were weighted by its estimated 1990 population. Note how the large data point at the upper right (the U.S.) "pulls" the regression line toward it.

One problem with using linear regression for this purpose is that the predicted rate in a fully exposed population (R_1) or in a fully non-exposed population (R_0) can be negative—which is, of course, impossible for a rate. In Figure 12–2, R_0 corresponds to the y-intercept of each regression line. In this instance, it is negative for the weighted regression, which might be the theoretically preferred model *a priori*. A negative value for R_0 also leads to a nonsensical negative estimate of relative risk.

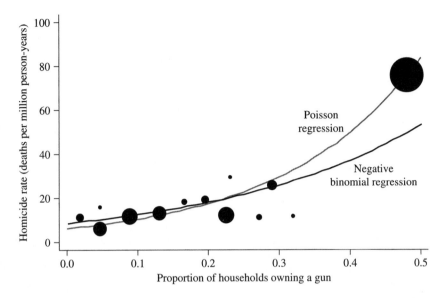

Figure 12-3. Poisson and Negative Binomial Regression Analyses of Ecological Data from Table 12-1.

The problem of impossible R_0 and R_1 values can be avoided by switching to a different form of regression. As described in Chapter 11, Poisson regression assumes a linear relation between log(rate) and the predictor variables (here, prevalence of gun ownership). Negative binomial regression posits a similar model form but also allows for extra-Poisson variation in rates. Both methods always lead to positive values for R_0 and R_1. Figure 12–3 shows Poisson regression and negative binomial regression curves fitted to the Killias study data. Plotted on the same arithmetic scale as before, the curves are exponential in shape.

Table 12–2 summarizes results from all four regression models. They all suggest a strong positive association between prevalence of gun ownership and homicide risk, but the estimates of relative and attributable risk vary greatly among models. Another look at Figures 12–2 and 12–3 clarifies why this is so. Relative risk and attributable risk depend on R_0 and R_1. We noted earlier that R_0 corresponds to the y-intercept. R_1 corresponds to the height of the regression curve where it crosses a vertical line at a gun-ownership prevalence of 1.0, which is far off to the right. This point lies well beyond the range of prevalence values actually observed in the 13 countries on which the regressions were based. Subtle differences in curve shape become greatly magnified when extrapolated that far, leading to very different predictions for R_1.

Because the number of population data points in an ecological study is often small, there may be very limited power to determine whether one model form

Table 12–2. Results from Ecological Regression Analyses of Data in Table 12–1

ANALYSIS	R_0	R_1	RELATIVE RISK[a]	ATTRIBUTABLE RISK[a]
Linear least-squares				
Unweighted	1.4	100.1	71.5	98.7
Weighted	−8.0	159.9	?	168.9
Poisson	6.1	1135.0	186.1	1128.9
Negative binomial	9.0	317.1	35.2	308.1

Rates shown as deaths per million person-years.

[a] Exposed = gun owner; non-exposed = gun non-owner.

fits significantly better than another (Greenland, 1992; Richardson et al., 1987). Accordingly, estimates of attributable and relative risk must often be viewed only as rough approximations. In this instance, a comparison of goodness-of-fit statistics (not shown) across models indicates that the negative binomial model fits the data best, suggesting that the bottom row of Table 12–2 may contain the most credible estimates of relative and attributable risk.

Pitfalls

Ecological studies of individual-level associations between exposure and disease are vulnerable to several potential sources of bias, some of which have no direct counterpart in studies of individuals.

To continue with the gun ownership and homicide example, so far several ways of viewing the data in Table 12–1 have led to the same general conclusion. Scatterplots, regression analyses, correlation coefficients, attributable risks, and relative risks have all basically suggested a positive association between gun ownership and homicide risk. But now consider the hypothetical data in Table 12–3 from an imaginary study, similar in design to the Killias study, but for simplicity confined to just four countries. As in the Killias study, at the country level, the homicide rate is positively associated with the prevalence of gun ownership. In fact, by construction, there is a perfect linear relation between these two country-level variables.

But the key feature of Table 12–3 is that we are allowed to peek at the individual-level data behind the country-specific homicide rates and prevalences of gun ownership on which the ecological analysis was based. Surprisingly, within each country, the homicide rate among gun owners is actually only *half* the rate among gun non-owners. The individual-level association is not even in the same direction as the association seen in the population-level data.

Table 12–3. Hypothetical Results of an Ecological Study of Gun Ownership and Homicide, Illustrating Cross-Level Bias

| | Ecological Data | | Individual-Level Data | | | | | | |
| | | | Gun Owners | | | Gun Non-Owners | | | |
COUNTRY	PREVALENCE OF GUN OWNERSHIP	HOMICIDE RATE[a]	HOMICIDES	POP. AT RISK[b]	HOMICIDE RATE[a]	HOMICIDES	POP. AT RISK[b]	HOMICIDE RATE[a]	RELATIVE RISK
A	.20	21.0	210	18	11.7	1680	72	23.3	0.50
B	.22	22.0	408	33	12.4	2892	117	24.7	0.50
C	.26	24.0	359	26	13.8	2041	74	27.6	0.50
D	.34	28.0	1147	68	16.9	4453	132	33.7	0.50

[a] Homicides per million person-years.
[b] In millions.

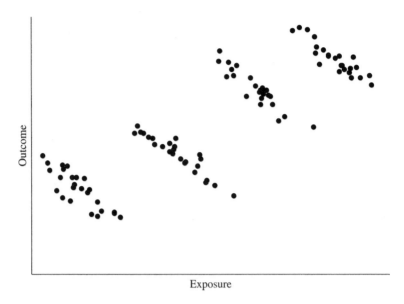

Figure 12–4. Example of Different Population-Level and Individual-Level Associations Between Continuous Exposure and Outcome Variables.

Figure 12–4 illustrates the same phenomenon graphically for continuous exposure and outcome variables. *Within* each of four populations, as exposure increases, outcome decreases. But *across* populations, as the mean exposure level increases, the mean level or rate of the outcome increases.

The hypothetical data in Table 12–3 and Figure 12–4 show that associations at the population level need not necessarily reflect associations of similar magnitude, or even of similar direction, at the individual level. The *ecological fallacy* occurs when a population-level association is erroneously taken to imply a similar individual-level association. It is an inferential pitfall long known to sociologists (Robinson, 1950). More generally, *cross-level bias* occurs when an association at one level of aggregation is assumed to represent the association at another level, when in fact the associations at the two levels are unequal.

Unfortunately, the kind of detailed individual-level data shown on the right side of Table 12–3 are seldom available in an ecological study. (If they were, the motivation for the ecological analysis might vanish altogether.) Hence there is usually no way to determine empirically whether cross-level bias is present and, if so, how large it is. Perhaps the best available defense is to understand situations that can lead to this bias, including:

- *Group-level association between exposure prevalence and baseline disease rate.* Here, "baseline" rate refers to the rate in *non-exposed* persons. For example, in Table 12–3, the prevalence of gun ownership rises steadily from .20 to .34 as we scan down the rows, while the homicide rate in gun *non*-owners rises steadily from 23.3 to 33.7 per million person-years. Thus, country itself is a group-level confounder: it is associated with both the outcome (in non-exposed persons) and with exposure level. This is an epidemiologic version of conditions first described by Firebaugh (1978) as necessary and sufficient to produce cross-level bias in sociological data.

Such a group-level association between exposure prevalence and baseline disease rate can, in turn, arise in several ways:

— The groups may differ on the distribution of one or more extraneous individual-level risk factors, such as age and gender. For example, if young males are likelier to own guns and are also at greater risk for homicide, then a country whose population is heavily weighted toward young males may have both a high prevalence of gun ownership and a high baseline homicide rate.

— An intrinsically group-level factor may be a confounder. For example, lax law enforcement could be associated both with widespread gun ownership and with high homicide rates in gun non-owners.

— The exposure itself may have effects at the group level above and beyond its effects at the individual level. In other words, an individual's risk may depend not only on his or her own exposure status, but also on the exposure status of other individuals in the group. For example, homicide risk to a gun non-owner may be greater in a country where owning a gun is common than where it is rare.

An important special case of this phenomenon in infectious disease epidemiology is *herd immunity*. A person's risk of developing a certain contagious disease can depend not only on his or her own immune status, but also on whether a large proportion of people with whom he or she comes in contact are immune (Fine, 1993). Higher prevalence of immunity can reduce the frequency of contacts between infectious individuals and susceptible individuals in the population. If the frequency of such contacts is lowered to the point that each new case transmits the disease to an average of less than one susceptible person, then the occurrence of new cases must decline over time, causing the epidemic to die out before all susceptibles have been infected. Based on this concept, mathematical modeling of disease spread has been used to try to estimate the critical prevalence of immunity needed to control an epidemic (Anderson and May, 1991).

- *Unequal distribution of an effect modifier across groups.* Greenland and Morgenstern (1989) present a hypothetical example in which esophageal cancer incidence in nonsmokers is the same across groups, but the incidence among smokers varies across groups because a characteristic that enhances smoking's harmful effect is more common in some groups than in others. In their example, an ecological analysis suggests a spurious inverse association between smoking and esophageal cancer, although more generally a bias in either direction could result. Piantadosi (1994) also discusses the statistical basis for this phenomenon.
- *Model misspecification.* For many graded exposures, the relationship between exposure and risk at the individual level is nonlinear. In an ecological study, the only available data may be the mean exposure level for each group, which cannot capture information about the distribution of individuals among different exposure levels. The same mean exposure level could result from most individuals falling near the mean, or from two subgroups at opposite ends of the exposure range. These two patterns could correspond to quite different expected overall disease rates. Moreover, in the ecological analysis, the number of groups available for study may be small. As a result, a simple linear or log-linear model between disease rate and mean exposure level may appear to fit the ecological data adequately, even though it is actually a poor reflection of the individual-level relationship of real interest (Greenland, 1992).

Measurement error and control of confounding factors also pose special challenges in ecological studies. As discussed in Chapter 10, in individual-level studies, nondifferential misclassification of exposure normally biases estimates of excess risk toward the null value. In ecological studies, however, nondifferential error in exposure measurement can have just the opposite effect, causing estimates of excess risk to be biased *away* from the null (Brenner et al., 1992). If sensitivity and specificity data for the measure of exposure are available, the size of this nonconservative bias can be estimated and a correction made (Greenland and Brenner, 1993).

Control over confounding factors can also be hard to achieve with ecological data. Confounders can operate at either the individual or the group level. Some may have nonlinear associations with disease risk at the individual level, making it difficult to remove confounding by them if only group-level means are available (Greenland and Morgenstern, 1989; Greenland, 1992; Greenland and Robins, 1994). For many of the diseases considered in Chapter 7, for example, nonlinear associations are seen between incidence or mortality and age. The possibility of nonlinear associations motivates using more finely detailed information about distribution of the confounder in each group, if this information is available. For example, rather than including just mean age in a group-level regression analysis in an attempt to remove confounding by age, better control may be gained by including several age-related variables, each of which reflects the proportion of group members falling into a particular age group (Greenland and Robins, 1994).

Rate standardization (see Chapter 11) can also be used to control confounding in ecological studies—for example, by using the age-adjusted rate, rather than the crude rate, for each group. It then becomes important to standardize the prevalence of exposure and of other covariates to the same reference population (Greenland and Robins, 1994).

Sometimes the researcher has choices in designing an ecological study, such as what kind of groups to study and on what basis to select those studied. Greenland (1992) notes that ecological studies should theoretically be less prone to bias when within-group variation in exposure is small but between-group variation in exposure prevalence is large. On the other hand, to prevent confounding, it is preferable that groups be similar to each other on potential confounders—a condition that can be hard to satisfy while simultaneously seeking to maximize exposure heterogeneity between groups.

In view of the many ways ecological studies can go wrong as a method of estimating individual-level associations, one might wonder why any self-respecting epidemiologist would choose to venture into such a minefield of possible biases. Indeed, some have argued that ecological studies should be used only for hypothesis generation (Piantadosi, 1994). Even that limited role would be hard to justify if these studies were just as likely to mislead as to point toward the truth.

Piantadosi and colleagues (1988) conducted one of the few studies in which the magnitude of ecological bias could be examined empirically with real data. They carried out parallel ecological and individual-level analyses of the associations between several pairs of variables in the Second National Health and Nutrition Examination Survey. Figure 12–5 plots the state-level correlation against the corresponding individual-level correlation for each of 13 pairs of variables: that is, the figure shows the correlation between correlations. While anomalies did occur in which the state-level and individual-level correlations had different signs (e.g., for race and weight), it is reassuring to note a general correspondence between associations at the two levels in their direction and magnitude. How generally this correspondence holds is, of course, unknown. For our earlier example of gun ownership and homicide, at least, individual-level case-control studies have also found a positive association between owning a gun and homicide risk (e.g., Kellermann et al., 1993), supporting one of the broad conclusions reached in the Killias study.

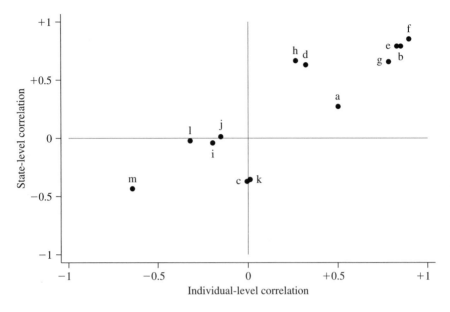

Key:

Point label	Variable #1	Variable #2
a	Height	Weight
b	Weight	Body mass index
c	Height	Body mass index
d	Age	Body mass index
e	Calories	Protein
f	Calories	Fat
g	Protein	Fat
h	Income	Education
i	Race	Income
j	Race	Education
k	Race	Weight
l	Sex	Weight
m	Sex	Height

Figure 12–5. Scatterplot of State-Level vs. Individual-Level Correlations for 13 Pairs of Variables in NHANES II (based on Piantadosi et al., 1988).

STUDYING EFFECTS OF GROUP-LEVEL EXPOSURES

A second main application of ecological designs in epidemiology is to study the health effects of group-level characteristics. One such use is to evaluate programs and policies that apply to entire populations.

Example: During the 1990s, several U.S. states passed laws making gun owners criminally liable if a child gained unsupervised access to a gun and injured him- or herself or someone else. Cummings and colleagues (1997) sought to determine whether the presence of such a law was associated with lower rates of firearm death in children.

The number of child suicides, homicides, and unintentional deaths due to firearms and the number of children at risk were obtained over the Internet from the National Center for Health Statistics for all possible groups formed by simultaneous stratification on age category, gender, race, state, and calendar year from 1979–1994. During this period, 12 states had enacted such laws, which took effect on various dates. Each group of children was considered exposed if a law was in effect in that state for six months or more of that calendar year; otherwise, the group was considered non-exposed. Negative binomial regression was used to model the number of firearm deaths as a function of the number of children at risk, state, calendar year, and the presence of a qualifying safe-firearm-storage law. Age, gender, and race were also examined as potential confounders but had little impact on the results once state and calendar year were included in the regression models.

When a safe-storage law was in effect, the incidence of unintentional firearm deaths among children under 15 years of age was 23% lower than expected ($RR = 0.77$, 95% C.I.: 0.63–0.94). Weaker negative associations were found with gun suicide ($RR = 0.81$, 95% C.I.: 0.66–1.01) and gun homicide ($RR = 0.89$, 95% C.I.: 0.76–1.05).

Here the exposure of interest was presence or absence of a safe-firearm-storage law—an intrinsically group-level characteristic that applied to all children in certain states in certain years. In a sense, this situation is a limiting case in which all of the variation in exposure is between groups, and none is within groups. We saw earlier that when ecological studies are used to study individual-level exposures by proxy, the need to extrapolate well beyond the exposure prevalences actually observed can lead to large errors in estimating relative risk and attributable risk. In happy contrast, when investigating group-level exposures, the study populations actually *were* either fully exposed or fully non-exposed, thus ameliorating this source of error. Cross-level bias is also of less concern, because the target level of inference is at the group level—the level at which such an exposure would be potentially modifiable. However, it is still possible for individual- or group-level confounding factors to bias the observed group-level association.

In this example, potential confounding was addressed by cross-classifying the study population by age, gender, race, state, and calendar time. Safe-storage laws were in effect for some of the resulting groups and not for others, but everyone in each group was either exposed or not exposed. Cross-classification permitted accounting for systematic variation in firearm mortality rates associated with the stratification factors, thus better isolating the remaining variation in rates associated with presence or absence of a law.

No doubt there were other unmeasured differences among groups that influenced firearm mortality rates, which contributed to extra-Poisson variation in rates (see Chapter 4). Negative binomial regression was used to account for this extra-Poisson variation, yielding wider but more defensible confidence limits around rate ratio estimates (McCullagh and Nelder, 1989; Gardner et al., 1995).

Ecological designs have been used to study health effects of a variety of other macro-level exposures, such as population income inequality in relation to mortality rates (Kaplan et al., 1996), vehicular traffic restrictions during the 1996 Olympic Games in relation to air quality and childhood asthma attacks (Friedman et al., 2001), and alcoholic beverage prices in relation to mortality from cirrhosis of the liver (Seeley, 1960). Blakely and Woodward (2000) have described several generic mechanisms by which ecological factors may affect individual health.

STUDYING EXPOSURES AT TWO OR MORE LEVELS AT ONCE

Broadly speaking, most diseases probably result from a complex "web" of risk factors operating at different levels. Even if an epidemiologic study focuses narrowly on a certain exposure, the researcher needs to consider other factors at the same or different levels as potential confounders or modifiers. Many ecological studies have only limited ability to do so because they rely on pre-existing group-level data. Individual-level studies may be carried out in only a single setting, or they may deliberately match or stratify study subjects on area of residence, thus controlling for neighborhood-level influences but precluding their study as exposures in their own right.

But in some situations, data are available or obtainable on factors at both the individual and the group levels. Proper analysis in such studies requires special statistical techniques, which fortunately are now quite widely available (Witte et al., 1998, 2000; Diez-Roux, 2000). Having information at more than one level can permit a richer and more complete conceptualization of how disease occurs, leading in turn to a wider range of opportunities for prevention (Diez-Roux, 1998; Susser, 1994a,b; Von Korff et al., 1992).

Example: Diez-Roux and colleagues (1997) studied associations between measures of neighborhood socioeconomic status and the prevalence of coronary heart disease (CHD), controlling for individual-level sociodemographic characteristics and known CHD risk factors. The investigators used data from the Atherosclerosis

Risk in Communities Study, which involved interviews and medical examinations on 12,601 adults aged 45–64 years in four U.S. communities (field centers) during 1987–1989. Each person's neighborhood was defined as the census block group in which he or she lived. Census block groups are predefined areas with about 1,000 inhabitants. Socioeconomic statistics were available from the 1990 U.S. census on each of the 567 block groups that included one or more study participants. For analysis, generalized linear mixed models for binary responses were used to model the presence or absence of CHD for each person as a function of individual- and neighborhood-level characteristics, all of which were included simultaneously in the regression models.

Table 12–4 shows results from three field centers in which most participants were white. In each row, the *OR* denotes the odds of CHD in a person

Table 12–4. Odds Ratios for Prevalent Coronary Heart Disease in Relation to Neighborhood Characteristics in Three Field Sites in the Atherosclerosis Risk in Communities Study

	Odds Ratios for 10th vs. 90th Percentile			
	Women		Men	
NEIGHBORHOOD CHARACTERISTIC	*OR*	(95% C.I.)	*OR*	(95% C.I.)
Adjusted for individual-level sociodemographic characteristics[a]				
Percent of adults who completed high school	1.88	(1.00–3.52)	0.82	(0.55–1.17)
Median household income	1.61	(1.11–2.87)	1.17	(0.88–1.53)
Median value of houses	2.17	(1.20–3.94)	1.15	(0.88–1.50)
Percent of persons in higher-class occupations	2.82	(1.29–6.16)	1.26	(0.92–1.71)
Adjusted for individual-level sociodemographic characteristics and CHD risk factors[b]				
Percent of adults who completed high school	2.54	(1.21–5.31)	0.89	(0.58–1.36)
Median household income	1.97	(1.07–3.62)	1.12	(0.81–1.56)
Median value of houses	2.58	(1.37–4.86)	1.11	(0.80–1.53)
Percent of persons in higher-class occupations	4.05	(1.56–10.40)	1.16	(0.81–1.66)

[a]Age, field center, individual indicators of social class, and interactions between field center and indicators of social class.

[b]LDL cholesterol, HDL cholesterol, cigarette smoking, systolic blood pressure, antihypertensive medication, diabetes, body mass index, Keys dietary score, leisure index, sports index, work index, and serum fibrinogen.

[*Source:* Adapted from Diez-Roux et al. (1997).]

whose neighborhood was at the 10th percentile on that characteristic (more disadvantaged), relative to the odds of CHD in a similar person whose neighborhood was at the 90th percentile on that characteristic (less disadvantaged). In the top part of the table, the ORs were adjusted only for individual-level sociodemographic characteristics and field center. In the bottom part, the ORs were adjusted also for several individual-level CHD risk factors, as identified in a footnote.

Among women, living in a disadvantaged neighborhood was associated with a 1.6-fold to 2.8-fold increased prevalence of CHD, after adjusting for individual-level sociodemographics and field center. These associations were even stronger after adjusting also for CHD risk factors. Among men, however, all of the associations with neighborhood socioeconomic factors were weaker and quite compatible with chance alone.

The individual-level risk factors had already been well studied and were not of main interest in this analysis, but multi-level modeling allowed the investigators to control for many such factors at once while examining associations with neighborhood characteristics. The differences in results between men and women in Table 12–4 suggest that gender may modify the association with neighborhood socioeconomic characteristics—an example of interaction across levels.

The analytic technique used in the Diez-Roux study is one of several methods that can be used for *multi-level* or *hierarchical* statistical modeling (Greenland, 2002; Diez-Roux, 2000; Witte et al., 2000, 1998; Bryk and Raudenbush, 1992). These techniques vary as to their statistical assumptions and modeling capabilities, but most importantly, they all allow for the possibility that observations on individuals within the same group may be correlated. Conventional multivariate analytic methods, such as those described in Chapter 11, assume independent observations. To the extent that this independence assumption is violated, the resulting regression coefficient estimates (or quantities derived from them, such as odds ratio estimates) and their confidence limits can be erroneous (Diez-Roux, 2000; O'Campo et al., 1995).

Pickett and Pearl (2001) summarized 25 studies in which both neighborhood-level and individual-level measures of socioeconomic status had been included in the same analysis as predictors of individual health outcomes. Their review identified many statistical approaches that have been used for multi-level analysis—unfortunately including some methods that are best avoided because they failed to account for non-independence of observations within neighborhoods. That limitation aside, Pickett and Pearl noted that in 23 of the 25 studies, significant associations with neighborhood socioeconomic status were found after adjusting for individual-level covariates, including individual socioeconomic status. This pattern lends empirical support to the concept of social context as a risk factor for ill health.

If such a group-level association is present, what might it represent? As in any observational study, the threat of a methodological artifact, such as measurement error or residual confounding, always lurks in the background. More substantive possibilities include:

- *Shared environmental exposures.* Living in a certain place can imply exposure to a physical and sociocultural environment that is common to everyone in that setting and that may influence disease risk.
- *Selection effects.* Living in a certain setting or belonging to a certain group can result instead from past self-selection. For example, people with asthma or allergies may relocate to a climate that they think offers cleaner, drier air free of allergens. To the extent that selective migration occurs, concentration of people with asthma or allergies in areas with clean, dry, allergen-free air should not imply that such a climate causes asthma or allergies.
- *Contagion.* For diseases that are transmissible from person to person— by any mechanism, including both biological and behavioral means—the prevalence of illness itself can affect the level of risk to susceptibles by influencing their chance of exposure. The disease becomes part of the environment. Prevalence can be a determinant of future incidence by other pathways as well, such as by influencing people's perceived vulnerability to disease and thereby altering their risk behavior.

CONCLUSION

Ecological studies have sometimes been disparaged as a relatively weak source of evidence in epidemiology because of their vulnerability to bias when group-level associations are studied as proxies for individual-level associations. As we have seen, that application of ecological studies is indeed based on strong and usually untestable assumptions, and cautious interpretation is warranted when the design is used for that purpose.

Yet many of those potential biases are greatly diminished or vanish altogether when ecological studies are used to study the effects of exposures that apply to an entire group. Accordingly, ecological studies can be a very useful tool for evaluating policies and programs—a theme to be explored further in Chapter 20.

In any case, our understanding of why certain people develop certain diseases can often be advanced by thinking about how people organize themselves into groups and how they interact within those groups. Ecological studies have a special role to play in translating those ideas into epidemiologic research.

EXERCISES

1. Researchers in England and Wales sought to investigate the relationship between vegetable consumption and risk of appendicitis (Barker et al., 1986). A National Food Survey had obtained detailed data on food purchases for about 150 households in each of 59 geographical areas for which data on hospital admissions for appendicitis were also available. Across these areas, the incidence of appendicitis was found to be negatively correlated with consumption of non-potato vegetables, chiefly green vegetables and tomatoes. The investigators noted that "Green vegetables and tomatoes may protect against appendicitis, possibly through an effect on the bacterial flora of the appendix."

   Based on the study design, what reservation might you have about concluding that if a person eats more green vegetables and tomatoes, his or her risk of developing appendicitis will be reduced?

2. Imagine an ecological study of the relationship between dietary intake of fish oil and mortality from coronary heart disease (CHD). For simplicity, suppose that only two communities are involved and that their populations are otherwise similar with regard to major risk factors for CHD. In Community A, 20% of the population has a diet high in fish oil, and CHD mortality is 100 deaths per 100,000 person-years. In Community B, 30% of the population has a high-fish-oil diet, and CHD mortality is 95 deaths per 100,000 person-years.

   (a) Assume that, at the population level, CHD mortality is linearly related to the prevalence of high fish oil consumption and that cross-level bias can be ignored. Estimate the relative risk and attributable risk of CHD mortality in relation to a high-fish-oil diet.

   (b) Now suppose that the *true* prevalence of a high-fish-oil diet is still 20% in Community A and 30% in Community B, but that these true prevalences cannot be measured directly. Instead, the prevalence of a high-fish-oil diet must be estimated in each community using a survey instrument that has sensitivity = 90% and specificity = 90% for such a diet. What would you expect the *observed* prevalence of a high-fish-oil diet to be in each community, based on the survey data?

   (c) Now recalculate the relative risk and attributable risk for CHD mortality in relation to a high-fish-oil diet, using the exposure prevalences you expect the survey to show. How do they compare to those calculated in part *(a)*?

3. Good information on socioeconomic status is sometimes unavailable from a data source that would otherwise be attractive for epidemiologic research.

"Geo-coding" is a technique that can sometimes be used to fill this gap when street addresses of study subjects are known. Geographic information systems are used to link each street address to a census tract, census block group, or other predefined area for which statistics on socioeconomic status are available from a recent census. For example, the median household income from the census block group in which an individual resides might be added to his or her data record as a proxy measure of income.

Suppose that a statewide case-control study of post-neonatal infant deaths is conducted, using birth certificates as the main source of controls and of exposure data. Geo-coding is used to impute household income. Address data on the mothers of all 150 cases and 150 controls are successfully linked to census block groups, and all mothers are found to have resided in different block groups.

Most of the study data would consist of individual-level characteristics gleaned from the birth certificates of cases and controls. But the imputed household income is actually a group-level measure pertaining to each subject's census block group. Would multi-level statistical methods be needed to do a proper analysis of data from this study?

ANSWERS

1. The study design was clearly ecological. We do not know that the specific people who got appendicitis were necessarily those who had diets low in green vegetables or tomatoes, only that they came from areas with low per capita consumption of these foodstuffs. The study could thus be vulnerable to the "ecological fallacy" (as well as confounding by other personal characteristics). The conclusion could, of course, be true, but studies on individuals would be desirable to confirm it.

2. (a) Because we are assuming a linear relation between CHD mortality and prevalence of a high-fish-oil diet, data from these two communities determine the slope and intercept of that line. In units of deaths per 100,000 person-years, its slope b is $(100 - 95)/(.20 - .30) = -50$. This value for b can then be applied to the data from either community to solve for the intercept a. Using data from Community A, $100 = a - 50(.20)$, so $a = 110$. The linear relation is thus

$$\text{CHD mortality} = 110 - (50 \times \text{prevalence})$$

Based on this equation, the predicted CHD mortality in a hypothetical community in which everyone followed a high-fish-oil diet would be

$R_1 = 110 - (50 \times 1) = 60$. CHD mortality in a community in which nobody followed such a diet would be $R_0 = 110 - (50 \times 0) = 110$. Hence the relative risk would be $R_1/R_0 = 60/110 = 0.55$, and the attributable risk would be $R_1 - R_0 = 60 - 110 = -50$ deaths per 100,000 person-years.

(b) Consider first Community A, in which the true prevalence of a high-fish-oil diet is 20%. In a random sample of, say, 100 people from Community A, there should be 20 people who truly followed a high-fish-oil diet and 80 who did not. If the dietary survey is 90% sensitive and 90% specific for a high-fish-oil diet, we would expect people in the sample to be distributed as follows:

| | True Intake | | |
SURVEY RESULT	HIGH	LOW	TOTAL
High	18	8	26
Low	2	72	74
Total	20	80	100

The observed prevalence of a high-fish-oil diet in the survey data should thus be $26/100 = 26\%$. Similar calculations for Community B yield an expected prevalence of 34%.

(c) Using the same method as in part (a) but with exposure prevalences of 0.26 and 0.34 instead, $b = -62.5$ and $a = 116.25$. This leads to $R_1 = 53.75$, $R_0 = 116.25$, relative risk = 0.46, and attributable risk = -62.5 deaths per 100,000 person-years.

Both measures of association fall farther from the null than do those obtained in part (a). As pointed out by Brenner and colleagues (1992), non-differential exposure misclassification in ecological studies leads to estimates of relative and attributable risk that are biased *away* from the null.

3. No. Although conceptually the data set includes measures derived from two levels of aggregation, group- and individual-level effects cannot be separated in this instance because each subject belongs to a different block group. There is no nesting of multiple subjects within the same block groups, which is when one might be concerned about non-independence of observations within the same block group. In this instance, the imputed income variable could be safely treated analytically as an individual-level measure, albeit one that undoubtedly involves measurement error.

REFERENCES

Advisory Committee to the Surgeon General. Smoking and health. Public Health Service Pub. No. 1103. Washington, D.C.: U.S. Department of Health, Education, and Welfare, 1964.

Anderson RM, May RM. Infectious diseases of humans: dynamics and control. New York: Oxford, 1991.

Barker DJP, Morris J, Nelson M. Vegetable consumption and acute appendicitis in 59 areas in England and Wales. BMJ 1986; 292:927–30.

Blakely TA, Woodward AJ. Ecological effects in multi-level studies. J Epidemiol Community Health 2000; 54:367–74.

Brenner H, Greenland S, Savitz DA. The effects of nondifferential exposure misclassification in ecologic studies. Am J Epidemiol 1992; 135:85–95.

Bryk AS, Raudenbush SW. Hierarchical linear models. Newbury Park, Calif.: Sage Publications, 1992.

COMMIT Research Group. Community Intervention Trial for Smoking Cessation (COMMIT): I. Cohort results from a four-year community intervention. Am J Public Health 1995a; 85:183–92.

COMMIT Research Group. Community Intervention Trial for Smoking Cessation (COMMIT): II. Changes in adult cigarette smoking prevalence. Am J Public Health 1995b; 85:193–200.

Cummings P, Grossman DC, Rivara FP, Koepsell TD. State gun safe storage laws and child mortality due to firearms. JAMA 1997; 278:1084–86.

Cummings P, Koepsell TD. Does owning a firearm increase or decrease the risk of death? JAMA 1998; 280:471–73.

Dean HT. Endemic fluorosis and its relation to dental caries. Public Health Rep 1938; 53:1443–52.

Diez-Roux AV. Bringing context back into epidemiology: variables and fallacies in multi-level analysis. Am J Public Health 1998; 88:216–22.

Diez-Roux AV. Multilevel analysis in public health research. Annu Rev Public Health 2000; 21:171–92.

Diez-Roux AV, Nieto FJ, Muntaner C, Tyroler HA, Comstock GW, Shahar E, et al. Neighborhood environments and coronary heart disease: a multilevel analysis. Am J Epidemiol 1997; 146:48–63.

Donne J. Devotions upon emergent occasions, no. 17. In: Gardner H, Healy T (eds.). Donne's selected prose. Oxford, England: Clarendon Press, 1967.

Fine PE. Herd immunity: history, theory, practice. Epidemiol Rev 1993; 15:265–302.

Firebaugh G. A rule for inferring individual-level relationships from aggregate data. Am Sociol Rev 1978; 43:557–72.

Friedman MS, Powell KE, Hutwagner L, Graham LM, Teague WG. Impact of changes in transportation and commuting behaviors during the 1996 Summer Olympic Games in Atlanta on air quality and childhood asthma. JAMA 2001; 285:897–905.

Frost CD, Law MR, Wald NJ. II—Analysis of observational data within populations. BMJ 1991; 302:815–18.

Gardner W, Mulvey EP, Shaw EC. Regression analyses of counts and rates: Poisson, overdispersed Poisson, and negative binomial models. Psychol Bull 1995; 118:392–404.

Goldberger J, Wheeler GA, Sydenstricker E. A study of the relation of family income and other economic factors to pellagra incidence in seven cotton-mill villages of South Carolina in 1916. Public Health Rep 1920; 35:2673–714.

Goodwin PJ, Boyd NF. Critical appraisal of the evidence that dietary fat intake is related to breast cancer risk in humans. JNCI 1987; 79:473–85.

Greenland S. Divergent biases in ecologic and individual-level studies. Stat Med 1992; 11:1209–23.

Greenland S. A review of multilevel theory for ecologic analyses. Stat Med 2002; 21:389–95.

Greenland S, Brenner H. Correcting for non-differential misclassification in ecologic analyses. Appl Stat 1993; 42:117–26.

Greenland S, Morgenstern H. Ecological bias, confounding, and effect modification. Int J Epidemiol 1989; 18:269–74.

Greenland S, Robins J. Invited commentary: ecological studies—biases, misconceptions, and counterexamples. Am J Epidemiol 1994; 139:747–60.

Jablon S, Hrubec Z, Boice JD. Cancer in populations living near nuclear facilities. A survey of mortality nationwide and incidence in two states. JAMA 1991; 265:1403–8.

Kaplan GA, Pamuk ER, Lynch JW, Cohen RD, Balfour JL. Inequality in income and mortality in the United States: analysis of mortality and potential pathways. BMJ 1996; 312:999–1003.

Kellermann AL, Rivara FP, Rushforth NB, Banton JG, Reay DT, Francisco JT, et al. Gun ownership as a risk factor for homicide in the home. N Engl J Med 1993; 329:1084–91.

Killias M. International correlations between gun ownership and rates of homicide and suicide. Can Med Assoc J 1993; 148:1721–5.

Kleck G, Gertz M. Armed resistance to crime: the prevalence and nature of self-defense with a gun. J Criminal Law Criminol 1995; 86:150–87.

Law MR, Frost CD, Wald NJ. By how much does dietary salt reduction lower blood pressure? I—Analysis of observational data among populations. BMJ 1991; 302:811–15.

Liu K, Cooper R, McKeever J, McKeever P, Byington R, Soltero I, et al. Assessment of the association between habitual salt intake and high blood presssure: methodological problems. Am J Epidemiol 1979; 110:219–26.

McCullagh P, Nelder JA. Generalized linear models (2nd ed.). London: Chapman and Hall, 1989.

Morgenstern H. Uses of ecologic analysis in epidemiologic research. Am J Public Health 1982; 72:1336–44.

Morgenstern H. Ecologic studies in epidemiology: concepts, principles, and methods. Annu Rev Public Health 1995; 16:61–82.

Morgenstern H. Ecologic studies. Chapter 23 in: Rothman KJ, Greenland S. Modern epidemiology (2nd ed.). Philadelphia: Lippincott-Raven, 1998.

O'Campo P, Gielen AC, Faden RR, Xue X, Kass N, Wang MC. Violence by male partners against women during the childbearing years: a contextual analysis. Am J Public Health 1995; 85:1092–97.

Piantadosi S. Invited commentary: ecologic biases. Am J Epidemiol 1994; 139:761–64.

Piantadosi S, Byar DP, Green SB. The ecological fallacy. Am J Epidemiol 1988; 127:893–904.

Pickett KE, Pearl M. Multilevel analyses of neighbourhood socioeconomic context and health outcomes: a critical review. J Epidemiol Community Health 2001; 55:111–22.

Prentice RL, Sheppard L. Aggregate data studies of disease risk factors. Biometrika 1995; 82:113–25.

Richardson S, Stücker I, Hémon D. Comparison of relative risks obtained in ecological and individual studies: methodological considerations. Int J Epidemiol 1987; 16:111–20.

Robinson WS. Ecological correlations and the behavior of individuals. Am Sociol Rev 1950; 15:351–57.

Rose G. Sick individuals and sick populations. Int J Epidemiol 1985; 6:1–8.

Seeley JR. Death by liver cirrhosis and the price of beverage alcohol. Can Med Assoc J 1960; 83:1361–66.

Selvin HC, Hagstrom WO. The empirical classification of formal groups. Am Sociol Rev 1963; 28:399–411.

Susser M. The logic in ecological: I. The logic of analysis. Am J Public Health 1994a; 84:825–29.

Susser M. The logic in ecological: II. The logic of design. Am J Public Health 1994b; 84:830–35.

Villaveces A, Cummings P, Espitia VE, Koepsell TD, McKnight B, Kellermann AL. Effect of a ban on carrying firearms on homicide rates in 2 Colombian cities. JAMA 2000; 283:1205–9.

Von Korff M, Koepsell T, Curry S, Diehr P. Multi-level analysis in epidemiologic research on health behaviors and outcomes. Am J Epidemiol 1992; 135:1077–82.

Walter SD. The ecologic method in the study of environmental health. I. Overview of the method. Environ Health Perspect 1991a; 94:61–65.

Walter SD. The ecologic method in the study of environmental health. II. Methodologic issues and feasibility. Environ Health Perspect 1991b; 94:67–73.

Witte JS, Greenland S, Kim LL. Software for hierarchical modeling of epidemiologic data. Epidemiology 1998; 9:563–66.

Witte JS, Greenland S, Kim LL, Arab L. Multilevel modeling in epidemiology with GLIMMIX. Epidemiology 2000; 11:684–88.

World almanac and book of facts. New York: Press Publishing, 1990.

13

RANDOMIZED TRIALS

AN INTRODUCTORY EXAMPLE

Lung cancer claims more lives in the U.S. than any other form of cancer (National Center for Health Statistics, 2000). In the early 1980s, several lines of evidence suggested that the naturally occurring compounds β-carotene and retinol (vitamin A) might be promising agents for chemoprevention of lung cancer (Prentice et al., 1985). Synthetic retinoids had been shown to prevent lung neoplasms in animals and to reverse pre-neoplastic changes in human bronchial epithelium. Cohort studies in humans had also found inverse associations between dietary intake of vitamin A and subsequent incidence of lung cancer. Although the exact mechanisms were unknown, it was felt plausible that β-carotene could prevent neoplastic transformation by functioning as an anti-oxidant, that vitamin A could promote differentiation of epithelial cells, and that these actions might be complementary (Omenn et al., 1994).

To determine whether a combination of β-carotene and retinol would be effective in preventing lung cancer in humans, Omenn and colleagues (1994; 1996a) initiated an intervention study called the Carotene and Retinol Efficacy Trial (CARET). Participants were sought from two high-risk groups: men with a history of occupational exposure to asbestos, and heavy smokers. Two pilot studies in Seattle were used to refine ways to recruit and follow study subjects, enhance compliance, and ascertain outcomes. Eventually, 18,314 participants were studied at six centers across the U.S. In the main phase, each newly enrolled subject was assigned at random with equal probability to take either a capsule containing 30 mg. of β-carotene and 25,000 IU of retinol, or a similar-appearing capsule containing an inactive substance (placebo). (During the pilot phase, heavy smokers were assigned in a 3:1 ratio to active treatment or placebo.) Neither participants themselves nor study staff who monitored participants during the trial were told which treatment group each participant was in.

During the trial, the CARET principal investigators met twice yearly with a Safety and Endpoints Monitoring Committee to review interim results. On January 11, 1996, the trial's steering committee halted the trial 21 months early. Lung cancer incidence through December 15, 1995, had been found to be 28%

higher in the active-treatment group than in the placebo group (95% confidence interval [CI]: 4%–57%), and deaths from all causes were 17% higher (95% CI: 3%–33%) with active treatment. In reporting these surprising results, the investigators noted:

> The results of the trial are troubling. There was no support for a beneficial effect of beta carotene or vitamin A, in spite of the large advantages inferred from observational epidemiologic comparisons. . . . We have no explanation for the possible adverse associations that we have observed to date.

The CARET study is an example of a *randomized trial*—a comparative study in which study subjects are assigned by a formal chance mechanism between two or more intervention strategies. Randomized trials occupy a special place among epidemiologic study designs because they have the potential to provide particularly strong evidence to support a hypothesis of a causal link between an exposure and an outcome. As in the CARET example, randomized-trial results may sometimes even reverse inferences drawn from non-randomized studies. As noted in Chapter 11, it is likely in retrospect that people who had chosen to take vitamin A or β-carotene in the earlier observational studies had other characteristics that placed them at relatively low risk for developing a malignancy, and the observational studies were unable to remove this confounding.

Why Randomize?

Above all, random assignment offers excellent protection against confounding. Confounding requires, at a minimum, that there be an association between exposure and the potential confounder. But randomization tends to distribute potential confounders similarly across exposure groups, thus removing—at least on average—this necessary precondition for confounding.

For example, in the CARET study, 1,558 (38.4%) of the 4,060 asbestos-exposed participants reported being current smokers when they entered the trial. Since smoking is such a strong risk factor for lung cancer, it was an important potential confounding factor. During randomization, each of those 1,558 current smokers had an equal chance of being assigned to active treatment or to placebo. It turned out that 781 current smokers were assigned by chance to active treatment, and 777 were assigned to placebo. The resulting prevalence of current smoking was $781/2,044 = .382$ in the active treatment group and $777/2,016 = .385$ in the placebo group—not equal, but very close indeed.

Randomization works in the same way to prevent confounding even by factors that have not been measured or that may be unknown to the investigator. In contrast, all other standard techniques for dealing with confounding—matching,

Table 13–1. Baseline Comparison of Active Treatment and Placebo Groups
in the CARET Study

CHARACTERISTIC	Asbestos Workers		Heavy Smokers	
	ACTIVE TREATMENT ($n = 2044$)	PLACEBO ($n = 2016$)	ACTIVE TREATMENT ($n = 7376^a$)	PLACEBO ($n = 6878^a$)
Age in years (mean ± s.d.)	57 ± 7	57 ± 7	58 ± 5	58 ± 5
Female gender (%)	0	0	43	45
Race/ethnicity (%)				
White	88	88	95	94
Black	7	8	1	2
Hispanic	2	2	1	1
Other/unknown	2	2	2	3
Smoking status (%)				
Never smoked	3	3	0	0
Former smoker	58	58	34	34
Current smoker	38	39	66	66
Cigarettes/day (mean ± s.d.)				
Former smokers	25 ± 12	25 ± 12	28 ± 11	28 ± 11
Current smokers	24 ± 10	25 ± 10	24 ± 9	24 ± 8
Pack-years of smoking (mean ± s.d.)	43 ± 24	42 ± 24	50 ± 21	49 ± 20
Years since quitting smoking (Ex-smokers only, mean ± s.d.)	10 ± 8	10 ± 8	3 ± 2	3 ± 2

[a] During pilot phase, participants were randomized to active treatment vs. placebo in a 3:1 ratio.
[*Source*: Omenn et al. (1996a).]

stratification, restriction, multivariate modeling—depend on having data on the potential confounders for each study subject, while randomization does not.

To illustrate randomization's ability to prevent confounding by many factors at once, Table 13–1 compares the active treatment and placebo groups within each of the two recruitment strata: asbestos-exposed workers and heavy smokers. On every factor, participants assigned to the two treatment arms proved to be very similar.

When Can a Randomized Trial Design Be Used?

Some exposure–disease relationships are more amenable than others to study with the randomized-trial design. Requirements that must generally be met in order for a randomized trial to be feasible and justifiable include the following:

1. *The exposure must be potentially modifiable.* Factors such as genotype, family history, and demographic characteristics cannot be altered, so their impact on disease occurrence must be studied with observational designs.
2. *The exposure must be potentially modifiable by the investigator.* Exposures such as occupation, marital status, and smoking habits can, in principle, be changed, but it is often impossible or impractical to assign people at random among the possible categories for research purposes.

   Even this limitation, however, does not preclude the use of a randomized trial in every instance, as is illustrated by the following example:

Example: In many observational studies, cigarette smoking during pregnancy has been associated with increased risk of having a low-birth-weight baby. Part of this association, however, could represent confounding by maternal risk factors associated with smoking. Sexton and Hebel (1984) randomly assigned 935 pregnant smokers to either a smoking-cessation intervention or a usual-care control group. By the eighth month of pregnancy, 57% of mothers in the intervention group still smoked, vs. 80% of mothers in the control group. The average birth weight of babies born to all intervention-group mothers was 92 grams higher than that in the control group ($p < .05$). These results suggested not only that the intervention was effective at helping pregnant mothers to stop smoking, but also that maternal smoking predisposed to low birth weight.

Here the exposure of main interest (smoking during pregnancy) was not the same as the randomized intervention actually studied (participation in a smoking-cessation program). Instead, the study compared groups that had been formed by random assignment but that had different proportions of members who continued to smoke. As discussed later in this chapter, an observed difference in outcomes from this kind of comparison can be expected to represent a "diluted" effect of exposure. It is biased away from finding a difference. But if an association is found nonetheless, as in this example, the case for a causal effect of exposure gains strong support.

3. *There is genuine uncertainty about which intervention strategy is superior.* Sometimes other available evidence already shows one intervention strategy to be clearly superior to another. If so, it would be unethical to offer people the probably inferior method in lieu of the probably superior one.

For example, it has often been observed that motorcyclists who wear a helmet are much less likely to die of a head injury in a motorcycle crash than are unhelmeted motorcyclists. There is little doubt that mechanical protection provided by the helmet is largely responsible for this difference. It would almost certainly be deemed unethical to withhold helmets at random for some motorcyclists in order to get further evidence that helmets actually do protect against fatal head injury.

4. *The primary outcomes are relatively common and occur relatively soon.* Randomized trials normally involve measuring the incidence of outcome events prospectively in two or more comparison groups. As shown later, the power of a trial to detect an intervention effect depends on how many outcome events occur. For this reason, randomized trials are less well suited to studying rare or long-delayed outcomes, because large samples or prolonged follow-up would be needed to get the necessary number of outcome events.

Randomized trials can be expensive, especially when a large number of participants is required, the period of follow-up is lengthy, or the identification of outcome events is costly. But the key distinguishing feature of a randomized trial is simply that the comparison groups be formed by a formal chance mechanism— a process that is technically quite easy and is neither costly nor time-consuming to carry out. Indeed, many randomized trials have been conducted speedily with little or no special funding when they concerned common, easily measured outcomes that occurred soon after the intervention was applied (Rosa et al., 1998).

Explanatory vs. Pragmatic Aims

Randomized trials are undertaken to determine whether one intervention strategy is better than another in some way. But why do we care? Sometimes it is because a potentially useful theory predicts the result, and the proposed experiment would test this theory. Trials designed for this reason are often called *explanatory* trials (Schwartz and Lellouch, 1967; Charlton, 1994). They are akin to basic research. The focus is on understanding causal mechanisms, and the main product is improved knowledge about a problem.

In other situations, we care which intervention strategy is better because a practical decision must be made between two or more possible courses of action. Time, money, lives, comfort, or other valued outcomes are at stake. Trials undertaken to guide decision-making in the "real world" are often called *pragmatic* trials. They are akin to applied research. The focus is on choosing between feasible alternatives that are potentially widely applicable. Whatever value the trial has as a test of theory is a happy byproduct.

Table 13–2. Influence of Explanatory vs. Pragmatic Orientations on Trial Design

FEATURE	EXPLANATORY	PRAGMATIC
Experimental intervention	What theory predicts should work best, whether practical for wider application or not	Strategy practical for use in real-world settings
Comparison intervention	Sharply defined, maximizing contrast between experimental and control conditions	Realistic practical alternative to experimental intervention, sometimes just "usual care"
Study subjects	Those in whom an effect of intervention is expected to be greatest, including highly compliant people	Relatively broad sample from the potential target population
Outcome variables	Variables most sensitive to effects predicted by theory	Outcomes most relevant to subjects and providers

Explanatory and pragmatic goals are both perfectly good reasons for carrying out a trial. Sometimes the same study can satisfy both kinds of aims well. But choices about specific features of trial design must often be made between mutually exclusive alternatives. These choices can involve trade-offs between testing a theory rigorously and maximizing relevance to practical decision-making. Table 13–2 lists aspects of trial design that can be influenced by which kind of goal takes precedence. A clear view of whether a trial's primary purpose is explanatory or pragmatic provides a consistent philosophy to guide these choices.

A related distinction is between the *efficacy* and the *effectiveness* of an intervention (Last, 2000; Haynes and Dantes, 1987). *Efficacy* refers to how well an intervention *can* work under ideal circumstances—i.e., when administered by well-trained experts and aimed at perfectly compliant recipients—even if those conditions are artificial and hard to mimic outside the research setting. *Effectiveness* refers to how well an intervention *does* work under "field conditions"—i.e., when administered by ordinary practitioners and offered to a relatively unselected target population.

In the CARET study, to be eligible for the trial, potential participants had to agree to limit their vitamin A intake to less than 5500 IU per day, to take no supplemental β-carotene, and to return to a study center annually for several years for an in-person examination. In addition, candidates were given a three-month supply of placebo at an initial visit and instructed to take a capsule daily on a trial basis. At a second visit three months later, only subjects who had taken at least 50% of the assigned number of placebo capsules were accepted into the trial and randomized. These study-design features suggest a mainly explanatory orientation: the trial's ability to detect an effect of active treatment was enhanced, possibly at the expense of some loss of generalizability to a broader potential target group.

TREATMENT ARMS

The alternative conditions or treatments participants are exposed to during a trial are often termed *arms* of the trial. A simple and common trial design involves just two arms: experimental and control. Other design variations are considered later.

Experimental

Interest in a particular intervention is usually what motivates a trial in the first place, and the trial is built around it. As noted above, the experimental intervention may need to be tailored to meet explanatory or pragmatic goals.

Control

Whether an experimental intervention is effective depends in part on what it is compared to. Possibilities include:

Nothing

If there is no widely accepted competitor for the experimental intervention, one option is to provide nothing at all to subjects in the control arm. For example, a randomized trial of low-dose aspirin for prevention of coronary heart disease was conducted among male British physicians, in which participants took either 500 mg. of aspirin daily or nothing (Peto et al., 1988). As one consequence of this design feature, the trial became an "open label" study, in which each participant knew full well whether he was in the aspirin group or in the control group.

Placebo

In drug trials, a *placebo* is a preparation that resembles the experimental drug to the senses but omits the active ingredient and thus is believed to have no true biological effect (Vickers and de Craen, 2000). Placebos have long been credited with having the potential to make patients feel better by inducing expectations of benefit, although evidence in support of this claim is mixed (Hrøbjartsson and Gøtzsche, 2001; Walsh et al., 2002). In a randomized trial, however, the main function of a placebo is to help keep subjects unaware of which treatment they are receiving— i.e., to preserve *blinding*—which in turn helps prevent bias in ascertainment of outcomes or from differential attrition in the two arms. The CARET study used placebo capsules for just this purpose.

In trials of non-pharmacological interventions, the same function can be served by a control intervention that appears similar to the experimental intervention but that lacks its active component.

Example: In the late 1950s, enthusiastic reports appeared in the lay press about internal mammary artery ligation as treatment for chest pain due to coronary heart disease (angina pectoris). To evaluate these claims, Cobb and colleagues (1959) randomly assigned 17 patients with angina pectoris to receive either internal mammary artery ligation or sham surgery. For all patients, two incisions were made in the chest under local anesthesia, and the left and right internal mammary arteries, which run just inside the chest wall, were located. Ligatures were placed around them but not tied. Then a sealed envelope was opened and, depending on the treatment-group assignment contained therein, the ligatures were either tied or removed. During follow-up, patients in the ligated group reported a sharp reduction in the average frequency of angina attacks following the operation. But so did those in the non-ligated group. Overall, outcomes differed very little between groups.

Other examples of non-drug "placebos" include sham hemodialysis in a trial of treatment for schizophrenia (Carpenter et al., 1983), placebo steam in a trial of moist air for relief of upper respiratory infections (Macknin et al., 1990), and sham electroconvulsive therapy in trials of treatment for for depression (Johnstone et al., 1980).

Active alternative

An older, established intervention may already be accepted as beneficial in comparison to nothing at all. If a new competitor then comes along, it is likely to be both more ethical and more relevant to compare the new intervention to the older one, rather than to compare the new one with a placebo or with nothing. For example, randomized trials done in the 1960s showed that treatment of high blood pressure with certain antihypertensive drugs could reduce the risk of cardiovascular complications, compared with the risk among those who received no such treatment (Veterans Administration Cooperative Study Group on Antihypertensive Agents, 1967). Nowadays, a new antihypertensive drug would need to be shown to be at least as good as older drugs of proven benefit if the new drug is to merit a role in clinical practice (ALLHAT Collaborative Research Group, 2000).

Usual care

A new intervention can be compared to what study subjects would otherwise receive. This option may be suitable when current practice is variable and hard to standardize, and when the trial is chiefly pragmatic in orientation. The researcher typically has little control over what happens to participants who are assigned to usual care, but what they actually receive can prove to be an important determinant of trial outcome.

Example: The Multiple Risk Factor Intervention Trial (MRFIT) sought to determine whether a multi-component intervention would reduce mortality from coronary heart disease (Multiple Risk Factor Intervention Trial Research Group, 1982). Some 12,866 high-risk men aged 35–57 years were randomized to either *(1)* a special intervention including hypertension control, smoking cessation, and/or dietary reduction of blood cholesterol; or *(2)* usual care. Risk-factor levels were evaluated through extensive testing during three baseline visits prior to randomization, and annually thereafter. For men in the special-intervention group, data from these visits were used to tailor the intervention to their individual needs. For men in the usual-care group, reports from these visits were sent to the participant's regular physician.

After an average of seven years, coronary heart disease mortality was slightly but not significantly lower (7%, 95% confidence interval: −15% to +25%) in the special-intervention group, while their mortality from all causes combined was actually slightly higher. Blood-pressure levels, cholesterol, and smoking prevalence had all declined in special-intervention group men, but declines were also observed in the usual-care group. Coronary heart disease mortality in both groups was much lower than had been expected when planning the trial. Possible explanations suggested for the trial's unexpected negative result included *(1)* the special intervention did not work; or *(2)* risk-factor changes in the usual-care group led to the trial's being unable to detect a modest relative benefit of the special intervention. A later report after ten years of follow-up found more convincing evidence of mortality reduction in special-intervention men (Multiple Risk Factor Intervention Trial Research Group, 1990).

SELECTION OF STUDY SUBJECTS

Eligibility

An important part of trial design is deciding who may qualify as a participant. Several factors come into play in setting eligibility criteria.

Internal validity

Some criteria for eligibility are motivated by a desire to protect the trial from potential biases. A trial's ability to reach a correct conclusion for subjects who actually take part is termed its *internal validity*. (The scope of generalizability of its findings to non-participants is termed *external validity*.) Criteria of this nature can address:

- *Subject retention*. People who expect to move away or who have an illness that may cut short their participation are often excluded.
- *Data quality*. People who do not share the native language of study personnel are often excluded because of the difficulty and expense of translating data instruments satisfactorily into other languages.
- *Compliance*. In trials that seek to determine efficacy, potential subjects may be excluded if they are unable or unwilling to comply with the intended treatment.

  One strategy for achieving high compliance is to screen potential subjects during a *run-in* phase (Lang, 1990; Pablos-Mendez et al., 1998). Before being accepted and randomized, screenees are asked to do on a test basis what they would be expected to do during the main trial, such as taking a drug or providing data. Only those who demonstrate compliance are accepted. In the CARET study, only potential participants who took at least half of the assigned placebo capsules during a three-month run-in phase were accepted into the trial (Thornquist et al., 1993).

Generalizability

The results of any study are most readily applied to people who would have qualified for the study. A pragmatic trial can thus be most useful if it includes a broadly representative sample of people for whom the practical decision addressed by the trial would arise. But the kinds of exclusions considered above, which seek to protect the trial's internal validity, often involve sacrificing generalizability.

The right balance between these competing goals depends in part on how much is already known about the experimental intervention. If there is uncertainty about whether it works even under favorable conditions, then establishing efficacy may need to take priority—without it, there is little reason to consider wide dissemination. But if previous studies have shown that the intervention can work, at least in certain settings, the emphasis may properly shift to evaluating whether, and how well, it works in a broader target population.

Risks and benefits to subjects

Finally, the experimental intervention or the control condition may pose unusual risks to certain kinds of people. A new vaccine that is prepared in eggs could be dangerous to someone with a known allergy to eggs, so she or he would almost certainly be excluded. An experimental treatment may be known to be highly toxic or risky, but the disease itself may be almost uniformly fatal. Eligibility for a trial of such a treatment may be open only to persons for whom other therapeutic options have been exhausted.

Any exclusion rule that stems from special risks or benefits posed by *one* of the treatment arms must nonetheless apply to *all* potential subjects. Bias can be introduced if such an exclusion is applied selectively after the outcome of randomization is known. Doing so would upset the similarity of the groups formed by random assignment, and thus potentially lose the key benefit of randomization.

Number of Study Subjects

A trial that involves too few study subjects or too short a period of follow-up is likely to be inconclusive. Even if the results suggest a large difference in outcomes between treatment arms, that difference may have such wide confidence limits that the results could easily be compatible with there being no true difference. Unfortunately, this problem has been found to be common (Moher et al., 1994). Yet an overly large trial wastes resources and time, and it can needlessly expose people to a treatment that turns out to be inferior.

Fortunately, statistical methods are available to help decide on a defensible target sample size (Wittes, 2002; Rosner, 1995; Lachin, 1981; Donner, 1984; Cohen, 1988; Kraemer, 1987; Hulley et al., 2001; Friedman et al., 1998). The specific method used depends on details of the study design and the primary outcome(s). Appendix 13A provides details for a common trial design that involves comparing two equal-sized groups on a binary outcome variable.

At a minimum, the researcher must specify in advance:

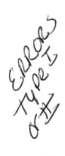

- How large a risk of reaching a wrong conclusion would be acceptable:
  - α, the largest acceptable probability of rejecting the null hypothesis if in fact it is true (a *Type I* error); and
  - β, the largest acceptable probability of accepting the null hypothesis if in fact a specified alternative hypothesis is true (a *Type II* error).
- The expected distribution of outcomes in each treatment arm if the experimental intervention works as hypothesized.

For some study designs, additional information is required.

Sometimes the available number of subjects is limited by external constraints, so that n is fixed. To help determine whether a trial is worth doing under those circumstances, formulas that are used to estimate sample size (e.g., equation 13.1 in Appendix 13A) can often be rearranged to solve for β. A decision on whether to proceed would be based on whether study power ($= 1 - \beta$) is judged to be high enough. Formulas are also available in references cited above to solve for the smallest detectable difference in outcome frequency, given specified values of the sample size, α, β, and possibly other design parameters.

Choices for α and β are more or less determined by statistical convention: $\alpha = .05$ and $\beta = .05, .10,$ or $.20$ are common, if somewhat arbitrary, choices. Other quantities needed in the calculations, such as the expected frequency of outcome events in the control group, must usually be estimated. Possible sources include published reports from other studies in similar populations, historical data from the proposed study setting, or a pilot study.

Specifying the size of the treatment effect—for example, the difference in incidence of outcome events between treatment arms—poses a special challenge. Uncertainty about the size of this effect is, after all, the main motivation for the trial in the first place, and it may seem circular to have to assume a value in order to plan the trial itself. This paradox can be resolved by thinking of the value specified for the treatment effect in sample-size calculations not as a prediction about what *will* happen, but as the smallest effect of treatment that the trial should be able to detect. Ideally, that threshold value would be motivated by theory in an explanatory trial (How big an effect would it take to confirm or refute the theory?), or by practical considerations in a pragmatic trial (How big a difference in outcomes would justify opting for one strategy over the other, given the other factors affecting that decision?).

In that vein, it can be hazardous to specify the target treatment effect based only on what was observed in a pilot study. This is because the small sample size of most pilot studies usually implies that the resulting estimate of treatment effect is quite imprecise. The pilot-study result may thus be far from the truth in either direction. A spuriously large value may spur enthusiasm for the intervention but cause the main trial to be badly underpowered, while a spuriously small value may cause a perfectly good intervention to be abandoned prematurely. Instead, a pilot study is best regarded as a small-scale evaluation of the feasibility of various aspects of study methodology, not as a preliminary test of the main hypothesis itself (Gore, 1981b; Wittes and Brittain, 1990).

In practice, setting a target sample size can be easier than achieving it. Recruitment into trials is a frequent problem (Hunninghake et al., 1987; Taylor et al., 1984). A pilot study can also be helpful to determine what recruitment problems may arise and to assure that the target number of subjects is realistic.

Informed Consent

Randomized trials funded by any U.S. government agency must meet strict standards concerning the involvement of human subjects (U.S. Department of Health and Human Services, 1991). Many research organizations apply these policies regardless of funding source. With rare exceptions, participants must give their informed consent to serve as research subjects. Required elements of informed consent include describing to subjects that they would be participating in research; the procedures that would be involved; the nature of risks and discomfort they might face; potential benefits to them and to others might result from their participation; alternative treatments or procedures that might be to their advantage; the extent to which information gathered will remain confidential; compensation available in event of injury, if more than minimal risk is involved; the name of the person to contact with questions about the research; and the fact that their participation in the research is voluntary and that they may withdraw without penalty or loss of benefits they might otherwise be entitled to. Ethical aspects of the conduct of randomized trials are discussed more fully by Sugarman (2002); Kahn et al. (1998); Kodish et al. (1990).

RANDOMIZATION

Allocation Method

A key element of randomization is the statistical method by which treatment-group assignments are made. Three common randomization schemes are described here: simple, blocked, and stratified. For simplicity, each method is described for a trial involving allocation of subjects between two treatment arms with equal probability, although each method is also adaptable for use with more elaborate designs. Other allocation methods are discussed in detail by Friedman et al. (1998); Lachin et al. (1988); Stout et al. (1994).

Simple randomization

Simple randomization is like flipping a coin for each study subject. In practice, however, it is preferable to create an "audit trail" to document that the process was done properly.

Simple randomization can be done without a computer by using a table of random numbers, available in most statistics books (Rosner, 1995; Gore, 1981c). The user decides on a rule that ties five of the ten decimal digits (e.g., 0–4) to the intervention group and the other five (e.g., 5–9) to the control group. Then the random number table is entered at an arbitrary spot. From that spot on, each digit in the table corresponds to a study subject—either in the order that subjects appear on a predefined list, or in the order that they enter the study—and the rule is applied to allocate each eligible participant.

Nowadays, randomization is more often done on a computer and can be carried out using a statistical analysis package or spreadsheet program with a built-in function that generates random (technically, pseudo-random) numbers. Appendix 13B describes an algorithm that can be used to implement simple randomization with such a program.

A disadvantage of simple randomization is that, although each subject has an equal chance of being assigned to either group, there is no guarantee that the groups will end up equal in size. This is not a serious problem if the total sample size is very large, as in the CARET study: by the laws of chance, the likelihood of a major difference in group sizes is low. But for smaller samples, the chance of getting badly unbalanced group sizes is greater. For example, with $n = 30$, the chance of getting a 11:19 split, or worse, in either direction is about 20% (Gore, 1981c). Such a lopsided allocation would not invalidate the trial, but it would reduce power and could be awkward to explain. One experienced trialist has suggested that simple randomization be used only if $n \geq 100$ (Gore, 1981c).

Blocked randomization

Blocked randomization is a way to guarantee that treatment group sizes will be equal, or nearly so. Starting with a list of study subjects, adjacent positions are grouped into *blocks*. For example, if a block size of four were used, positions 1–4 would comprise the first block, positions 5–8 the second block, etc. For a two-arm trial, the block size is normally chosen to be an even number. Within each block, half of the subjects are then chosen at random to go to the intervention group, and the rest go to the control group. An algorithm for blocked randomization by computer is described in Appendix 13B.

In principle, any block size that is a multiple of the number of treatment arms can be used. If recruitment ends halfway through a block, all participants in the first part of that final block may have gone to the same treatment group, making the group sizes unequal. This could be a reason for choosing a small block size, perhaps only two per block for a two-arm trial. On the other hand, if subjects enter the trial one at a time, it is also important to keep the treatment-group assignment of the next study subject as unpredictable as possible. Larger block sizes help attain this goal. Block size can be varied at random to promote unpredictability, as was done in the CARET trial (Thornquist et al., 1993).

A special case of blocked randomization can be used if the total number of subjects is known in advance—for example, if all trial participants have already been identified at the start of the trial, and all are to be randomized at once. Then all subjects on the list can be regarded as belonging to one big block. The list can then be "shuffled" into random order by sorting on a random number. Subjects who end up in the top half of the sorted list then go to the intervention group, and the rest go to the control group.

Stratified randomization

Stratified randomization is used to guarantee balance on a few key characteristics (Kernan et al., 1999). The usual process is simple:

1. Divide up study subjects according to strata.
2. Within each stratum, use blocked randomization to assign subjects to treatment arms.

A major reason to use stratification is to prevent confounding by some key factor in trials with a small number of participants. For example, in a British randomized trial of drug treatments for persons aged 65 to 74 years with high blood pressure, randomization was done separately for men and women using blocks of size eight within each stratum (MRC Working Party, 1992). The purpose of this procedure was to assure that the gender composition of the groups assigned to different treatment arms would be similar. Mortality proved to be nearly twice as great among men as among women, confirming the importance of gender as a potential confounder.

Because there may be many potential confounders, it can be tempting to try to stratify simultaneously on lots of them. Unfortunately, this strategy soon becomes self-defeating. Within each stratum, blocked randomization only assures equal allocation of subjects to treatment arms at the completion of a block. If there are numerous small strata, many of them may contain unfilled blocks when recruitment ends, so it is likely that the desired balance will not have been achieved. Hence, if stratified randomization is used, the number of strata is best kept small (Kernan et al., 1999).

Allocation Concealment

When subjects enter a trial over time, a system is needed to keep treatment-group assignments unpredictable until each subject has been officially enrolled and allocated to a group. Otherwise, study subjects or the caregivers who are referring potential subjects to the trial may be tempted to "game" the system by waiting until they think the chances are good of being assigned to whichever group they prefer. Unfortunately, subversion of the randomization scheme does occur (Schulz, 1995), and inadequate concealment appears to bias trial results (Schulz et al., 1995; Chalmers et al., 1983).

Fortunately, this form of bias is largely preventable. Studies that use blocked randomization can avoid very small block sizes or vary the block size to reduce predictability of the assignment sequence. Treatment-group assignments are often best done at a central study office by trained personnel whose primary responsibility is to preserve study validity. For example, the study coordinating center can be telephoned whenever a potential subject has been identified. Eligibility is checked, and if the candidate passes the check, he or she is officially logged in and the caller is given the treatment-group assignment over the telephone. Other systems include using sequentially numbered, sealed, opaque envelopes containing treatment-group assignments; or sequentially numbered, pre-randomized medication containers (Schulz et al., 1995; Friedman et al., 1998).

Blinding

Blinding (or *masking*) refers to keeping persons involved in a trial unaware of which study subjects are in which treatment arm. The main reasons for this deliberate withholding of information are to prevent bias in ascertainment of outcomes and to minimize differential attrition of subjects. A trial is *double-blind* if both the study subjects and the research staff members responsible for measuring outcomes are kept unaware of treatment-group assignments. A trial is *single-blind* if only one of these parties (usually study subjects) is kept unaware.

Blinding can also be extended to people who play other roles. In clinical trials, a patient's caregiver may not be the person who measures outcomes, but the caregiver's actions can nonetheless influence outcomes and be influenced by knowing which intervention the patient is receiving. The study protocol may therefore keep caregivers blinded, but provide a way to remove the blinding if knowing which arm of the study the patient has been assigned to becomes important for delivery of good care. Even the statistician(s) responsible for day-to-day data analysis may be kept blinded to the identity of the intervention being received by each of the study groups, because it may be hard for a statistician who is in regular contact with other members of a research team to remain completely neutral about the expected outcome. Almost all large trials create an independent Data Safety and Monitoring Board, and only members of such a board have access to information about which group is which. These people are charged with deciding whether any differences in outcomes across study groups justify breaking the blinding and halting the trial, as in the CARET study.

Blinding is not always possible. In community trials, for example, the intervention may involve a mass-media campaign to influence health behavior (Koepsell, 1998), which is clearly at odds with keeping people unaware of which treatment arm they are in. Even when blinding is attempted, it may be only partly successful because it is difficult to design a perfect placebo. Certain characteristic side effects, for example, may be hard to mimic. The success of blinding can often be evaluated at trial's end simply by asking people to guess which treatment they received. Experience has shown that attempts at blinding can fall well short of their goal (Byington et al., 1985; Howard et al., 1982). Nonetheless, even if some trial participants correctly judge the nature of the intervention arm they have been assigned to, removing some of the potential bias is likely to be better than removing none at all.

DATA COLLECTION

Baseline Characteristics

Information to characterize study subjects upon entry into a trial is usually collected for at least one of the following reasons:

- *To verify eligibility.* Data must be gathered about study subjects to confirm that they qualify for entry according to the study's eligibility criteria. This information also serves to describe the study population and helps consumers of the results to judge the scope of generalizability.
- *To assess potential confounding.* Although randomization works well *on average* at creating balanced treatment groups, "accidents of randomization" do occur. Often one of the first tables in a published report of a randomized trial compares the groups formed by randomization (Altman and Dore, 1990; Assmann et al., 2000). Table 13–1 is an example. Such a table describes the study population and permits a check on the degree to which randomization balanced the groups. Characteristics that are known determinants of the trial's main outcomes are of special importance, because any imbalance between treatment arms would make these factors confounders. Information on potential confounders may also be needed for use in stratified or blocked randomization.
- *To identify planned subgroups.* Some trials have a priori hypotheses about variation in the size of treatment effects across different subgroups (effect modification). Hence, baseline information is needed to place study subjects in the relevant subgroup for later analysis. For example, in the Multiple Risk Factor Intervention Trial, the investigators hypothesized in advance that men with a normal baseline electrocardiogram would benefit the most from intervention (Multiple Risk Factor Intervention Trial Research Group, 1982).
- *To enhance study power.* If a study outcome is also a characteristic that can be measured at baseline—e.g., blood pressure, body weight, or bone density—then a trial's statistical power can often be enhanced by including

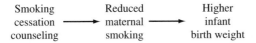

Figure 13-1. Hypothesized Mechanism for Effect of Smoking Cessation Intervention (based on Sexton and Hebel, 1984).

each subject's baseline value in the analysis of later outcomes (Fleiss, 1986). To the extent that baseline and follow-up values are correlated within subjects, including the baseline value in the analysis can remove a source of between-subject variation that would otherwise be treated as part of random variation in outcomes.

Outcomes

Outcome measures of primary interest usually follow from a trial's objectives. Whether it has chiefly explanatory or pragmatic aims can guide the choice of measures: effects that matter in testing theory may matter less in guiding practice, and vice versa (Table 13–2).

Investigators often have in mind a causal model under which an intervention should produce certain effects in a certain order. For example, the randomized trial of smoking cessation counseling to prevent low birth weight in infants born to smoking mothers described earlier was based on the model in Figure 13–1. This model led to measuring two outcomes: *(1)* whether pregnant smokers stopped smoking, and *(2)* infant birth weight. Maternal smoking behavior was an *intermediate* outcome. In this instance, more than twice as many pregnant smokers in the intervention group as in the control group quit smoking (43% vs. 20%), and babies born to intervention-group mothers averaged 92 grams heavier. Together, these findings suggested that the intervention did indeed work as intended.

But suppose there had been no difference in mean birth weight between groups. We might then have wondered whether the intervention had been ineffective in getting pregnant mothers to stop smoking, or the causal link between smoking in pregnancy and low infant birth weight was not as strong as had been supposed. Knowing whether maternal smoking behavior differed between groups would have provided a useful clue about where the hypothesized causal chain was broken.

While intermediate outcomes can help shed light on causal mechanisms, it can be risky to rely on these measures by themselves to evaluate intervention effects (Fleming and DeMets, 1996; Psaty et al., 1999).

Example: The Cardiac Arrhythmia Suppression Trial (CAST) (Echt et al., 1991) was motivated by two observations: *(1)* myocardial infarction survivors whose

Table 13–3. Mortality Experience in the Cardiac
Arrhythmia Suppression Trial

	ENCAINIDE OR FLECAINIDE	PLACEBO
No. of patients	755	743
No. of deaths:		
Fatal arrhythmia	43	16
Other cardiac	17	5
Non-cardiac	3	5
Total	63	26

[*Source:* Adapted from Echt et al. (1991).]

electrocardiogram showed frequent premature ventricular contractions (PVCs) had
an increased risk of sudden cardiac death, and *(2)* anti-arrhythmic drugs could
reduce the frequency of PVCs in these patients. In early testing, two drugs—
encainide and flecainide—were found to be particularly effective in suppressing
PVCs (Cardiac Arrhythmia Pilot Study (CAPS) Investigators, 1988). The main
CAST trial was then mounted to assess the ability of these drugs to save lives.
After 10 months, the results shown in Table 13–3 were obtained, and the trial was
stopped. Unexpectedly, both arrhythmic and non-arrhythmic cardiac deaths were
more common among patients who received encainide or flecainide than among
those who received placebo. Although the precise mechanisms for the observed
excess deaths remain unclear, these drugs evidently have important cardiac side-
effects beyond their ability to suppress PVCs. Using PVC suppression alone as
an intermediate endpoint to measure effectiveness would have been dangerously
misleading.

More broadly, to be a valid surrogate endpoint for assessing effectiveness,
an intermediate or short-term outcome measure must *fully* capture the effects of
treatment on the clinical endpoint (Prentice, 1989)—a requirement that is very
difficult to satisfy in practice.

Like cohort studies, randomized trials can lend themselves to study of multiple outcomes of a given exposure or intervention. Once the treatment groups
are established, it is often easy to add secondary outcome measures to the data
collection plan. The CARET study, for example, provided a convenient setting in
which to examine the effects of β-carotene and vitamin A on endpoints other than
lung cancer, including coronary heart disease (Omenn et al., 1996a).

ANALYSIS

Intent-to-Treat Principle

An important potential pitfall in the analysis and interpretation of randomized trials is perhaps best introduced by an example:

Example: The Coronary Drug Project was a multi-center, randomized, double-blind, placebo-controlled trial to determine whether treatment with lipid-altering agents, including clofibrate, could reduce mortality from coronary heart disease (Coronary Drug Project Research Group, 1980). Among trial participants who actually took 80% or more of the clofibrate dispensed, five-year mortality was 15.0%, compared to 24.6% among patients who were less compliant ($p = .00011$). It is tempting to infer that clofibrate worked well but that it could not benefit patients who failed to take it. Among patients who were 80%+ compliant *with placebo*, however, five-year mortality was 15.1%, compared with 28.3% among those who were less compliant *with placebo* ($p < 5 \times 10^{-16}$). Multivariate adjustment for 40 baseline characteristics had little effect on these findings. Overall, five-year mortality among patients randomized to clofibrate was 20.0%, compared to 20.9% among those randomized to placebo ($p = .55$), suggesting that use of clofibrate itself had little effect.

Under the intent-to-treat principle, the primary analysis in a randomized trial should compare outcomes *between the groups formed by randomization*. In other words, each participant is categorized according to what intervention he or she was intended to receive. The main reason for using the randomized-trial design in the first place is to form groups that can be assumed similar, even with regard to unmeasured factors that may affect outcomes. If the composition of one or more of those groups is altered, this property of randomization is lost. A study that began as a randomized trial would, in effect, be converted into an observational study in which confounding may be present.

Several circumstances can tempt investigators to depart from the intent-to-treat principle:

- *Non-compliance* with the intended treatment can occur, as in the Coronary Drug Project.
- *Crossing over* can occur if persons who were originally randomized to one treatment end up receiving the other. For example, in the Veterans Administration Cooperative Study of medical vs. surgical treatment for coronary heart disease, one patient in four who was randomized to medical therapy ultimately ended up receiving surgery (Peduzzi et al., 1991).

- *Late exclusions* can occur if participants are dropped from analysis after randomization. For example, in the Joint Study of Extracranial Arterial Occlusion (Sackett and Gent, 1979), the risk of recurrent transient ischemic attack, stroke, or death was reportedly reduced 27% ($p = .02$) in patients who had surgery to bypass an arterial occlusion when the analysis was based on those "available for follow-up." However, this analysis excluded 15 patients who had been randomized to surgery but who died early or had perioperative strokes, while only one patient who had been randomized to medical treatment was excluded after randomization. In an intent-to-treat analysis, patients who were assigned to undergo surgery had only a 16% reduction in risk ($p = .09$).

The price paid for keeping the benefits of randomization in an intent-to-treat analysis is typically a diluted treatment effect. (Exclusions after randomization can, of course, shift the results in either direction depending on the reasons for exclusion.) In an *effectiveness* trial, this dilution may be a good reflection of what to expect under real-world conditions and thus may be consistent with trial goals. In an *efficacy* trial, a diluted treatment effect is unwanted, but at least the direction of bias is generally predictable, toward finding no difference. Any treatment effect found in an intent-to-treat analysis is thus likely to be a conservative estimate of efficacy.

But suppose that little or no treatment effect is found in an intent-to-treat analysis when non-compliance or cross-overs were common. It may be impossible to distinguish between an inefficacious treatment and a Type II error. Some features of trial design can help avoid this dilemma. As noted earlier, non-compliance can be reduced by accepting only subjects who demonstrate compliance in a run-in phase or by other special efforts during the main trial (Haynes and Dantes, 1987). Late exclusions can be reduced by delaying randomization until as late as possible, so that some persons who are destined to drop out do so before randomization.

Subgroup Analyses

In most trials, the primary aim is to determine whether one strategy is superior to another among all participants combined. But sometimes larger treatment effects are expected in some subgroups than in others. For example, in the CARET study, the investigators anticipated that participants who had low serum β-carotene levels at baseline might benefit more from active treatment than those who had high baseline β-carotene levels (Omenn et al., 1996b).

Because there are always many ways to divide up a study population, subgroup analyses can quickly present a *multiple-comparisons problem* (Oxman and Guyatt, 1992; Yusuf et al., 1991). The more ways one looks for subgroup differences, the more likely it is that some "statistically significant" ones will be found, even if they reflect only the play of chance. Methods exist to "correct" p-values for the number of comparisons done, but their use remains controversial (Savitz and Olshan, 1995). Some investigators seek to limit the severity of this problem by specifying a very limited number of planned subgroup comparisons in advance (Yusuf et al., 1991), as in the Multiple Risk Factor Intervention Trial. The issues surrounding the interpretation of associations whose presence or size varies within subgroups of the study population are not confined to randomized trials, as will be discussed in Chapter 17.

Because each subgroup is smaller than the full study population, statistical tests for a treatment effect within subgroups have less power. If certain subgroups are of enough scientific importance, trial size can be increased accordingly during the planning phase. For example, Caritis and colleagues (1998) studied low-dose aspirin for prevention of pre-eclampsia in pregnant women. Four high-risk groups were identified in advance (women with pregestational diabetes, hypertension, multiple fetuses, or previous pre-eclampsia), and the trial was designed to be large enough to detect a 50% reduction in pre-eclampsia in each high-risk subgroup considered by itself.

Another problem can arise if subgroups are formed according to characteristics that were determined after randomization. Whether a trial participant ends up in a certain subgroup may then depend on the treatment group he or she was assigned to. In the Coronary Drug Project example, one might be tempted to try to circumvent the "dilution" of treatment effects that would occur in an intent-to-treat analysis by comparing outcomes only among patients who were compliant with their assigned treatment. But compliance was determined only after randomization and may well have depended on the particular treatment received. A patient who was compliant with a placebo regimen might not have complied with clofibrate, and vice versa. Hence, this analysis cannot be considered a true randomized comparison.

Peduzzi et al. (2002) discuss in more detail these and other issues that arise in analysis of data from randomized trials.

DESIGN VARIATIONS

Randomized trials comprise a large family of study designs, a few other members of which are introduced briefly here.

Factorial Design

Another randomized trial that sought to determine whether taking β-carotene would reduce the incidence of cancer was the Physicians' Health Study, conducted among more than 22,000 male U.S. physicians (Steering Committee of the

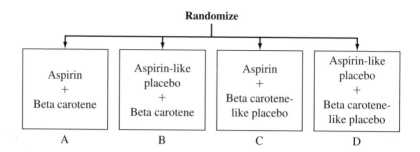

Figure 13–2. Physicians' Health Study as a Factorial Trial.

Physicians' Health Study Research Group, 1988). This study also had a second primary aim, however: namely, to determine whether taking 325 mg. of aspirin every other day would reduce the risk of a myocardial infarction. The aspirin and beta-carotene questions were essentially unrelated scientifically, but both were issues that could be well studied in a large sample of middle-aged male physician volunteers. The trial therefore used a 2 × 2 *factorial* design, as shown in Figure 13–2. It had four arms, representing all possible combinations of (1) either aspirin or an aspirin-like placebo, and (2) either beta carotene or a beta carotene-like placebo. Each participant was asked to take two kinds of pills, but he was not told what was in either kind.

To see why the factorial design was attractive here, consider two other possible trial designs. First, the investigators could have mounted two separate studies, one on aspirin and the other on beta carotene. If each such trial had required 22,000 participants (roughly the number actually studied), then the two separate trials would have required 44,000 physicians in all.

Second, recognizing that both aspirin and beta carotene were to be taken once every other day, it might have been possible to join these two separate trials by having the placebo group do double duty. The same placebo arm could serve as a control for both the aspirin and beta carotene arms. The study would now be a three-arm trial with 33,000 participants.

Under the design actually used, the investigators effectively did both studies for little more than the cost of doing one. Referring to Figure 13–2, the aspirin question could be studied by comparing outcomes in groups A + C combined vs. groups B + D combined. The beta carotene question could be studied by comparing outcomes in groups A + B combined vs. groups C + D combined. Each question could thus be addressed using the full study population.

But what if the effect of aspirin had differed depending on whether the participant was taking beta carotene? If so, this kind of effect modification might have been important to know about, because predictions about the effects of one drug would then depend on whether a man also took the other drug. Neither the two-separate-trials design nor the three-arm design could furnish this information, but the factorial design could. In this instance, no such pharmacological interaction was expected or observed (Steering Committee of the Physicians' Health Study Research Group, 1989).

In general, if synergy or antagonism between two interventions could be important scientifically, a factorial design provides a good opportunity to study it. If *no* synergy or antagonism is expected, a factorial design can be an attractive way to do two studies in one (Green, 2002; Stampfer et al., 1985).

Sequential Trials

For both ethical and economic reasons, it is desirable to end a trial early if the accumulated evidence shows that one treatment strategy is clearly superior. The CARET study was stopped almost two years early when it became clear that lung cancer incidence was unexpectedly greater in the active-treatment group. The CAST study was stopped early when it became clear that encainide and flecainide had unexpectedly increased cardiovascular mortality. Trials that involve continuous or periodic comparisons of outcomes as the study proceeds are termed *sequential* trials.

The design and analysis of sequential trials must account for multiple "looks" at the results, which again pose a kind of multiple-comparisons problem. Without special measures, repeated statistical testing would inflate the probability of a Type I error beyond the specified level. Fortunately, biostatistical methods are available to deal with this problem (Whitehead, 1999). It is even technically possible to re-analyze the data each time a new outcome event has occurred. But in practice it is usually more feasible to plan a few interim analyses at regular intervals for review by a data monitoring committee (Fleming and Watelet, 1989; DeMets, 1987).

Randomizing within Individuals

So far we have considered conventional trial designs in which individual people are randomized to different treatments. But entities smaller in scale than individual people can be randomized as well. For example:

- *Body parts* can be randomized within the same individual. One such trial sought to determine whether laser photocoagulation treatments could slow the progression of retinal complications of diabetes (Blankenship, 1979). For each eligible diabetic patient, one eye was chosen at random to be treated with laser photocoagulation, while the other eye served as a matched control.

- The *order of exposure* to alternative treatments is randomized in a *crossover* study. To determine the efficacy of hemodialysis as treatment for schizophrenia, Carpenter and colleagues (1983) used a crossover trial design in which half of the participants received real hemodialysis twice weekly for eight weeks, followed by sham hemodialysis twice weekly for another eight weeks. The other half of the patient sample received the same two treatments, but in the opposite order. A crossover design is most suitable when the expected effects of treatment occur promptly after treatment is begun and taper off promptly after it is stopped.
- *Intervals of time* can be randomized to different treatments within the same individual. This design is a generalization of the crossover design, with participants switching back and forth between treatments repeatedly. As a special case, a so-called *n-of-1* trial involves only one patient, for whom randomization is used to help guide a clinical decision about optimal therapy (Guyatt et al., 1986, 1988; Larson et al., 1993).

Analysis of results for this family of designs involves within-person comparisons between alternative treatments. Being able to make this kind of comparison offers two main advantages. First, patient-level characteristics that may influence outcomes, such as overall disease severity and symptom perceptions, apply in common to both intervention and control conditions. Hence the potential for confounding by these characteristics is greatly reduced or eliminated. Second, statistical power is usually enhanced because the variability in responses within the same individual tends to be smaller than the variability in responses between different individuals (Hills and Armitage, 1979; Gore, 1981a). Accordingly, when these designs can be used, they often require fewer participants than a parallel-groups design in which each person receives only one treatment.

Randomizing Groups of Individuals

The design variation just discussed involved randomizing something smaller than an individual. Another useful variation involves randomizing aggregates of individuals. Such a *group-randomized* design is worth considering when:

- By its nature, the experimental intervention applies non-selectively to an entire group. For example, fluoridation of a community's water supply or broadcasting health promotion messages via the mass media would affect nearly everyone in a community, so randomizing individuals to receive or not to receive such interventions would be difficult or impossible.

- Intervention effects are thought to be transmissible from person to person. For example, Peterson and colleagues (2000) randomized 40 school districts either to implement a smoking-prevention intervention or to serve as controls. The intervention sought to change norms about the desirability of smoking, so that schoolchildren would reinforce each other's decisions not to smoke. The intervention mechanism itself thus depended on interactions between individuals within a school. In other contexts, transmissibility of intervention effects may instead be a potential source of unwanted contamination of controls if individuals were randomized (Torgerson, 2001). That contamination may be largely avoidable if groups that are not in close communication with each other are randomized instead.

Study planning and data analysis for a group-randomized trial are typically more complex than when individuals are randomized (Atienza and King, 2002; Koepsell, 1998). Because outcome measurements on people within the same group are often correlated, analyzing the data as if individuals had been randomized tends to exaggerate statistical significance (Donner et al., 1981; Koepsell et al., 1991; Simpson et al., 1995). Avoiding this non-conservative bias requires taking both individual-level and group-level random variation within a treatment arm into account (Murray, 1998; Donner and Klar, 2000). The total sample size of individuals needed to achieve a certain level of statistical power is usually greater in a group-randomized study than in an individual-randomized study of the same topic.

CONCLUSION

Most of the time, epidemiologists must rely on non-randomized study designs. These methods provide us with many ways to detect and quantify associations. There is broad consensus (though by no means unanimity!) about how evidence from observational studies can be interpreted to support or refute causal inferences. Nonetheless, an association observed in a randomized trial provides perhaps the sturdiest bridge we have from association to causation. On several occasions, results from a randomized trial have ended up contradicting a theory that had been built on multiple prior observational studies (Omenn et al., 1996a; Hulley et al., 1998; Heart Outcomes Prevention Evaluation Study Investigators, 2000). These surprises ought to keep us humble when we seek to interpret the results of observational studies. They also show why randomized trials deserve a special place in our set of research tools and why well-trained epidemiologists need to know when and how to use them.

APPENDIX 13A

Estimating Sample Size Requirements for a Two-Arm Trial with a Binary Outcome

For a trial comparing two equal-sized groups on a binary outcome variable, the following formula can be used to estimate the number of study subjects (n) needed in *each* of the two arms (Friedman et al., 1998):

$$n = \frac{2(Z_\alpha + Z_\beta)^2 \bar{p}(1 - \bar{p})}{(p_0 - p_1)^2} \tag{13.1}$$

where:

α is the maximum acceptable risk of a *Type I error*—i.e., of concluding that the effects of the two treatments on outcomes differ, when in fact they do not. A standard choice is $\alpha = .05$.

Z_α is a standard normal deviate (z-score) corresponding to the chosen level of α and whether one- or two-tailed significance testing will be done. The value of Z_α is 1.96 for two-tailed significance testing at $\alpha = .05$.

β is the maximum acceptable risk of a *Type II error*—i.e., of concluding that the effects of the two treatments on outcomes are the same, when in truth they differ by a specified amount. Values chosen for β are less standardized by convention than for α, but common choices are .05, .10, or .20. Statistical *power* is defined as $1 - \beta$.

Z_β is a standard normal deviate for the chosen level of β (using one tail only). Common values are $Z_\beta = 1.645$ for $\beta = .05$, $Z_\beta = 1.28$ for $\beta = .10$, and $Z_\beta = .84$ for $\beta = .20$.

p_0 is the projected cumulative incidence of the outcome among control-arm participants.

p_1 is the projected cumulative incidence of the outcome among intervention-arm participants, assuming that the intervention works as hypothesized.

$\bar{p}$ is the projected cumulative incidence of the outcome in both arms combined, which is $(p_1 + p_0)/2$.

Example: For many years, it was standard obstetrical practice in some settings to admit a woman pregnant with twins to the hospital when she reached 32 weeks gestation, in the belief that bed rest would reduce the risk of pre-term delivery. Faced with a shortage of hospital beds and of empirical evidence in support this practice, Saunders and colleagues (1985) conducted a randomized trial in Harare, Zimbabwe. From historical data, they estimated that 30% of such women would deliver before 37 weeks. They hypothesized that bed rest might reduce this percentage to 20%. If they chose $\alpha = .05$ (two-tailed) and $\beta = .20$, then $Z_\alpha = 1.96$, $Z_\beta = 0.84$, $p_0 = 0.30$, $p_1 = .20$, $\overline{p} = .25$, and the necessary sample size in each arm would be:

$$n = \frac{2(1.96 + .84)^2(.25)(1 - .25)}{(.30 - .20)^2}$$

$$= 294.$$

(To their surprise, pre-term delivery turned out to be significantly *more* common among electively hospitalized mothers—30% vs. 19%—so they were wise to have used a two-tailed test!)

APPENDIX 13B

Methods for Randomization by Computer

The methods below assume that the computer program used for randomization provides a function for generating random numbers with a uniform distribution from 0 to 1. They also assume that study subjects are to be assigned to either of two groups with equal probability.

Simple Randomization

1. Start with a list of study subjects. If subjects will be recruited later and their identities are not yet known, the list can be just a list of consecutive integers that denote the sequence in which subjects will enter the study. Each sequence number later gets matched to a specific person as recruitment proceeds.
2. Add a new variable (column) called R to the list, and fill in its values using the random-number function.
3. Assign each position on the list with $R < 0.5$ to intervention, and each position on the list with $R \geq 0.5$ to control.

The rule used in the last step is arbitrary but simple, yields the desired allocation probabilities, and was specified in advance.

Blocked Randomization

For blocks of size k, where k is an integer multiple of the number of treatment arms (e.g., k is an even number for a two-arm trial):

1. Start with a numbered list of study subjects. As with simple randomization, spaces on the list for identifiers may be empty at first, to be filled in sequentially later as subjects enter the study.
2. Add a variable R, containing a different random number value for each subject on the list.
3. Sort the list by R within block number.
4. Within each block, assign the $k/2$ subjects now listed earliest in the sorted list to the intervention group. The rest go to the control group.

After the last step, the list can be re-sorted into the original sequence if desired. The rule in the last step can easily be modified for studies with more than two treatment arms, or to allocate subjects in a ratio other than 1:1.

EXERCISES

1. Internal mammary artery ligation enjoyed brief popularity in the 1950s for treatment of coronary artery disease, until randomized trials showed no appreciable benefit from the procedure compared to sham surgery. A key study by Cobb and colleagues (1959) was described in this chapter and involved a total of twelve men and five women.

   (a) According to the published report, all five of the women were randomly assigned to the ligated group. But the probability that all of the women would be assigned to the new procedure by chance alone is only about .03. Does this imply tampering with the randomization scheme?

   (b) Under what circumstances would the resulting imbalance in the sex composition of the two treatment groups bias the outcome of the study?

   (c) Is there any way by which the investigators could have prevented the gender imbalance, yet still allocate subjects at random to the two groups? If so, how?

   (d) During 3 to 15 months of follow-up, patients who received sham surgery tended to report marked improvement in their symptoms and reduced need for nitroglycerin tablets to control their angina attacks. Does this indicate that sham surgery is effective for relieving angina? Why or why not?

2. The Heart and Estrogen/progestin Replacement Study (HERS) sought to confirm many prior non-randomized studies that observed a lower risk of coronary heart disease associated with use of estrogens by postmenopausal women
(Hulley et al., 1998). Among other effects, estrogens are thought to lower LDL
cholesterol and to raise HDL cholesterol. The HERS trial involved randomizing
2763 women with a history of coronary heart disease to either *(a)* 0.625 mg./day
of conjugated estrogens plus 0.25 mg./day of medroxyprogesterone acetate; or
(b) placebo. During an average follow-up of 4.1 years, the incidence of the combined endpoint, myocardial infarction or death from coronary heart disease, was
almost identical in the two groups (relative risk = 0.99, 95% confidence interval
= 0.80–1.22).

(a) The HERS trial's primary aim was to test the efficacy of postmenopausal
hormone therapy for preventing CHD. But it also sought to evaluate the
safety of this regimen in terms of the incidence of other health conditions.
In what way might a randomized trial be limited in its ability to establish
safety in comparison to other epidemiologic study designs?

(b) After the study was published, a critic contended that the results may have
been biased because diagnostic tests were not performed at the outset of
the trial to ascertain the extent of coronary and other vascular disease in
participants. Would you agree that this was a flaw?

(c) Lipid-lowering drugs turned out to be used more often during the course
of the trial by placebo recipients than by estrogen/progestin recipients.
Should this differential use be considered a potential confounding factor
in evaluating the effectiveness of these hormones for preventing coronary
heart disease?

3. Falls are common in older adults. Kannus and colleagues (2000) conducted
a randomized trial of thin, inexpensive pads that can be positioned over the
greater femoral trochanter and worn under clothing. If the wearer falls, the
hip pad is intended to cushion the blow and keep the upper femur from
breaking.

The trial involved 1,801 ambulatory adults who resided in 20 Finnish geri-
atric treatment units. The treatment units were randomly allocated in a 1:2 ratio
to be either a hip-pad unit or a control unit.

(a) In principle, each individual adult could have been randomized either to
wear hip pads or to serve as a control. Why do you suppose the investigators
chose to randomize treatment units instead?

(b) The published trial report contains a table comparing the baseline characteristics of residents of units assigned to the hip-pad and control groups,
from which the results shown in Table 13–4 are excerpted.

Table 13–4. Baseline Characteristics of Residents in the Intervention
and Control Groups in a Randomized Trial of Hip Pads

| | Percent or mean ± s.d. | | |
| | HIP-PAD GROUP | CONTROL GROUP | |
CHARACTERISTIC	$(n = 653)$	$(n = 1148)$	p-VALUE
Sex			.41
Female	77%	79%	
Male	23%	21%	
Age (years)	81 ± 6	82 ± 6	.006
Weight (kg.)	63.1 ± 11.8	65.5 ± 13.1	<.001
Medical conditions			
Heart disease	52%	51%	.46
Dementia	33%	26%	.001
Hypertension	20%	23%	.13
Past stroke	21%	15%	.002
Mental status			<.001
Normal	39%	42%	
Mild impairment	19%	25%	
Moderate impairment	22%	22%	
Severe impairment	21%	12%	
Walking ability			.001
Independently	39%	35%	
With cane or walker	49%	57%	
With help	12%	8%	

[*Source:* Adapted from Kannus et al. (2000).]

We normally expect only about 5% of baseline comparisons to be
statistically significant at the .05 level. Why do you think so many of the
differences shown in this table resulted in such small p-values?

(c) After the treatment units had been randomized, older adults on each unit
were asked whether they would be willing to take part in the study. Some
31% of patients on hip-pad units declined, vs. 9% of patients on control
units. Could this difference have led to bias? If so, how might it have been
avoidable by designing the trial differently?

(d) Suppose that you are thinking about conducting a confirmatory trial in
which older adults in assisted-living settings would be individually randomized with equal probability to hip-pad or control conditions and then
followed for 18 months. Drawing on the Finnish study results, you consider

it reasonable to assume that the 18-month cumulative incidence of hip fracture among controls should be about 7.5%. You would like the study to have
80% power to detect a 50% reduction in hip-fracture incidence in the hip-
pad group. You plan to test the results for statistical significance with a
two-tailed test at the .05 level. Assume that dropouts will be negligible.
How many subjects would be needed in each arm?

ANSWERS

1. *(a)* *Imply* is too strong a word. Even under a fair random allocation process,
   all five women could be assigned to the ligated group with probability
   $1/2 \times 1/2 \times 1/2 \times 1/2 \times 1/2 = 1/32$—an unusual but not impossible
   outcome of random allocation. After all, people do win the lottery.

   (b) Because of the apparent "accident of randomization," gender was strongly
   associated with exposure (whether the internal mammary artery was ligated). If gender itself were associated with any of the outcomes under study,
   then it would become a confounding factor. The results were not reported
   separately by gender, however, so we cannot actually compare outcomes
   between men and women within the ligated group.

   (c) They could have used randomly permuted blocks within each gender group.
   For example, if blocks of size two were used, the first two men recruited for
   study would be considered to belong to the same block. A random number
   would then be chosen to decide which of the two men would be assigned to
   the ligated group, with the other man automatically going to the non-ligated
   group.

   (d) No. This was only a before-after comparison. Symptoms of coronary heart
   disease tend to vary over time within an individual, waxing and waning
   in severity. Patients would be unlikely to consider surgery at a time when
   their symptoms were relatively mild or improving; instead, they would be
   looking for new therapeutic options when their symptoms were relatively
   severe for them. Even in the absence of any therapeutic benefit, we might
   expect such patients' symptom severity to improve over time as they regress
   to their respective mean severity levels. More convincing evidence of the
   effectiveness of sham surgery would come from a randomized comparison
   group that did not undergo sham surgery.

2. *(a)* Randomized trials are not statistically efficient for detecting rare or delayed,
   but nonetheless serious, unintended effects of a therapy. For example, the
   investigators noted that the HERS trial had insufficient power to determine

whether long-term use of hormones would affect the risk of breast cancer, given that "only" 2763 women were included and that the total length of the study was only 4.1 years.

(b) Given the large sample size, it is reasonable to assume that randomization balanced the groups well on unknown or unmeasured potential confounders, including the nature and extent of pre-existing coronary heart disease.

(c) No. The lower prevalence of lipid-lowering drug use among placebo recipients was probably due to a true biological effect of estrogens on lipids; a placebo would have no such effect. But because lipid-lowering drug use would be causally "downstream" from the treatment assigned at random, it would not be a true confounder. Part of the overall effect of hormone replacement on heart disease risk may include making it less likely that the recipient would receive other lipid-lowering drugs.

3. (a) They feared that randomizing individual patients within a unit would pose too great a risk of "contamination" if those who were randomized to the control group felt short-changed, got access to hip pads, and started wearing them.

(b) Randomization was conducted at the treatment-unit level, but the statistical testing for this table was apparently done as if individual patients had been randomized. (Note that the n's atop the columns total to 1801, not 20.) The mix of patients was evidently quite variable among treatment units, with some units catering to older adults, some to adults with dementia, etc. When entire treatment units were randomized, all adults in a unit that served generally older people or people with dementia were assigned *en bloc* to one of the treatment groups.

Randomizing clusters generally does not balance the treatment arms as evenly as randomizing individuals, because fewer units are randomly allocated. Proper statistical significance testing must account for the cluster randomization and would no doubt have shown many fewer baseline comparisons to be statistically significant in this instance.

(c) Yes, it could have led to bias. Many control-group participants probably would have declined participation had they been assigned to the hip-pad group, but they remained in the study. No comparable subjects remained in the hip-pad group—they declined to take part. Hence selection bias occurring after randomization may have rendered two groups of participants dissimilar.

This bias might have been avoided if potential participants had been asked *first* if they would be willing to be randomized to either a hip-pad group or a control group. Only those who consented would then have been randomized and taken part in the rest of the study.

(d) For power $= 80\%$, $\beta = 0.2$, which corresponds to $Z_\beta = .84$. For a two-tailed test at $\alpha = .05$, $Z_\beta = 1.96$.

$$p_0 = \text{cumulative incidence in controls}$$
$$= .075$$
$$p_1 = \text{cumulative incidence in hip-pad group}$$
$$= .075 \times 0.5 = .0375$$
$$\overline{p} = \frac{p_0 + p_1}{2}$$
$$= .05625$$
$$n = \frac{2(Z_\alpha + Z_\beta)^2 \overline{p}(1 - \overline{p})}{(p_0 - p_1)^2}$$
$$= \frac{2(1.96 + .84)^2(.05625)(1 - .05625)}{(.075 - .0375)^2}$$
$$= 592$$

REFERENCES

ALLHAT Collaborative Research Group. Major cardiovascular events in hypertensive patients randomized to doxazosin vs chlorthalidone: the antihypertensive and lipid-lowering treatment to prevent heart attack trial (ALLHAT). JAMA 2000; 283:1967–75.

Altman DG, Dore CJ. Randomisation and baseline comparisons in clinical trials. Lancet 1990; 335:149–53.

Assmann SF, Pocock SJ, Enos LE, Kasten LE. Subgroup analysis and other (mis)uses of baseline data in clinical trials. Lancet 2000; 355:1064–69.

Atienza AA, King AC. Community-based health intervention trials: an overview of methodological issues. Epidemiol Rev 2002; 24:72–79.

Blankenship GW. Diabetic macular edema and argon laser photocoagulation: a prospective randomized study. Ophthalmology 1979; 86:69–78.

Byington RP, Curb JD, Mattson ME. Assessment of double-blindness at the conclusion of the β-Blocker Heart Attack Trial. JAMA 1985; 253:1733–36.

Cardiac Arrhythmia Pilot Study (CAPS) Investigators. Effects of encainide, flecainide, imipramine and moricizine on ventricular arrhythmias during the year after acute myocardial infarction: the CAPS. The Cardiac Arrhythmia Pilot Study (CAPS). Am J Cardiol 1988; 61:501–9.

Caritis S, Sibae B, Hauth J, Lindheimer MD, Klebanoff M, Thom E, et al. Low-dose aspirin to prevent pre-eclampsia in women at high risk. N Engl J Med 1998; 338:701–5.

Carpenter WT, Sadler JH, Light PD, Hanlon TE, Kurland AA, Penna MW, et al. The therapeutic efficacy of hemodialysis in schizophrenia. N Engl J Med 1983; 308:669–75.

Chalmers TC, Celano P, Sacks HS, Smith H Jr. Bias in treatment assignment in controlled clinical trials. N Engl J Med 1983; 309:1358–61.

Charlton BG. Understanding randomized controlled trials: explanatory or pragmatic? Fam Pract 1994; 11:243–44.

Cobb LA, Thomas GI, Dillard DH, Merendino KA, Bruce RA. An evaluation of internal-mammary-artery ligation by a double-blind technic. N Engl J Med 1959; 260:1115–18.

Cohen J. Statistical power analysis for the behavioral sciences (2nd ed.). Hillsdale, N.J.: Lawrence Erlbaum Associates, 1988.

Coronary Drug Project Research Group. Influence of adherence to treatment and response of cholesterol on mortality in the Coronary Drug Project. N Engl J Med 1980; 303:1038–41.

DeMets DL. Practical aspects in data monitoring: a brief review. Stat Med 1987; 6:753–60.

Donner A. Approaches to sample size estimation in the design of clinical trials—a review. Stat Med 1984; 3:199–214.

Donner A, Birkett N, Buck C. Randomisation by cluster: sample size requirements and analysis. Am J Epidemiol 1981; 114:906–14.

Donner A, Klar N. Design and analysis of cluster randomisation trials in health research. New York: Edward Arnold, 2000.

Echt DS, Liebson PR, Mitchell LB, Peters RW, Obias-Manno D, Barker AH, et al. Mortality and morbidity in patients receiving encainide, flecainide, or placebo. The Cardiac Arrhythmia Suppression Trial. N Engl J Med 1991; 324:781–88.

Fleiss JL. The design and analysis of clinical experiments. New York: Wiley and Sons, 1986.

Fleming TR, DeMets DL. Surrogate end points in clinical trials: are we being misled? Ann Intern Med 1996; 125:605–13.

Fleming TR, Watelet LF. Approaches to monitoring clinical trials. J Natl Cancer Inst 1989; 81:188–93.

Friedman LM, Furberg CD, DeMets DL. Fundamentals of clinical trials (3rd ed.). New York: Springer-Verlag, 1998.

Gore SM. Assessing clinical trials—design I. BMJ 1981a; 282:1780–81.

Gore SM. Assessing clinical trials—first steps. BMJ 1981b; 282:1605–7.

Gore SM. Assessing clinical trials—simple randomisation. BMJ 1981c; 282: 2036–39.

Green S. Design of randomized trials. Epidemiol Rev 2002; 24:4–11.

Guyatt G, Sackett D, Adachi J, Roberts R, Chong J, Rosenbloom D, et al. A clinician's guide for conducting randomized trials in individual patients. CMAJ 1988; 139:497–503.

Guyatt G, Sackett D, Taylor DW, Chong J, Roberts R, Pugsley S. Determining optimal therapy—randomized trials in individual patients. N Engl J Med 1986; 314:889–92.

Haynes RB, Dantes R. Patient compliance and the conduct and interpretation of therapeutic trials. Control Clin Trials 1987; 8:12–19.

Heart Outcomes Prevention Evaluation Study Investigators. Vitamin E supplementation and cardiovascular events in high-risk patients. N Engl J Med 2000; 342:154–60.

Hills M, Armitage P. The two-period cross-over clinical trial. Br J Clin Pharmacol 1979; 8:7–20.

Howard J, Whittemore AS, Hoover JJ, Panos M. How blind was the patient blind in AMIS? Clin Pharmacol Ther 1982; 32:543–53.

Hrøbjartsson A, Gøtzsche PC. Is the placebo powerless? An analysis of clinical trials comparing placebo with no treatment. N Engl J Med 2001; 344:1594–602.

Hulley S, Grady D, Bush T, Furberg C, Herrington D, Riggs B, et al. Randomized trial of estrogen plus progestin for secondary prevention of coronary heart disease in post-menopausal women. JAMA 1998; 280:605–13.

Hulley SB, Cummings SR, Browner WS, Grady D, Hearst N, Newman TB. Designing clinical research: an epidemiologic approach (2nd ed.). Baltimore: Lippincott, Williams & Wilkins, 2001.

Hunninghake DB, Darby CA, Probstfield JL. Recruitment experience in clinical trials: literature summary and annotated bibliography. Control Clin Trials 1987; 8:6S–30S.

Johnstone EC, Drakin JFW, Lawler P, Frith CD, Stevens M, McPherson K, et al. The Northwick Park electroconvulsive therapy trial. Lancet 1980; 2:1317–20.

Kahn JP, Mastroianni AC, Sugarman J. Beyond consent: seeking justice in research. New York: Oxford, 1998.

Kannus P, Parkkari J, Niemi S, Paganen M, Palvanen M, Jarvinen M, et al. Prevention of hip fracture in elderly people with use of a hip protector. N Engl J Med 2000; 343:1506–13.

Kernan WN, Viscoli CM, Makuch RW, Brass LM, Horwitz RI. Stratified randomization for clinical trials. J Clin Epidemiol 1999; 52:19–26.

Kodish E, Lantos JD, Siegler M. Ethical considerations in randomized controlled clinical trials. Cancer 1990; 65:2400–4.

Koepsell TD. "Epidemiologic issues in design of community intervention trials." Chapter 6 in Brownson RC, Petitti D (eds.). Applied epidemiology. New York: Oxford, 1998.

Koepsell TD, Martin DC, Diehr PH, Psaty BM, Wagner EH, Perrin EB, et al. Data analysis and sample size issues in evaluations of community-based health promotion and disease prevention programs: a mixed-model analysis of variance approach. J Clin Epidemiol 1991; 44:701–13.

Kraemer HC. How many subjects? Statistical power analysis in research. Newbury Park, Calif.: Sage Publications, 1987.

Lachin JM. Introduction to sample size determination and power analysis for clinical trials. Control Clin Trials 1981; 2:93–113.

Lachin JM, Matts JP, Wei LJ. Randomization in clinical trials: conclusions and recommendations. Control Clin Trials 1988; 9:365–74.

Lang JM. The use of a run-in to enhance compliance. Stat Med 1990; 9:87–95.

Larson EB, Ellsworth AJ, Oas J. Randomized clinical trials in single patients during a 2-year period. JAMA 1993; 270:2708–12.

Last JM. A dictionary of epidemiology (4th ed.). New York: Oxford University Press, 2000.

Macknin ML, Mathew S, Medendorp SV. Effect of inhaling heated vapor on symptoms of the common cold. JAMA 1990; 264:989–91.

Moher D, Dulberg CS, Wells GA. Statistical power, sample size, and their reporting in randomized controlled trials. JAMA 1994; 272:122–24.

MRC Working Party. Medical Research Council trial of treatment of hypertension in older adults: principal results. BMJ 1992; 304:405–12.

Multiple Risk Factor Intervention Trial Research Group. Multiple Risk Factor Intervention Trial. Risk factor changes and mortality results. JAMA 1982; 248:1465–77.

Multiple Risk Factor Intervention Trial Research Group. Mortality rates after 10.5 years for participants in the Multiple Risk Factor Intervention Trial. Findings related to a priori hypotheses of the trial. JAMA 1990; 263:1795–801.

Murray DM. Design and analysis of group-randomized trials. New York: Oxford, 1998.

National Center for Health Statistics. Health, United States, 2000, with adolescent chartbook. Hyattsville, Md.: National Center for Health Statistics, 2000.

Omenn GS, Goodman GE, Thornquist MD, Balmes J, Cullen MR, Glass A, et al. Effects of a combination of beta-carotene and vitamin A on lung cancer and cardiovascular disease. N Engl J Med 1996a; 334:1150–55.

Omenn GS, Goodman GE, Thornquist MD, Balmes J, Cullen MR, Glass A, et al. Risk factors for lung cancer and for intervention effects in CARET, the beta-Carotene and Retinol Efficacy Trial. J Natl Cancer Inst 1996b; 88:1550–59.

Omenn GS, Goodman GE, Thornquist MD, Grizzle J, Rosenstock L, Barnhart S, et al. The β-Carotene and Retinol Efficacy Trial (CARET) for chemoprevention of lung cancer in high risk populations: smokers and asbestos-exposed workers. Cancer Res 1994; 43 (suppl.):2038s–2043s.

Oxman AD, Guyatt GH. A consumer's guide to subgroup analyses. Ann Intern Med 1992; 116:78–84.

Pablos-Mendez A, Barr RG, Shea S. Run-in periods in randomized trials. Implications for the application of results in clinical practice. JAMA 1998; 279:222–25.

Peduzzi P, Detre K, Wittes J, Holford T. Intent-to-treat analysis and the problem of crossovers. J Thorac Cardiovasc Surg 1991; 101:481–87.

Peduzzi P, Henderson W, Hartigan P, Lavori P. Analysis of randomized controlled trials. Epidemiol Rev 2002; 24:26–38.

Peterson AV Jr, Kealey KA, Mann SL, Marek PM, Sarason IG. Hutchinson Smoking Prevention Project: long-term randomized trial in school-based tobacco use prevention—results on smoking. J Natl Cancer Inst 2000; 92:1979–91.

Peto R, Gray R, Collins R, Wheatley K, Hennekens C, Jamrozik K, et al. Randomised trial of prophylactic daily aspirin in British male doctors. BMJ 1988; 296:313–16.

Prentice RL. Surrogate endpoints in clinical trials: definition and operational criteria. Stat Med 1989; 8:431–40.

Prentice RL, Omenn GS, Goodman GE, Chu J, Henderson MM, Feigl P, et al. Rationale and design of cancer chemoprevention studies in Seattle. NCI Monogr 1985; 69:249–58.

Psaty BM, Weiss NS, Furberg CD, Koepsell TD, Siscovick DS, Rosendaal FR, et al. Surrogate end points, health outcomes, and the drug-approval process for the treatment of risk factors for cardiovascular disease. JAMA 1999; 282:786–90.

Rosa L, Rosa E, Sarner L, Barrett S. A close look at therapeutic touch. JAMA 1998; 279:1005–10.

Rosner B. Fundamentals of biostatistics (4th edition). New York: Duxbury Press, 1995.

Sackett DL, Gent M. Controversy in counting and attributing events in clinical trials. N Engl J Med 1979; 301:1410–12.

Saunders MC, Dick JS, Brown IM, McPherson K, Chalmers I. The effects of hospital admission for bed rest on the duration of twin pregnancy: a randomised trial. Lancet 1985; 2:793–95.

Savitz DA, Olshan AF. Multiple comparisons and related issues in the interpretation of epidemiologic data. Am J Epidemiol 1995; 142:904–8.

Schulz KF. Subverting randomization in controlled trials. JAMA 1995; 274: 1456–58.

Schulz KF, Chalmers I, Hayes RJ, Altman DG. Empirical evidence of bias. Dimensions of methodological quality associated with estimates of treatment effects in controlled trials. JAMA 1995; 273:408–12.

Schwartz D, Lellouch J. Explanatory and pragmatic attitudes in therapeutical trials. J Chron Dis 1967; 20:637–48.

Sexton M, Hebel JR. A clinical trial of change in maternal smoking and its effect on birth weight. JAMA 1984; 251:911–15.

Simpson JM, Klar N, Donner A. Accounting for cluster randomization: a review of primary prevention trials, 1990 through 1993. Am J Public Health 1995; 85:1378–83.

Stampfer MJ, Buring JE, Willett W, Rosner B, Eberlein K, Hennekens CH. The 2 × 2 factorial design: its application to a randomized trial of aspirin and carotene in U.S. physicians. Stat Med 1985; 4:111–16.

Steering Committee of the Physicians' Health Study Research Group. Preliminary report: findings from the aspirin component of the ongoing Physicians' Health Study. N Engl J Med 1988; 318:262–64.

Steering Committee of the Physicians' Health Study Research Group. Final report on the aspirin component of the ongoing Physicians' Health Study. N Engl J Med 1989; 321: 129–35.

Stout RL, Wirtz PW, Carbonari JP, Boca FKD. Ensuring balanced distribution of prognostic factors in treatment outcome research. J Stud Alcohol 1994; 12:70–75.

Sugarman J. Ethics in the design and conduct of clinical trials. Epidemiol Rev 2002; 24: 54–58.

Taylor KM, Margolese RG, Soskolne CL. Physicians' reasons for not entering eligible patients in a randomized clinical trial of surgery for breast cancer. N Engl J Med 1984; 310:1363–67.

Thornquist MD, Omenn GS, Goodman GE, Grizzle JE, Rosenstock L, Barnhart S, et al. Statistical design and monitoring of the Carotene and Retinol Efficacy Trial (CARET). Control Clin Trials 1993; 14:308–24.

Torgerson DJ. Contamination in trials: is cluster randomisation the answer? BMJ 2001; 322:355–57.

US Department of Health and Human Services. 45 Code of Federal Regulations 46. Fed Reg 1991; 56:28012.

Veterans Administration Cooperative Study Group on Antihypertensive Agents. Effects of treatment on morbidity in hypertension. Results in patients with diastolic blood pressures averaging 115 through 129 mmHg. JAMA 1967; 202:116–22.

Vickers AJ, de Craen AJ. Why use placebos in clinical trials? A narrative review of the methodological literature. J Clin Epidemiol 2000; 53:157–61.

Walsh BT, Seidman SN, Sysko R, Gould M. Placebo response in studies of major depression: variable, substantial, and growing. JAMA 2002; 287:1840–47.

Whitehead J. A unified theory for sequential clinical trials. Stat Med 1999; 18:2271–86.

Wittes J. Sample size calculations for randomized controlled trials. Epidemiol Rev 2002; 24:39–53.

Wittes J, Brittain E. The role of internal pilot studies in increasing the efficiency of clinical trials. Stat Med 1990; 9:65–72.

Yusuf S, Wittes J, Probstfield J, Tyroler HA. Analysis and interpretation of treatment effects in subgroups of patients in randomized clinical trials. JAMA 1991; 266:93–8.

14

COHORT STUDIES

Cohort studies, sometimes called follow-up studies, compare the subsequent occurrence of illness, injury, or death among groups of people whose exposure status differs "naturally," i.e., not as the result of random assignment. Sometimes the "exposure" to be studied is an exogenous one, such as infection with hepatitis B virus or consumption of dietary fiber. Other times it is a characteristic of persons, such as ABO blood type or their height and weight. The exposure or characteristics under study can be present as discrete categories, such as blood type O, A, B, or AB, or as a gradient on a continuous scale (such as fiber intake) when no natural categories exist.

The follow-up of study subjects for the occurrence of illness, injury, or death may already have occurred prior to the time of the initiation of the study. For example, many studies of the possible relationship of occupational exposures to health identify persons employed in earlier years and monitor the mortality rates of these workers up until the time the study is initiated. These are often called "retrospective" cohort studies. Alternatively, a cohort study may ascertain exposure status at the outset with follow-up to occur in the future. Studies of this type are "prospective" cohort studies. In either case, the studies are able to determine cumulative incidence or incidence rates directly from the experience of the study subjects, which sets them apart from most case-control studies. What sets cohort studies apart from randomized controlled trials, of course, is that in them something other than chance alone led an individual study subject to receive a particular exposure or to possess a particular characteristic. Therefore, in contrast to the interpretation of randomized controlled trials, the interpretation of the results of cohort studies must consider the reason for the person's being exposed or not (or the reason underlying their level of exposure) as a possible explanation for the results seen.

COHORT IDENTIFICATION

Some cohort studies seek to enlist as participants a sample of persons who reside in a defined geographical area. From those who agree to take part in the study, exposure information and health outcomes are ascertained. During the second half of the twentieth century in the United States, studies of this type have taken place in such locations as Framingham, Massachusetts; Tecumseh, Michigan; Evans County, Georgia; and Washington County, Maryland. More commonly, however, cohort studies are fashioned around persons who have distinctive and measurable exposures, or among groups of people for which there are special resources that allow for either cohort identification and/or cohort follow-up.

Cohort Studies Initiated Because of the Presence of a Distinctive Exposure

Assessments of the potential impact of ionizing radiation on the incidence of cancer have exploited the presence of identifiable groups of persons who had been exposed to such radiation in various contexts. Specifically, epidemiologists have conducted studies of cancer incidence among survivors of the atomic detonations in Hiroshima and Nagasaki (Shimizu et al., 1990); Israeli children who received scalp irradiation for tinea capitis (Ron et al., 1988); British patients with ankylosing spondylitis who underwent radiation therapy (Court-Brown and Doll, 1957); persons exposed to radiation on the job [such as radiologists (Seltser and Sartwell, 1965) and uranium miners (Darby et al., 1995)]; and children who, while in utero, had been exposed to diagnostic X-rays given to their mothers (Harvey et al., 1985). Most of what we know about the health effects of irradiation on human beings comes from studies such as these.

Special Resources for Cohort Identification and/or Follow-up

Some cohort studies have been mounted among persons enrolled in life insurance plans, since follow-up for mortality in such persons can be achieved with nearly complete success by monitoring claims submitted by beneficiaries of cohort members. For example, one of the earliest cohort studies of smoking and mortality involved the mailing of brief questionnaires to former World War II servicemen who held government life insurance policies (Kahn, 1966). Subsequent mortality rates from lung cancer and other conditions could then be compared between men who had and had not reported being cigarette smokers.

Similarly, the strong incentive for members of prepaid health care plans to receive medical care from within the plan enables cohort studies to be conducted in such individuals at relatively low cost. Studies done in these settings can determine if the incidence of various illnesses that generally require medical treatment among health plan members differs according to the presence of various antecedent medical conditions or the use of prescription drugs, since these can be ascertained through the records of many prepaid health care plans as well.

Finally, it is also relatively easy to do cohort studies among women seeking prenatal care, since the large majority of them will continue to seek care from the same provider through the time of the delivery of their child. This allows for relatively complete access to information on pregnancy outcomes that occur among patients of a given provider of prenatal care.

Occasionally, investigators have at their disposal an unusual ability to collect follow-up information on potential cohort members, allowing a cohort study to take place that would not otherwise be feasible. For example, prior to the advent of the National Death Index in the United States, the American Cancer Society conducted a large cohort study (Hammond, 1966) that utilized the very large number of Cancer Society volunteers to both identify potential cohort members and help monitor their whereabouts and vital status. Also, several studies of college alumni have been conducted (Lee and Paffenbarger RS Jr, 1998; Sesso et al., 1998) because of the existence of alumni association records that maintain a listing of their members' addresses. In each of these instances, the cohort study was done prospectively, with a questionnaire being sent out to potential cohort members at the outset and the follow-up for mortality occurring subsequently.

Increasingly, with the advent of population-based disease registries, it has been possible to follow cohort members for the occurrence of diseases that are ascertained by these registries. Thus, the follow-up of cancer incidence among Israeli children treated with scalp irradiation was done simply by linking the identity of the irradiated children with those who later appeared in the records of the Israel Tumor Registry (Ron et al., 1988).

METHODS OF ASCERTAINMENT OF EXPOSURE STATUS

Records

Records, of one sort or another, serve as the means of characterizing the exposure status of study participants in many cohort studies. Occupational records, available from employers or unions, can identify the fact of employment in a job or industry in which a particular exposure is known to be (or to have been) present. Often, additional relevant information is available from this source as well, such as the duration and recency of employment, as well as the type of job held and the location(s) of that job within the work environment. A discussion of the ascertainment of occupational exposures, along with other aspects of occupational cohort studies, can be found in Checkoway and Eisen (1998).

The availability of *medical* and *pharmacy* records over a period of years on members of prepaid health care plans, or enrollees in government health insurance programs, has allowed many cohort studies to be conducted. Examples include the evaluation of the possible influence of vasectomy on the incidence of coronary heart disease (Walker et al., 1981; Petitti et al., 1983; Nienhuis et al., 1992) and of the use of appetite-suppressant drugs on the incidence of valvular heart disease (Jick et al., 1998).

Some cohort studies have been made feasible because of "exposure" information contained in *vital* records. For example, women who underwent elective induction of labor were identified from birth certificates of the state of Washington during 1989 through 1993, and the occurrence of caesarean section and selected unfavorable pregnancy outcomes was compared between them and otherwise comparable women delivering a child whose labor had not been induced (Dublin et al., 2000). In some countries *census* records can be used to characterize employment status. This has permitted an examination of the possible influence of occupation on health outcomes (e.g., cancer incidence) that are routinely ascertained for residents of those countries (Lynge and Thygesen, 1990).

Interviews or Questionnaires

The principal advantage of most prospective cohort studies, relative to retrospective cohort studies, is the ability to obtain information on current and past exposures from the study participants who are to be enrolled for follow-up, and to do so in a way that directly fits the aim(s) of the study. For example, in one cohort study, a questionnaire was returned by 51,529 male dentists, veterinarians, and other health professionals, which provided information on a number of prior and present health conditions and exposures. Health outcomes were monitored in this group by means of follow-up questionnaires sent every two years, with medical records obtained pertinent to illnesses that were reported. The information contained in these questionnaires permitted the investigators to characterize exposures in some detail (e.g., a history of vasectomy *and* the age at which that operation occurred). For an outcome of particular interest, prostate cancer, it also allowed them to assess other factors (such as race) that could confound the examination of a possible association with vasectomy (Giovanucci et al., 1993).

Some cohort studies seek interviews or questionnaires from participants only at the outset of follow-up, whereas others seek to update some or all of that information periodically. If it is believed that the action of the exposure in causing or preventing an illness could be relatively short-term, clearly it is desirable to have updated information.

Example: The Nurses' Health Study enrolled registered nurses in 11 states of the U.S. in a prospective cohort study in 1976. Detailed information on use of postmenopausal hormones was first collected in 1978, then updated every two years as part of a questionnaire sent to participants that inquired about health outcomes (and also about changes in other exposures and characteristics). Analyses of the incidence of coronary heart disease among members of this cohort (Grodstein et al., 1996) compared users of hormones as of the most recent questionnaire to women who had never used hormones, since, because of several relatively short-term physiological changes that result from hormone use (Guetta and Cannon, 1996), relatively recent use is likely to be particularly relevant to the occurrence of coronary heart disease.

Direct Measurements Made on Cohort Members

Many exposures of interest cannot be determined with any accuracy, or perhaps at all, for individual study subjects from either records or interviews, but can be determined by direct measurement. For example, blood samples were obtained from civil servants in Taiwan and tested for the presence of the hepatitis B surface antigen (an indicator of chronic active hepatitis B infection). During the next several years, those who tested positive had an incidence of primary liver cancer that was some 200 times that of persons who tested negative (Beasley et al., 1981). As other examples:

- In a number of cohort studies the incidence of vascular disease has been compared among persons who differ in terms of their levels of serum cholesterol and other lipids (Dawber et al., 1963; Tyroler et al., 1971; Klag et al., 1993).
- Investigators at the Portsmouth Naval Shipyard mounted a retrospective cohort study in which each participant's exposure to occupational radiation was assessed by reading the dose recorded on that person's radiation film badge (Rinsky et al., 1981).
- The results of psychiatric evaluations of Swedish military recruits during 1969–1970 were examined as possible predictors of the incidence of suicide among these men during the subsequent 13 years (Allebeck et al., 1988).

If the characteristic being measured exhibits short-term variability (e.g., serum cholesterol or systolic blood pressure, which can vary hour-to-hour), the value obtained will not necessarily reflect the study participant's long-term mean level. The impact of this misclassification will be to dull the study's ability to assess the degree of association between the characteristic and a given health outcome, resulting in what has been termed "regression dilution" bias (Clarke et al., 1999). For characteristics that do vary, it is desirable (although not always practical) to obtain repeated measurements as a way of minimizing this bias. Thus, most cohort studies that obtain a blood pressure reading do so several times on each participant during the study examination. If the cohort is to be followed for health outcomes over an extended period and the characteristic exhibits long-term changes (e.g., weight, blood pressure), then remeasurement of that characteristic during the course of followup may be important as well. Additional discussion of the issue of remeasurement of exposure status, as well as other exposure measurement questions that arise in the conduct of prospective cohort studies, can be found in White et al. (1998).

ESTIMATING THE EXPECTED OCCURRENCE OF DISEASE AMONG "EXPOSED" COHORT MEMBERS

In cohort studies in which there is heterogeneity of exposure status among study participants, the occurrence of disease can be contrasted between persons who have or who have not been exposed, or across levels of exposure. For example, in a group of 715 monozygotic twins, all of whom had served in the American armed forces during 1965 to 1975, the prevalence of post-traumatic stress disorder in 1987 was compared between those who had and had not served in southeast Asia (Goldberg et al., 1990). In the Framingham study, the incidence of heart attack was calculated for persons in each fourth of the distribution of serum cholesterol (Kannel et al., 1971). In the Nurses' Health study, women in the lowest fifth of the distribution of body mass index (BMI)—weight in kilograms divided by the square of the height in meters, a measure of obesity—served as the reference category for women in each of the other fifths of the distribution in terms of the incidence of coronary heart disease (Manson et al., 1990).

When every member of the cohort under study has sustained the exposure of interest, however, then some external basis for the expected rate must be found. One possibility is the rate of the health outcome(s) of interest in members of cohorts who sustained other exposures, ones that are believed not to influence the health outcome. For example, the mortality rate from lung cancer in asbestos textile workers was compared in one of several analyses to that of cotton textile workers (Gardner, 1986). Cancer mortality among American radiologists was compared to that of a sample of physicians in other specialties (Seltser and Sartwell, 1965).

Another basis for comparison is the rate of the health outcome present in the geographic population in which cohort members reside. This approach commonly is used when death is the outcome of concern, given the availability of mortality statistics for most geographic populations. For other health outcomes, such as cancer incidence and birth defects, data may be available for the relevant geographical area or, if not, rates may be "borrowed" from another area if it is felt that they are likely to reflect the rates that would have prevailed in the appropriate population.

Each approach for generating the "expected" mortality or morbidity among exposed cohort members has potential strengths and weaknesses. The rates among non-exposed persons within the cohort itself, when available, are generally to be preferred, since for both exposed and non-exposed persons, the means of cohort identification and follow-up for illness outcomes should then be comparable. Also, the distribution of demographic and other potentially confounding factors often is similar between these two groups. But when the size of the non-exposed group is relatively small, and the outcome of interest is relatively uncommon, then this choice might provide but a flimsy statistical basis for estimating the expected rate among exposed persons.

Example: Blair et al. (1998) sought to assess the possibility that occupational exposure to trichloroethylene (TCE), a carcinogen in some animal experiments, was associated with an increased incidence of one or more forms of cancer in humans. They identified a cohort of persons who had been employed in an aircraft maintenance facility in Utah during 1952–1956, and monitored their mortality experience through 1990. Based on a review of each individual's job title(s), about 7000 persons were characterized as having been exposed to TCE, about 3300 as being exposed to one or more other industrial chemicals but not TCE, and about 3700 as not being exposed to chemicals in the workplace.

The primary comparison was site-specific mortality from cancer between TCE-exposed persons and persons not exposed to chemicals. For relatively common cancers, this comparison most likely was a valid one, more so than a comparison of the TCE-exposed cohort to an external population. For relatively uncommon cancers, however, this strategy led to problems. For example, 10 deaths from esophageal cancer occurred in TCE-exposed persons, corresponding to a rate 5.6 times that of persons with no known chemical exposure. But the rate in non-exposed persons was based on but a single death from esophageal cancer, so the 95% confidence interval around the relative risk of 5.6 was very wide (0.7–44.5), severely restricting the interpretation of this association. Since the mortality rate from esophageal cancer among the entire cohort of 14,000 was actually slightly below that of the population as a whole, it is highly unlikely that esophageal cancer mortality in persons with TCE exposures similar to the 7000 TCE-exposed persons in this study is truly elevated by a factor of 5.6; most or all of the apparent excess must be attributable to an atypically *low* rate in non-exposed persons, which, given the low frequency of esophageal cancer, could easily have occurred by chance.

When a comparison internal to the study is not available, there may be advantages in selecting the experience of a group of individuals who have sustained different sorts of exposures than the one of interest. Comparing the mortality of radiologists in the U.S. to that of other physicians (Seltser and Sartwell, 1965) was likely to provide a more valid contrast than a comparison with mortality rates for the population in general. By choosing the experience of non-radiologist physicians, it was possible to achieve a greater degree of comparability with respect to a number of social and economic factors that bear on the risk of developing and dying from a variety of causes (and that might bear on the likelihood that the cause of death was correctly classified). Nonetheless, the success of the above strategy is contingent on the comparison cohort's not having their own exposure(s) that have an impact on the health outcomes of interest. If, for example, the mortality from a given cancer among TCE-exposed workers were compared only to that of workers with other chemical exposures, and no differences were found, it could mean either that:

- there is no association between exposure to TCE and the occurrence of that cancer; or that
- exposure to TCE as well as to one or more other chemicals used in aircraft maintenance is associated with an altered cancer risk to a similar degree.

Example: In a cohort of American asbestos textile workers, 24 deaths from lung cancer occurred (Gardner, 1986). This was exactly twice the number expected based on U.S. mortality rates (95% confidence interval = 1.3–3.0), but was 7.4 times the number predicted when the death rates among cotton textile workers served as a basis for comparison (95% confidence interval = 3.1–20.3). Which of these estimates of the relative risk is likely to be closer to the truth? While the use of population rates as a source for the expected number of deaths is likely to produce a figure that is spuriously high (and therefore a relative risk that is too low—see below), the magnitude of that bias is generally modest. Alternatively, the relative risk of 7.4 could be spuriously high if the occupational exposures sustained by cotton textile workers provided them some protection against the development of lung cancer. Given that the mortality rate from lung cancer in cotton textile workers was but 27 percent of the U.S. population rate, this appears to be a credible hypothesis. The true relative risk of lung cancer in the American asbestos textile workers probably was considerably closer to 2.0 than to 7.4.

In summary, there may be instances in which the experience of a comparison group of persons exposed to something other than the agent of interest will reflect that of nonexposed persons who are otherwise comparable to the exposed cohort, and thus provide a valid result. The use of such a comparison group, however, can also lead to a potentially large bias in either direction. If possible, rates of illness in parallel cohorts should be supplemented by rates available for the broader defined population in which the cohort is situated.

Many cohort studies employ population rates as a basis for comparison to the illness or mortality experience of a particular cohort of exposed individuals. These rates generally are based on a sizeable number of events and so are, statistically speaking, quite precise. Nonetheless, some care must be used when interpreting the results of such a comparison. Specifically, it is necessary to address the following questions:

1. *Have the outcome events under study been ascertained comparably between the exposed cohort and the general population?* For events that are identified by means of linkage with death or other registries, under-ascertainment in the cohort can occur more readily than in the general population, since only in the former group do specific persons have to be followed over time and the occurrence of illness or death be linked to their identity. For example, a cohort study of possible adverse effects of cosmetic breast implants compared the incidence of breast cancer among women in Alberta, Canada, who had received these implants (and who had no prior history of breast cancer) with that of all adult female Alberta residents (Berkel et al., 1992). The study observed a modest deficit of breast cancer among cohort members, but one possible explanation lay in the fact that follow-up for the occurrence of breast cancer relied on linkage of the identities of these women to the records of the population-based cancer registry serving Alberta. The investigators did not monitor individual cohort members for migration outside the province, or for changes in surname, and so a number of breast cancers diagnosed in these women could have been missed.

   The criteria for defining outcome events need to be comparable between the exposed cohort and general population as well. When for both groups the same source of information is used to characterize the events, such as a statement of cause of death on a death certificate or a report in a cancer or a congenital malformations registry, this comparability is easily achieved. But problems can arise when the information available differs between the groups.

Example: In a cohort mortality study of U.S. insulation workers, Selikoff et al. (1980) were particularly interested in deaths from mesothelioma. Yet during the period of follow-up in that study, 1967–1976, this malignancy was only beginning to be recognized as such, and it was suspected that some mesothelioma deaths were being attributed to other causes. To address this concern, the investigators sought to obtain medical and pathology records of cohort members who died of cancer, so that they might identify possibly undiagnosed cases of mesothelioma. This strategy did, in fact, uncover nearly one additional mesothelioma death for every one actually listed as such on the death certificate. Nonetheless, since the assessment of excess mortality from mesothelioma was obliged to rely on a comparison of the rates in the cohort with rates in the population as a whole, and since the deaths that comprised the numerator of the latter rates did not undergo the same intensive re-evaluation, the authors' primary analysis used death certificate information only. The goal of comparability of outcome ascertainment in exposed and unexposed groups was given priority, properly so, over the goal of accuracy of classification of outcome status in just one of the two groups. Use of the revised assignment of cause of death in the insulation workers would be appropriate only for estimating their *absolute* mortality rate from mesothelioma.

2. *To what extent has the rate of illness in the exposed cohort influenced the size of the rate for the population as a whole?* Cohort studies seek to contrast the incidence of illness and/or death in exposed and non-exposed individuals. In most cohort studies that use population rates as a basis for comparison, the contribution of events in exposed persons to the total number in the general population is so small that the population's rate is very similar to that of non-exposed persons. However, if more than a small proportion of the population has been exposed, and if the relative risk associated with exposure is very high, then an appreciable degree of bias can be produced by the use of general population rates as a basis for comparison. Figure 14–1 (taken from Jones and Swerdlow, 1998) illustrates this bias and the circumstances that produce it. If the observed standardized mortality ratio (i.e., relative risk) is below 1.5, little relative bias is present no matter how common the exposure. If the prevalence of the exposure in the population is less than five percent, only for observed standardized mortality ratios of more than five does the bias exceed 25%.

3. *On average, are cohort members different from the general population in ways that bear on disease incidence or mortality, beyond differences in those demographic characteristics that are measured in both groups and for which statistical adjustment can be performed?* This question was of

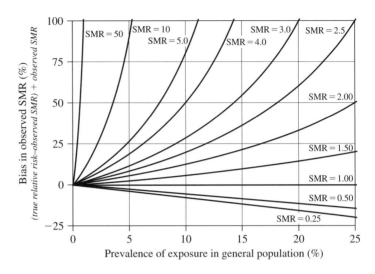

Figure 14–1. Bias in Observed Standardized Mortality Ratio (SMR) in Relation to Population Prevalence of Exposure (based on Jones and Swerdlow, 1998).

concern to William Farr of the British General Register Office, who in the mid-nineteenth century wished to determine if, during peacetime, British soldiers suffered an atypically high mortality rate (Farr, 1979). During 1839–1853, the annual mortality among soldiers averaged 33.0 per 1000, whereas for men of corresponding ages in England and Wales it was but 9.2 per 1000. Farr pointed out that this difference of nearly 24 per 1000 actually had to be an *under*estimate of the adverse impact on mortality of being a soldier in peacetime Britain, since

> ... the mortality of the troops in peacetime ought to be lower than that of civilians. First of all, there was a process of selection involved. Soldiers were "picked lives." They had passed a medical examination at the time of recruitment, while those who failed remained in the general population. Furthermore, men who developed chronic diseases in the army were discharged and reappeared in the civilian ranks.

This incomparability between British soldiers and British men as a whole with regard to their underlying risk of death would nowadays be viewed as an example of confounding. It arises to at least some degree in most occupational cohort mortality studies that use population death rates for comparison, and has been termed the "healthy worker" bias (McMichael, 1976). The two components of this bias that Farr noted—selective recruitment and selective retention—have been given their own designations as well; i.e., "healthy hire effect" and "healthy worker survivor effect" (Arrighi and Hertz-Picciotto, 1996). In the absence of a workplace exposure that has an influence on mortality, persons who are employed would be expected to have a lower death rate than the population in general because, in order to obtain and retain a job, a certain level of health generally is required. The magnitude of this bias differs among the various causes of death, being greatest for those illnesses for which there is a long interval between the onset of disability and death (such as might be true for chronic obstructive lung disease or multiple sclerosis), and smallest for those that typically produce death rapidly (such as pulmonary embolism). While it is possible for healthy worker bias to be present in cohort studies of disease incidence, in general its magnitude will be considerably smaller than in mortality studies, since hiring and retention are not often strongly influenced by the presence of risk factors for disease incidence. So, for example, while persons disabled by lung cancer or chronic lung disease may be preferentially excluded from many types of employment, generally persons with only a predisposition to these conditions, by virtue of their being cigarette smokers, would not.

If studies of mortality in relation to occupation are based on a comparison of death rates between retirees and the population at large, a bias akin to the healthy worker bias can emerge, though in the opposite direction. This results from the fact that some people retire because they have developed a condition that can prove fatal, so members of the retired cohort below the typical retirement age will be over-represented in that condition compared to the demographically comparable population as a whole. In the absence of any negative impact of a particular occupation on mortality, death rates among people who have retired from that occupation will tend to be higher than those of the population in which they reside.

Example: In a cohort mortality study intended to estimate potential hazards from asbestos exposure, Enterline et al. (1987) ascertained deaths among white men who had retired during 1941–1967 after having been production or maintenance employees of a U.S. asbestos products company. Cause-specific mortality rates were compared to those of American white men as a whole. In order to minimize bias that probably would arise from an over-representation in the exposed group of men who had retired due to ill health, the investigators restricted their analysis to the person-time that accrued in each of the men after he had turned 65 years of age. This was the age that retirement would have been anticipated for all men in this industry, healthy or not.

When rates of illness or death are compared between patients who have received a specific medical intervention and the population as a whole—perhaps to assess the presence of adverse effects associated with that intervention—two particular sources of potential bias commonly must be considered:

1. *Could the condition that necessitated the treatment itself have an impact on the incidence of the disease(s) being studied?* Solely from a comparison of treated patients and the population in general, it would not be possible to disentangle the impact of the treatment from that of the illness that necessitated the treatment. So, for example, when mortality from a variety of causes was observed to be higher in British patients who were prescribed an H2 blocker, cimetidine, during the first year after the drug had been prescribed, relative to mortality rates in demographically comparable persons in England and Wales (Colin-Jones et al., 1983), the interpretation was ambiguous: Either the drug, or the conditions that led to the drug's being prescribed, or both, could have been responsible. If confounding of this sort (known as "confounding by indication") is likely to be present, it is necessary for the comparison group to comprise persons who have the same condition(s) as the treated cohort, but who are treated in a different way or not treated at all (Weiss, 1996).

2. *At the time treatment was being considered, were members of the treated group evaluated for the presence of a condition, with only those* not *having the condition allowed to receive the treatment?* A comparison of the subsequent incidence of this condition between the treated patients and the population at large—most of whom probably would not have received such an evaluation—would give rise to "healthy screenee bias," i.e., a spuriously low rate in the patient group (Weiss and Rossing, 1996). For example, women who receive cosmetic breast implants would be expected to have a lower incidence of breast cancer following implantation than women in general, even if this treatment had no anti-carcinogenic effect at all. This would result from the fact that all the treated women, but only some in the comparison group, would have had a thorough breast evaluation around the time the implant was being considered, and only those believed not to have breast cancer could go on to have (by definition) a "cosmetic" implant.

Because population rates as a basis for comparison have some attractive features—and, often, because there is no better alternative available!—epidemiologists have developed strategies to minimize the healthy worker and healthy screenee biases. The primary one involves omitting from the analysis that part of the follow-up experience of exposed individuals that is most susceptible to these biases; i.e., that which accrues relatively soon after exposure status is defined. The actual length of time chosen will differ from study to study, depending on the suspected duration of the incomparability between the exposed cohort and the comparison population. For example, most screen-detectable breast cancers (which are likely to be more prevalent among women in general than in women who just received a cosmetic breast implant) are expected to progress to clinically evident disease within two to three years. Thus, a comparison with population rates that is more likely to be valid (assuming no other forms of bias are present) would tabulate rates of breast cancer among cosmetic implant recipients starting about three years after their surgery. In an occupational cohort mortality study, either a shorter (e.g., one year) or a longer period of time after the criteria for exposure have been met could be deleted from the analysis, depending on the typical duration of disability prior to death from those causes of death of particular interest.

FOLLOW-UP OF COHORT MEMBERS

Ideally, a cohort study will be able to completely enumerate all relevant health outcomes that occur among study participants, and also determine for all participants whether follow-up has been truncated (due to death or to migration beyond the reach of the follow-up mechanisms). If the duration of follow-up is quite short—e.g., a few hours, perhaps during an assessment of rapidly developing adverse effects of various anesthetic agents—then it might be possible to meet this ideal. In most cohort studies, however, when the period of follow-up extends from months to decades, ascertainment both of the numerator and denominator of the rate of illness or death will be incomplete to at least some extent, allowing for the possibility of bias. If the degree of under-ascertainment is relatively modest, and is present to a comparable extent for exposed and non-exposed persons, the bias will be small or absent. But as the degree of under-ascertainment grows—especially if it is present for just exposed individuals, as in a study that compares the morbidity or mortality of these persons to that of the population as a whole—then the validity of the results will be increasingly threatened.

The means by which outcome events are enumerated in cohort members depends upon the specific outcome(s) of interest and the resources available in the setting in which the study is done. In the U.S., deaths in 1979 and later among study subjects can be identified by means of linkage with the National Death Index (Bilgrad, 1990), whereas in some parts of the world, death certificates are not made available for health research. In Scandinavia, cohort studies of cancer incidence routinely rely on population-based registries to determine the development of cancer in specified individuals. In contrast, the *absence* of cancer registries that serve the entire population in which cohort members reside for most or all of the period of follow-up has obliged cohort studies done in many other parts of the world to rely on cancer mortality as an outcome, rather than incidence. The occurrence of a number of outcomes of potential interest (e.g., urinary tract infections, rheumatic diseases, smoking cessation) are not ascertained routinely by any sort of registry. Their identification would require conducting a review of medical records, or an interview with or measurement upon, individual cohort members. Studies that utilize records, interviews, or measurements as means of assessing illness occurrence need to take particular care to develop standardized criteria for the presence of outcome events, and need to apply these criteria without knowledge of each subject's exposure status.

Example: As part of a prospective cohort study of 115,886 American nurses, Manson et al. (1990) examined the possible influence of obesity on the incidence of coronary heart disease. After enrollment in 1976, participants were queried every two years regarding the development of a myocardial infarction or angina pectoris. (The occurrence of fatal cases was ascertained by means of the National Death Index.) Medical records were sought for each woman who responded affirmatively regarding one or both conditions. Using these records, physicians (who were blinded to the presence or absence of a women's weight and other possible risk factors) applied a standard set of criteria to judge whether a woman had sustained a myocardial infarction or had developed angina pectoris.

In order to determine for each cohort member the amount of person-time that she or he is contributing to the denominator of the incidence rate, in many studies it is necessary to periodically monitor that person's whereabouts. In the Nurses' Health Study, the return of the biennial questionnaire serves to ascertain not only the development of relevant outcomes, but also that the woman is still reachable to report such outcomes if they were to occur. (As mentioned earlier, this questionnaire also elicits updated information on exposure status.) There are instances in which it is likely that all outcomes that occur in cohort members will be ascertained through a reliable linkage procedure with a database that covers a geographic area outside of which migration is expected to be minimal; e.g., the US National Death Index or a cancer registry in a Nordic country. In such an instance, no additional follow-up is needed beyond the linkage procedure. But there are other circumstances in which considerable resources need to be devoted to tracking study participants:

Example: Hagan et al. (2001) sought to assess determinants of the acquisition of hepatitis C virus (HCV) infection among intravenous drug users (IDUs). They obtained information on patterns of drug use and other potential risk factors from a group of HCV-seronegative IDUs. Cohort members then were followed for a period of one year, at which time a blood sample and additional interview information was to be obtained. To arrange for the blood draw and re-interview, letters were mailed to the address given at the outset, but if there was no response, the investigators tried calling the participant and (if necessary) persons whose phone numbers had been provided by the participant at the beginning of the study. In addition, censuses of the county jail and of drug treatment facilities were checked for the presence of any cohort members, as were state prison and death records.

On occasion, criteria for eligibility of persons to serve as cohort members are tailored to maximize the likelihood of successful followup. For example, in the cohort study of aircraft maintenance workers in Utah referred to earlier (see Blair et al. example earlier in chapter), persons who had been employed at the facility for less than one year were not included. Such persons would be expected to be relatively mobile, residentially, and thus the most likely to have left the state during the follow-up period. Since one of the means of identifying health outcomes in this study was the Utah Cancer Registry, including the short-term workers would have led, for cancer incidence, to a relatively lower level of follow-up. Restriction of the cohort to aircraft maintenance workers of one year or longer also had the desirable feature of excluding workers whose cumulative exposures to TCE would very likely have been quite low.

NATURE OF THE ILLNESS OUTCOME: PREVALENCE VERSUS INCIDENCE

Some studies compare, not the occurrence of an illness between persons who have and have not had a given exposure, but rather the presence of that condition at a specified point in time. Such studies (termed "cross-sectional" because they have no longitudinal component) often are done to investigate possible harmful effects of a work environment by examining employed persons with different levels or types of exposure on the job. Examples are studies of lung function in pipe coverers in 1940s shipyards who had been exposed to asbestos to varying degrees (Fleischer et al., 1946), or studies of musculo-skeletal disorders in persons whose work requires repetitive and/or forceful movements of the hand and wrist (Silverstein et al., 1987). A cross-sectional study, however, will not give a valid result if persons whose health has been impaired by their occupational exposure(s) are no longer employed when the study is done. For example, the investigation conducted in the shipyard (Fleischer et al., 1946) observed the prevalence of asbestosis was not elevated among pipe coverers who had sustained a substantial exposure to asbestos. It is highly likely that selective retirement of men whose health already had been compromised by their asbestos exposure led to a result that falsely minimized the occurrence of asbestosis associated with this occupation.

ISSUES IN THE ANALYSIS AND INTERPRETATION OF COHORT STUDIES

For Purposes of Analysis, How Soon After Exposure Should Outcome Events That Occur in Cohort Members Begin To Be Counted?

Generally, the answer to this question is "immediately," in order to capture the full range of consequences of the exposure. An exception would be made if "healthy worker" bias or "healthy screenee" bias were anticipated (see pp. 356–358). Another exception would be made if there were reasons to believe that persons for whom the diagnosis was made very early in the follow-up period had that disease present in an occult form before exposure commenced. While the presence of the disease in those persons could not have been affected by the exposure, it could possibly have influenced the likelihood of receipt of exposure, or the presence or level of a characteristic under study. In this situation, a more valid analysis would exclude cases (and the associated person-time) for a long enough period of time after the beginning of follow-up to allow for most or all of these prevalent-but-undetected cases to have been diagnosed.

Example: A number of studies have observed the incidence of colon cancer to be relatively high among persons with relatively low levels of serum cholesterol. Yet in an analysis of the combined results of these studies (Law and Thompson, 1991), the increased risk was confined to the first two years of follow-up: No association was present once cases diagnosed in the first two years after the serum sample had been drawn were excluded. Since it is unlikely that an elevated serum cholesterol value could influence the development of a colon tumor so rapidly, and then not over the longer term, it seems more probable that the presence of the tumor or its antecedent pathology led to metabolic changes that resulted in,

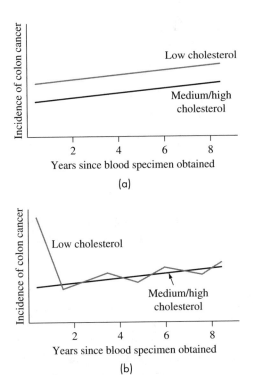

Figure 14–2. Does a Low Serum Cholesterol Predispose to Colon Cancer, or Does the Presence of Cancer Cause a Lowering of Serum Cholesterol?
(a) Pattern of results in support of an etiologic role for serum cholesterol.
(b) Pattern of results in support of the hypothesis that colon cancer depresses serum cholesterol.

on average, a reduction in serum cholesterol. Figure 14–2 depicts the patterns of results that would and would not tend to support the hypothesis that a low serum cholesterol (or another metabolic characteristic it is correlated with) is a cause of colon cancer. To avoid being influenced by "reverse causality," an analysis would simply ignore diagnoses and person-time that accrued during the early part of the period of follow-up.

Example: Because administration of phenobarbital was known to lead to tumor development in mice, Clemmesen and Hjalgrim-Jensen (1981) sought to determine the impact of long-term use of this drug in humans. They identified 8,077 Danes who had been hospitalized for treatment with an anticonvulsive agent during 1933–1963, most of whom would have received phenobarbital while hospitalized and for a long period of time thereafter. With the help of records from the Danish tumor registry, they sought to identify brain tumors that arose in cohort members through 1976. The following table describes the results of the study:

TIME SINCE FIRST HOSPITALIZATION (YRS.)	Malignant Brain Tumors		RELATIVE RISK
	OBSERVED	EXPECTED	
<10	45	3.87	11.6
10–14	13	2.42	5.4
15–19	4	2.28	1.8
>20	9	4.79	1.9

While the observed association was very strong during the first 10 to 15 years of follow-up, it is unlikely that much of it reflects a causal role of phenobarbital in the development of brain tumors: (1) It would be an unusual carcinogen that predisposed to a brain tumor in the first 10 to 15 years after exposure but scarcely at all after that time; and (2) An alternative, non-causal hypothesis is highly plausible— that the presence of an undiagnosed brain tumor led to a seizure disorder, which in turn led to treatment with anticonvulsants. In the era before intracranial imaging techniques became available, often seizure patients not treated with phenobarbital would have a brain tumor identified as the likely basis for the disorder some years after the onset of the seizures. There would be some uncertainty regarding precisely what period of time after initiating anticonvulsant medication should be excluded from the interpretation of these data. Nonetheless, it seems likely that the relative risks observed 15 to 19 and more than 20 years (1.8 and 1.9, respectively) are a better indication of the possible capacity of phenobarbital use to cause brain tumors in humans than the relative risk of 11.6 observed during the first decade of follow-up.

How Are Changes in the Exposure Status of Cohort Members Handled?

Persons with a history of long-term occupational exposure to asbestos are at a sharply increased risk of mesothelioma. It has been observed in cohort studies that several decades are required for the inhalation of asbestos fibers (and the body's response to them) to lead to the development of mesothelioma. Additional asbestos inhalation by persons whose occupational exposure had begun several decades earlier does not appear to contribute to risk in any substantial way during his or her maximum lifespan (Peto et al., 1982). In retrospect, if no attempt had been made to characterize asbestos exposure once the criteria for "long-term" exposure had been met, the validity of studies of the incidence of mesothelioma among these persons would not have been compromised to any appreciable degree. In contrast, if in this same cohort one had been studying the impact of the combination of cigarette smoking and asbestos exposure on the risk of lung cancer, it would have been important to obtain updated information on smoking status during entire the period of follow-up. This is because of the beneficial influence that smoking cessation exerts on lung cancer incidence among cigarette smokers without a history of occupational exposure to asbestos (Hammond, 1966).

Some cohort studies ascertain exposure status only when subjects are first enrolled, and so they are not able to consider the issue of changes in the presence or level of exposure. For example, some 1.2 million persons were enrolled in a cohort study conducted by the American Cancer Society, in which mortality rates during a 14-year followup period were related to characteristics and exposures reported on a questionnaire at the start of the study. Using these data, Calle et al. (1999) examined the association of BMI with mortality from all causes combined. Other cohort studies of body mass index and disease have obtained updated information on exposure status during the followup period, and conducted analyses that took account of this additional information. For example, in the Nurses' Health Study, participants were asked about their weight and height every two years, and in their analysis of the relationship of BMI to the incidence of coronary heart disease Manson et al. (1990) re-categorized women after each additional questionnaire was returned. Thus, the person-time contribution of a woman to the denominator of the incidence rate (and to the numerator, if coronary disease occurred) could be made to more than one BMI category as the follow-up continued. For characteristics such as BMI that do change over time, and for outcome events whose occurrence is sensitive to relatively recent exposure status, being able to take into account the updated data can serve to reduce exposure misclassification. [If there is a suspected "lag" between the presence of an exposure and its impact on disease occurrence, analyses also can be done in which the suspected induction time is ignored—see Rothman and Greenland (1998, pp. 82–88) for details.]

Among exposed cohort members, duration of exposure often increases with continuing follow-up. For example, among a group of persons with a given occupational exposure whose death rates are being monitored, those who continue on the job generally will increase their duration of exposure to one or more agents present in that workplace, while those who quit or retire will not. Duration of exposure is a central feature of the analysis of many cohort studies, but some care must be taken in order not to bias that analysis. Specifically, cohort members can not be permitted to contribute events to the numerator of a rate, nor person-time to the denominator, until they meet the criteria for a particular category of duration. If, for example, one wished to determine the mortality rate from a particular disease in employees of at least 10 years duration, only illnesses and person-time that took place beginning at 10 years from first employment would enter the calculation. Person-time in these individuals would not begin at the time of first employment since, by definition, none of these persons could have died during the ensuing 10 years! In a comparison of mortality in workers with an occupational exposure of <10 and ≥10 years duration, only data gathered beginning 10 years after the date of first employment of *any* study subject would enter into the analysis.

CONCLUSION

To the extent that they can ascertain exposure status prior to disease occurrence, cohort studies have been and will remain indispensable for evaluating the impact of exposures whose presence or magnitude cannot be retrospectively ascertained in a valid way. Despite the complexities that sometimes arise in the design and conduct of cohort studies, their longitudinal nature—begin with exposure status, then document disease occurrence—makes them relatively easy to understand.

Because this longitudinal character is shared with randomized controlled trials, epidemiologists reporting the results of these studies have an obligation to remind their audience (and themselves!) of the limitations of their study that are imposed by the absence of randomization. They must not lose sight of the fact that associations between exposure and disease that are observed in cohort studies, even when it is clear that the exposure has preceded the presence of disease, are not necessarily causal associations.

Example: Greenberg et al. (1996) conducted a randomized controlled trial in which 1,720 patients with nonmelanotic skin cancer were assigned to receive either 50 mg. per day of beta-carotene or a placebo. During the follow-up period (median of 4.3 years), total mortality was identical in the two groups (relative risk = 1.0, 95% confidence interval = 0.8–1.3), as was mortality from the two major cause-of-death categories, cardiovascular disease and cancer. Plasma beta-carotene measured at entry into the study, however, was inversely related to mortality: Relative to the death rate of subjects in the lowest fourth of the distribution of plasma beta-carotene, mortality among persons in the second, third, and upper fourth was 0.7, 0.6, and 0.6, respectively, adjusted for age, sex, BMI, and history of cigarette smoking. These estimates were reasonably statistically precise; for example, the 95% confidence interval of the relative risk for persons in the highest fourth of the distribution was 0.4–0.9. Since the dose of beta-carotene use in the study produced approximately a tenfold increase in the beta-carotene levels compared to those prior to treatment, and since the administration of beta-carotene clearly had no impact on mortality rates, it seems almost certain that the association observed between low levels of beta-carotene and mortality does not reflect a cause–effect relation, at least in the short term. After seeing the results of their study, Greenberg et al. concluded as follows: "Although the possibility exists that beta-carotene supplementation produces benefits that are too small or too delayed to have been detected in this study, non-causal explanations should be sought for the association between plasma concentrations of beta-carotene and diminished death."

EXERCISES

1. Roscoe et al. (1995) enumerated deaths during 1960–90 among 757 Navajo uranium miners in the southwestern U.S. They estimated standardized mortality ratios, using the combined New Mexico and Arizona non-white mortality rates as a basis for comparison. In this study, there was a low standardized mortality ratio not only for cirrhosis of the liver (0.5, 95% confidence interval = 0.2–0.7), usually an alcohol-related disease, but for alcoholism (SMR = 0.4, 95% confidence interval = 0.1–1.1), as well. What do you believe to be the most likely explanation for the reduced mortality from these two causes among the Navajo uranium miners?

2. Among 22,597 Swedish women to whom non-contraceptive hormone therapy had been prescribed during 1977–1980 and who had not previously been diagnosed with cancer, Persson et al. (1996) found that 102 died from breast cancer through 1991. Based on the mortality rate from breast cancer among the Swedish female population of the same ages during the same period of time, 195.9 breast cancer deaths would have been expected (relative risk = 0.5, 95% confidence interval = 0.4–0.6).

   It is likely that this study underestimated the size of the true relative risk relating hormone use to mortality from breast cancer. Why?

3. Most epidemiologists seeking to assess the impact of the cessation of cigarette smoking on a person's risk of death have excluded from consideration both deaths and person-time during the first year after a study participant stops smoking. What do you believe to be the rationale behind this?

4. The following is excerpted from an investigation of the possible influence of pregnancy following breast cancer in young women on the likelihood of survival:

   > One or more pregnancies occurred in approximately one-quarter of our patients. The age distributions of women who did and did not have a subsequent pregnancy were similar. Patients with subsequent pregnancies had an excellent prognosis (see Table 14–1).

   Beyond the possible beneficial influence of pregnancy itself on survival, what are the two likeliest explanations for the observed association?

5. The following is a portion of an abstract of an article (Bender et al., 1999), along with Table 14–2, derived from that article.

Table 14–1. Survival from Breast Cancer by Number of Subsequent Pregnancies

NO. OF PREGNANCIES FOLLOWING DIAGNOSIS	NO. OF PATIENTS	%	Survival (%)*		
			3 YEARS	5 YEARS	10 YEARS
0	83	76.2	86.7	72.8	58.5
1+	26	23.8	96.2	96.2	84.1
Total	109	100.0	89.0	78.5	64.7

*Survival from date of diagnosis of breast cancer.

Table 14–2. Standardized Mortality Ratio in Patients Hospitalized for Obesity

GENDER	AGE RANGE	PERSON-YEARS	NO. OF DEATHS	SMR	95% CI	p-VALUE
Men	18–29	5109	36	2.46	1.72–3.41	<.001
	30–39	3425	63	2.30	1.77–2.95	<.001
	40–49	3297	105	1.99	1.62–2.40	<.001
	50–74	7483	161	1.31	1.11–1.52	.001
	TOTAL	19,314	365	1.67	1.51–1.85	<.001
Women	18–29	13,661	31	1.81	1.23–2.57	.003
	30–39	10,139	85	2.10	1.68–2.60	<.001
	40–49	10,916	176	1.70	1.46–1.97	<.001
	50–74	25,305	371	1.26	1.13–1.39	<.001
	TOTAL	60,021	663	1.45	1.34–1.57	<.001

[*Source:* based on Bender et al. (1999).]

Context: The effect of age on excess mortality from all causes associated with obesity is controversial. Few studies have investigated the association between body mass index (BMI), age, and mortality, with sufficient numbers of subjects at all levels of obesity.

Objective: To assess the effect of age on the excess mortality associated with all degrees of obesity.

Design: Prospective cohort study.

Setting and Participants: A total of 6,193 obese patients with mean (SD) BMI of 36.6 (6.1) kg/m^2 and mean ($\pm$SD) age of 40.4 (12.9) years who had been referred to the obesity clinic of Heinrich-Heine University, Dusseldorf, Germany, between 1961 and 1994. Median follow-up time was 14.8 years.

Main Outcome Measure: All-cause mortality through 1994 among 6,053 patients for whom follow-up data were available (1,028 deaths) analyzed as standardized mortality ratios (SMRs) using the male-female population of the geographic region (North Rhine Westphalia) as reference.

Results: The cohort was grouped into approximate quartiles according to age (18–29, 30–39, 40–49, and 50–74 years) and BMI (25 to <32, 32 to <36, 36 to <40, and >40 kg/m^2) at baseline. The SMRs showed a significant excess mortality with an SMR for men of 1.67 (95% confidence interval, 1.51–1.85; $p < .001$) and an SMR for women of 1.45 (95% confidence interval, 1.34–1.57; $p < .001$). The excess mortality associated with obesity declined with age. For men, the SMRs of the four age groups were 2.46, 2.30, 1.99, and 1.31, respectively; for women, they were 1.81, 2.10, 1.70, and 1.26, respectively (Poisson trend test, $p < .001$).

(a) There are features of the choice of exposed and comparison cohorts that could lead to bias. Among persons of all ages (combined), how is it possible that this study could have overestimated the association between obesity and mortality? How is it possible that the association could have been underestimated? (Assume that the SMRs that were calculated have eliminated potential confounding by age and other demographic characteristics.)

(b) The authors concluded the paper by stating that "the excess mortality associated with obesity declined considerably with age." Assuming for the moment that the results of this study are valid, is the mortality burden associated with obesity greater in 18–29-year-olds than 50–74-year-olds? Provide your answer in quantitative terms.

ANSWERS

1. Alcoholism and cirrhosis almost certainly are less prevalent in Navajos who initiate or maintain employment in uranium mines than in Navajos who do not. The presence of this "healthy worker" bias is the most plausible explanation for the observed reduced mortality among these miners, certainly more so than a beneficial effect of underground exposure to uranium.

   Nonetheless, being employed in any manner probably reduces one's risk of becoming or staying an alcoholic, and it is possible that this accounts for a portion of the low SMRs for cirrhosis and alcoholism as well.

2. Women diagnosed with breast cancer prior to 1977–1980 are absent from the cohort of hormone users. In contrast, the breast cancer mortality rates in the women against whom the hormone users are being compared—Swedish women in general—are based on deaths that occurred during 1977–1991, irrespective of when a given woman's diagnosis took place. Therefore, even if hormone use had no bearing on mortality from breast cancer, an apparent deficit would be seen among the hormone users due to this lack of comparability.

3. Many people with smoking-related conditions stop smoking once that condition is diagnosed. Because of this, in the short term, persons who stop smoking actually have a higher mortality rate than continuing smokers. In studies in which the reason for smoking cessation is not ascertained (or is not ascertained

reliably), the potential beneficial impact of stopping smoking is most validly measured by excluding that period of time during which the diseases that caused the smoking cessation in study participants lead to death. While some of these fatal diseases last longer than one year, excluding the first year after cessation probably removes much of the bias.

4. (a) Women with high probability of survival—that is, those with no recurrence of their tumor—may be those most likely to seek to become pregnant, and also able to become pregnant. This would be an example of confounding.

   (b) The way this analysis has been constructed guarantees that, even in the absence of a true benefit of pregnancy on survival, one will be observed. Having a pregnancy assures that a woman has survived until that time—no such "advantage" is conferred to nonpregnant cases of breast cancer. In other words, the calculated mortality rate is spuriously low among women who had a pregnancy, and thus the estimated survival is spuriously high, because these women were allowed to accrue person-time prior to the pregnancy without the possibility of a death occurring.

   In order to overcome these sources of bias it is necessary to select, as a bias for comparison to each of those who become pregnant, one or more other women with breast cancer who are similar to them with regard to predictors of survival (e.g., time since breast cancer diagnosis, history of a recurrence) at the time of the pregnancy. Deaths and person-years would be tabulated for women in both groups only from the date the pregnancy begins (Velentgas et al., 1999).

5. (a) The observed association between obesity and mortality could have been overestimated if there had been selective referral to the clinic of obese persons in ill health. It also could be underestimated, however, due to inclusion of persons with obesity in the comparison cohort.

   (b) Table 14–3 can be constructed from the data. In both men and women, the mortality burden associated with obesity—when viewed as a difference rather than as a ratio—is, if anything, greater at older ages, not smaller.

Table 14–3. Mortality Difference between Obesity Clinic Patients and General Population, by Gender and Age

| SEX | AGE | Mortality per 1000 Person-Years | | MORTALITY DIFFERENCE |
		CLINIC PATIENTS	POPULATION	
Male	18–29	$36/5,109 = 7.05$	$7.05 \div 2.46 = 2.86$	$7.05 - 2.86 = 4.19$
Male	50–74	$161/7,483 = 21.52$	$21.52 \div 1.31 = 16.42$	$21.5 - 16.4 = 5.10$
Female	18–29	$31/13,661 = 2.27$	$2.27 \div 1.81 = 1.25$	$2.27 - 1.25 = 1.02$
Female	50–74	$371/25,305 = 14.66$	$14.66 \div 1.26 = 11.64$	$14.66 - 11.64 = 3.02$

REFERENCES

Allebeck P, Allgulander C, Fisher LD. Predictors of completed suicide in a cohort of 50,465 young men: role of personality and deviant behavior. BMJ 1988; 297:76–78.

Arrighi HM, Hertz-Picciotto IH. Controlling the healthy worker survivor effect: an example of arsenic exposure and respiratory cancer. Occup Environ Med 1996; 53:455–62.

Beasley RP, Lin CC, Hwang LY, Chen CS. Hepatocellular carcinoma and hepatitis B virus. Lancet 1981; 2:1129–33.

Bender R, Jockel KH, Trautner C, Spraul M, Berger M. Effect of age on excess mortality in obesity. JAMA 1999; 281:1498–504.

Berkel H, Birdsell DC, Jenkins H. Breast augmentation: a risk factor for breast cancer? N Engl J Med 1992; 326:1649–53.

Bilgrad R. National Death Index User's Manual. DHHS Pub. No. (PHS) 90-1148. Washington, D.C.: U.S. Department of Health and Human Services, 1990.

Blair A, Hartge P, Stewart PA, McAdams M, Lubin J. Mortality and cancer incidence of aircraft maintenance workers exposed to trichloroethylene and other organic solvents and chemicals: extended follow up. Occup Environ Med 1998; 55:161–71.

Calle EE, Thun MJ, Petrelli JM, Rodriguez C, Heath CW Jr. Body-mass index and mortality in a prospective cohort of U.S. adults. N Engl J Med 1999; 341:1097–1105.

Checkoway H, Eisen EA. Developments in occupational cohort studies. Epidemiol Rev 1998; 20:100–11.

Clarke R, Shipley M, Lewington S, Youngman L, Collins R, Marmot M, et al. Underestimation of risk associations due to regression dilution in long-term follow-up of prospective studies. Am J Epidemiol 1999; 150:341–53.

Clemmesen J, Hjalgrim-Jensen S. Does phenobarbital cause intracranial tumors? A follow-up through 35 years. Ecotoxicol Environ Saf 1981; 5:255–60.

Colin-Jones DG, Langman MJ, Lawson DH, Vessey MP. Postmarketing surveillance of the safety of cimetidine: 12-month mortality report. BMJ (Clin Res Ed) 1983; 286:1713–16.

Court-Brown WM, Doll R. Leukemia and aplastic anaemia in patients irradiated for ankylosing spondylitis. Medical Research Council Special Report Series No. 295. London: Her Majesty's Stationery Office, 1957.

Darby SC, Whitley E, Howe GR, Hutchins SJ, Kuisiak RA, Lubin JH, et al. Radon and cancers other than lung cancer in underground miners: a collaborative analysis of 11 studies. J Natl Cancer Inst 1995; 87:378–84.

Dawber TR, Kannel WB, Lyell LP. An approach to longitudinal studies in a community: The Framingham Study. Ann NY Acad Sci 1963; 107:539–56.

Dublin S, Lydon-Rochelle M, Kaplan RC, Watts DH, Critchlow CW. Maternal and neonatal outcomes after induction of labor without an identified indication. Am J Obstet Gynecol 2000; 183:986–94.

Enterline PE, Hartley J, Henderson V. Asbestos and cancer: a cohort followed up to death. Br J Ind Med 1987; 44:396–401.

Farr W. Quoted in: Eyler EM. Victorian social medicine. Baltimore: Johns Hopkins University Press, 1979.

Fleischer WE, Viles FJ, Gode RL. A health survey of pipe covering occupations in construction naval vessels. J Ind Hyg Toxicol 1946; 28:9–16.

Gardner MJ. Considerations in the choice of expected numbers for appropriate comparisons in occupational cohort studies. Med Lav 1986; 77:23–47.

Giovanucci E, Ascherio A, Rimm EB, Colditz GA, Stampfer MJ, Willett WC. A prospective cohort study of vasectomy and prostate cancer in U.S. men. JAMA 1993; 269:873–77.

Goldberg J, True WR, Eisen SA, Henderson WG. A twin study of the effects of the Vietnam War on posttraumatic stress disorder. JAMA 1990; 263: 1227–32.

Greenberg ER, Baron JA, Karagas MR, Stukel TA, Nierenberg DW, Stevens MM, et al. Mortality associated with low plasma concentration of beta carotene and the effect of oral supplementation. JAMA 1996; 275:699–703.

Grodstein F, Stampfer MJ, Manson JE, Colditz GA, Willett WC, Rosner B, et al. Postmenopausal estrogen and progestin use and the risk of cardiovascular disease. N Engl J Med 1996; 335:453–61.

Guetta V, Cannon RO. Cardiovascular effects of estrogen and lipid-lowering therapies in postmenopausal women. Circulation 1996; 93:1928–37.

Hagan H, Thiede H, Weiss NS, Hopkins SG, Duchin JS, Alexander ER. Sharing of drug preparation equipment as a risk factor for hepatitis C virus incidence. Am J Public Health 2001; 91:23–27.

Hammond EC. Smoking in relation to the death rates of one million men and women. J Natl Cancer Inst 1966; Monograph #19:127–204.

Harvey EB, Boice JD, Honeyman M, Flannery JT. Prenatal X-ray exposure and childhood cancer in twins. N Engl J Med 1985; 312:541–45.

Jick H, Vasilakis C, Weinrauchand LA, Meier CR, Jick SS, Derby LE. A population-based study of appetite-suppressant drugs and the risk of cardiac-valve regurgitation. N Engl J Med 1998; 339:719–27.

Jones ME, Swerdlow AJ. Bias in the standardized mortality ratio when using general population rates to estimate expected number of deaths. Am J Epidemiol 1998; 148:1012–17.

Kannel WB, Castelli WP, Gordon T, McNamara PM. Serum cholesterol, lipoproteins, and the risk of coronary heart disease. The Framingham Study. Ann Intern Med 1971; 74:1–12.

Klag MJ, Ford DE, Mead LA, He J, Whelton PK, Liang KY, et al. Serum cholesterol in young men and subsequent cardiovascular disease. N Engl J Med 1993; 328:313–18.

Law MR, Thompson SG. Low serum cholesterol and the risk of cancer: an analysis of the published prospective studies. Cancer Causes Control 1991; 2:253–61.

Lee IM, Paffenbarger RS Jr. Physical activity and stroke incidence: the Harvard Alumni Health Study. Stroke 1998; 29:2049–54.

Lynge E, Thygesen L. Primary liver cancer among women in laundry and dry cleaning work in Denmark. Scand J Work Environ Health 1990; 16:108–12.

Manson JE, Colditz GA, Stampfer MJ, Willett WC, Rosner B, Monson R, et al. A prospective study of obesity and risk of coronary heart disease. N Engl J Med 1990; 322:882–89.

McMichael AJ. Standardized mortality ratios and the "healthy worker effect": scratching below the surface. J Occup Med 1976; 18:165–68.

Nienhuis H, Goldacre M, Seagroatt V, Gill L, Veseey M. Incidence of disease after vasectomy: a record linkage retrospective cohort study. BMJ 1992; 304: 743–46.

Persson I, Yuen J, Bergkvist L, Schairer C. Cancer incidence and mortality in women receiving estrogen and estrogen-progestin replacement therapy. Int J Cancer 1996; 67:327–32.

Petitti DB, Klein R, Kipp H, Friedman GD. Vasectomy and the incidence of hospitalized illness. J Urology 1983; 129:760–62.

Peto J, Seidman H, Selikoff IJ. Mesothelioma mortality in asbestos workers: Implications for models of carcinogenesis and risk assessment. Br J Cancer 1982; 45:124–35.

Rinsky RA, Zumwalder RD, Waxweiler RJ, Murray WE, Bierman PJ, Landrigand PJ, et al. Cancer mortality at a naval nuclear shipyard. Lancet 1981; 1:231–35.

Ron E, Modan B, Boice JD Jr. Mortality from cancer and other causes following radiotherapy for ringworm of the scalp. Am J Epidemiol 1988; 127:713–25.

Roscoe RJ, Deddens JA, Salvan A, Schnorr TM. Mortality among Navajo uranium miners. Am J Public Health 1995; 85:535–40.

Rothman KJ, Greenland S. Modern epidemiology (2nd ed.). Philadelphia: Lippincott-Raven, 1998.

Selikoff IJ, Hammond EC, Seidman H. Latency of asbestos disease among insulation workers in the United States and Canada. Cancer 1980; 46:2736–40.

Seltser R, Sartwell PE. The influence of occupational exposure to radiation on the mortality of American radiologists and other medical specialists. Am J Epidemiol 1965; 81:2–22.

Sesso HD, Paffenbarger RS Jr, Lee IM. Physical activity and breast cancer risk in the College Alumni Health Study (United States). Cancer Causes Control 1998; 9:433–39.

Shimizu Y, Kato H, Schull WJ. Studies of the mortality of A-bomb survivors. 1950–1985. Part 2. Cancer mortality based on the recently revised doses. Radiation Res 1990; 121:120–41.

Silverstein BA, Fine LJ, Armstrong TJ. Occupational factors and carpal tunnel syndrome. Am J Ind Med 1987; 11:343–58.

Tyroler HA, Heyden S, Bartel A, Cassel J, Cornoni JC, Hames CG, et al. Blood pressure and cholesterol as coronary heart disease risk factors. Arch Intern Med 1971; 128:907–14.

Velentgas P, Daling JR, Malone KE, Weiss NS, Williams MA, Self SG, et al. Pregnancy after breast carcinoma: outcomes and influence on mortality. Cancer 1999; 85:2424–32.

Walker AM, Jick H, Hunter JR, Danford A, Rothman KJ. Hospitalization rates in vasectomized men. JAMA 1981; 245:2315–17.

Weiss NS. Clinical epidemiology: the study of the outcome of illness (2nd ed.). New York: Oxford, 1996.

Weiss NS, Rossing MA. Healthy screenee bias in epidemiologic studies of cancer incidence. Epidemiology 1996; 7:319–22.

White E, Hunt JR, Casso D. Exposure measurement in cohort studies: the challenges of prospective data collection. Epidemiol Rev 1998; 20:43–56.

15

CASE-CONTROL STUDIES

In 1971, Herbst et al. (1971) reported that the mothers of seven of eight teenage girls diagnosed with clear cell adenocarcinoma of the vagina in Boston during 1966–1969 reported having taken a synthetic hormone, diethylstilbestrol (DES), while that child was in utero. None of the mothers of 32 girls without vaginal adenocarcinoma, matched to the mothers of cases with regard to hospital and date of birth, had taken DES during the corresponding pregnancy. Within a year, a New York study of five cases and eight girls without vaginal cancer obtained similar results (Greenwald et al., 1971). The introduction of prenatal DES use into obstetrical practice in the U.S. during the 1940s and 1950s, followed by the appearance of this hitherto unseen form of cancer some 20 years later, supported a causal connection between in utero exposure to DES and vaginal adenocarcinoma. The means by which in utero DES exposure might predispose to the occurrence of clear cell vaginal adenocarcinoma was unknown in 1971. Nonetheless, a causal inference was made at that time by the Food and Drug Administration, which specified pregnancy as a contraindication for DES use. (At present, it is believed that DES acts by interfering with the normal development of the female genital tract, resulting in the persistence into puberty of vaginal adenosis in which adenocarcinoma can arise [Ulfelder and Robboy, 1976]).

The investigation by Herbst et al. was a case-control study: a comparison of prior exposures or characteristics of ill persons (cases) with those of persons at risk of developing the illness. Generally, the prior experience of persons at risk is estimated from observations of a sample of them (controls). A difference in the frequency or levels of exposure between cases and controls—i.e., an association—may be a reflection of a causal link.

At first glance, the case-control approach appears to proceed backwards, from consequence to potential cause. Nonetheless, if a case-control study enrolls cases and controls from the same underlying population at risk of the outcome, and can measure exposure status validly in them, the results obtained will closely resemble those from a properly done cohort study. A case-control, cohort, or any other form of non-randomized study does have the potential to observe a spurious association because of the influence of some other factor associated with both exposure and outcome. Even so, the evidence that is provided by well-done case-control studies can carry great weight when evaluating the validity of a causal hypothesis. Indeed, a number of causal inferences have been based largely on the results of case-control studies. These include, in addition to the DES–vaginal adenocarcinoma relationship, the connection between aspirin use in children and the development of Reye's syndrome (Hurwitz et al., 1985), and the use of absorbent tampons and the incidence of toxic shock syndrome (Stallones, 1982).

One of the criteria used to assess the validity of a causal hypothesis is the strength of the association between exposure and disease, usually as measured by the ratio of the incidence rate in exposed and nonexposed persons. In most case-control studies, it is not possible to measure incidence rates in either of these groups. Nonetheless, from the frequency of exposure observed in cases and controls, it is usually possible to estimate closely the ratio of the incidence rates. The way this is done—through the use of the odds ratio—as well as the underlying rationale were discussed in Chapter 9.

RETROSPECTIVE ASCERTAINMENT OF EXPOSURE STATUS IN CASES AND CONTROLS

Epidemiologic studies seek to obtain information on exposures present during an etiologically relevant period of time. That period varies across etiologic relationships. For example, excess consumption of alcohol predisposes to motor vehicle injuries within minutes to hours, but it predisposes to cirrhosis of the liver only after a number of years. Most case-control studies are required to consider explicitly how best to assess, in retrospect, subjects' exposure status during a period of time in which an exposure might have been acting to influence disease risk. Possible sources of data an exposure status include interviews or questionnaires, available records, or physical or laboratory measurements.

Interviews/Questionnaires

For many exposures, a subject's memory is an excellent window to the past. A number of important etiologic relationships have been identified through interview-based case-control studies. As a general rule, study participants will report longer-term and more recent experiences with the greatest accuracy. Attention to the ways in which questions are asked (Armstrong et al., 1992) will maximize the accuracy of the information received, along with the use of visual aids when appropriate (e.g., pictures of medicines, or of containers of household products; calendars for important life events to enhance recall of the timing of other exposures). This type of attention, together with the use of the same questions for cases and controls asked in the same way, will also minimize the potential for bias that could result from the subject's or interviewer's awareness of case or control status.

One virtue of exposure ascertainment via interview or questionnaire is that information can be sought for several points in time. It is possible that a given exposure plays an etiologic role only if present at a certain age, for a certain duration, or at a certain time in the past. Because there is often little guidance before a study starts to suggest the most relevant age, length, or recency, key exposures are often elicited throughout much of the subject's lifetime. Still, care must be taken not to include exposures that took place after the illness began.

Example: Victora et al. (1989) conducted a case-control study of infant death from diarrhea in relation to type of feeding. They asked mothers of cases whether their child was or was not being breast-fed immediately prior to the onset of the fatal illness. Mothers of controls were queried about type of feeding prior to a comparable point in time. Mothers were also asked if subsequent to the onset of the illness there had been any changes in type of feeding: following the development of diarrhea, many breast-fed children are supplemented with formula and cow's milk. Relative to infants who were solely breast-fed, those who also drank powdered or cow's milk prior to their illness had about four times the risk of diarrheal death. The authors showed, however, that if one inappropriately considered the feeding method that was present during the illness, about a 13-fold increase in risk associated with supplementation would have been estimated.

Records

Case-control studies have exploited vital, registry, employment, medical and pharmacy records, to name only some, as a means of obtaining information on exposures. But because the information contained in the records usually has been assembled for purposes other than epidemiologic research, it may not provide precisely the information desired by the epidemiologist. For example, a death certificate or an occupational record may state an individual's job, but often not her or his actual exposure to the substance(s) of interest to the study. Or a pharmacy record will indicate a prescription's having been filled, but not whether the patient took the medication on a given day or took it at all. This sort of imprecision will impair a study's ability to discern a true association between an exposure and a disease; the greater the imprecision, the greater the impairment. Nonetheless, some very strong associations have been identified through record-based case-control studies. For example (and as described more fully in Chapter 10), in a study based entirely on tumor registry records Daling et al. (1982) observed that men with anal cancer were substantially less likely to be married than men with other types of cancer. This served as a stimulus to conduct interview-based studies that could elicit information regarding receptive anal intercourse, the exposure suspected to underlie the association with never having been married. The latter studies showed an exceedingly strong association with a history of receptive anal intercourse among men, an odds ratio of 50 (Daling et al., 1987).

In case-control studies in which medical records are used to characterize exposure status, care must be taken to restrict the information obtained to that which preceded the case's diagnosis and the presence of symptoms, if any, that led to the diagnosis. The records of controls must be truncated at similar points in time. Without this safeguard, it is possible that bias will arise from there being systematically more complete information available to review on cases than on controls: the case's illness may have stimulated an inquiry by medical personnel into his or her past, whereas no corresponding inquiry would necessarily have occurred for control subjects.

Example: Weinmann et al. (1994) conducted a case-control study of renal cell cancer in relation to antecedent use of antihypertensive medications within the membership of Kaiser-Permanente Northwest. For cases and their matched controls (demographically similar members of the health care plan without this disease), outpatient and inpatient medical records were reviewed for information regarding medication use up to a date three months prior to the case's diagnosis. By selectively not including the last three months in the data collection period, the investigators sought to minimize differences between cases and controls regarding the quantity of information contained in the records on prior medication use. Also, they felt it implausible that use of a drug during such a relatively short time as the three months prior to diagnosis would have had an influence on the development of that patient's renal cell cancer.

Physical and Laboratory Measurements

The recognized limitations of interviews and records in characterizing a variety of potentially relevant exposures have stimulated the conduct of epidemiologic studies that use laboratory and other methods of measurement. A woman cannot tell an investigator the level of her reproductive hormones, the concentration of various micronutrients in her blood, or whether her cervix is infected with human papillomavirus, while laboratory tests can. Unfortunately, such tests tell us only what these things are at the time the specimens have been obtained. For some exposures, there will be a high correlation between the measured level following case and control identification and that present during the etiologically relevant time period. For example, lead enters and does not leave the dentine of teeth. Therefore, in young school-age children, lead dentine levels are an indicator of cumulative lead exposure, a good portion of which could be relevant to the development of intellectual impairment and other adverse neurologic outcomes (Needleman et al., 1990). For another example, in a case-control study of vaccine efficacy against tuberculosis, the presence of a BCG vaccination scar is just as reliable an indicator of exposure status when measured after illness is present than had it been possible to assess the presence of a scar earlier in time (Rodrigues and Smith, 1999). In contrast, one would not rely on serum levels of reproductive hormones of post-menopausal women with breast cancer and controls to indicate what their premenopausal levels were, much less the hormonal status during their very early reproductive years (at which time it is plausible that hormones can exert the greatest impact on future risk of breast cancer).

Example: Green et al. (1999) compared 88 children who had been diagnosed with leukemia and 133 controls regarding exposure to magnetic fields. During a two-day period that took place an average of 2.5 years after the diagnosis had been made, study participants wore a personal monitoring device that assessed these fields once each minute. (The study was restricted to children who continued to live in the same residence as the one they had in the 6 to 12 months prior to the time of diagnosis.) Earlier studies of the possible association between magnetic field exposure and leukemia typically had estimated exposures based on the electric wire configuration of the household, or on direct measures within the household itself, but had not used personal monitors. The study of Green, et al. observed a substantially stronger association between exposure to magnetic fields and leukemia than nearly all prior studies of this question. While it is possible that this stronger association is genuine—a result of a relatively more accurate means of assessing exposure status—it is also possible that some bias has been introduced by having to rely on magnetic field measurements obtained several years after each child's leukemia had been diagnosed, or by behavioral changes produced by the leukemia.

Some case-control studies are nested within cohort studies in which specimens (e.g. blood, urine) have been obtained prior to diagnosis on all cohort members, but have not yet been analyzed for the exposure(s) in question. At a later time, measurements are made upon the specimens from cohort members who developed a particular illness (cases) and on controls sampled from: *(1)* the cohort as a whole (case-cohort studies); or *(2)* cohort members who did not develop the illness as of the date of diagnosis of their respective cases (nested case-control studies) (Wacholder, 1991). The results obtained from studies of this type cannot be influenced by metabolic and other changes that occur following the diagnosis of the illness. However, the results can be influenced by changes that take place between the time the illness first develops and the time it is diagnosed as such. So, in order to lessen the chance that occult illness in cases has influenced levels of a suspected etiologic factor, many studies of this type exclude from the analyses specimens obtained within the period prior to diagnosis that might correspond to the duration of the preclinical stage of disease.

Also, among the large majority of case-control studies in which exposure status is not measured until the illness or injury has been diagnosed, some are concerned only with an exposure or characteristic that would have been the same at all times in a person's life. This is true for a genetically determined characteristic such as ABO blood type, or the absence of glutathione transferase M1 activity (an enzyme that metabolizes several potentially carcinogenic constituents of cigarette smoke). Clearly, these studies are no less valid for having had to measure exposure in retrospect.

CASE DEFINITION

Ideally, the cases in a case-control study would comprise all (or a representative sample of) members of a defined population who develop a given health outcome during a given period of time. For studies of disease etiology, that outcome is disease occurrence. For studies that seek to determine the efficacy of early disease detection or treatment, the outcome generally is mortality or the onset of complications of the disease; such studies have been described in detail elsewhere (Selby, 1994; Weiss, 1994) and will not be covered any further here.

The population from which cases are to be drawn may be defined geographically, or it may be defined on the basis of other characteristics, such as membership in a prepaid health care plan or an occupational group. The identification of all newly ill persons in a defined population can be facilitated by the presence of a reporting system, such as a cancer or malformation registry, that seeks to accomplish this identification for other purposes. On occasion, care for the condition being studied may be centralized, so that it would be necessary to review the records of only one or a few institutions to identify all cases in the population in which those institutions are located. In many instances, however, it is not feasible to identify all cases that occur in a given population, so case-control studies are often based on but a portion of them, perhaps cases identified from hospital records or from the records of selected providers from whom patients had sought health care. The study of Herbst et al. (1971) of vaginal adenocarcinoma was of this type. Whether or not the cases are derived from a defined population, it is necessary that they be drawn in an unselected manner with regard to exposure status; e.g., by including in the study all eligible cases diagnosed or receiving care during a defined time period.

While the goal of a case-control study of etiology is to enroll incident cases, under some circumstances it may be necessary to enroll prevalent cases at a particular point in time, irrespective of when each one's illness had begun. For some conditions, the date of occurrence may simply not be known. For example, in the absence of very close sero-monitoring, one generally cannot determine when a person acquired an HIV infection. Second, for uncommon diseases of long duration, an incidence series may yield too few cases for meaningful analysis. The disadvantages of using prevalent cases in a case-control study relate in part to the added problems of accurate exposure ascertainment. For prevalent conditions whose date of diagnosis is known, pre-illness exposure information on study subjects must be obtained for more distant points in the past, on average, than would be necessary for an incident series. For prevalent conditions whose date of occurrence is unknown (e.g., HIV infection), there will be uncertainty about the best point in time before which one should elicit exposure information. Also, by studying persons remaining alive with a given condition, one is studying at the same time not only etiologic factors, but factors that influence the duration of the condition, including those associated with survival.

Ideally, the criteria used to identify and select individual cases for study should be objective, and also have a high sensitivity and specificity for the disease. Specificity is of particular concern, since the inadvertent inclusion of persons without disease in the case group will generally obscure any true association with exposure (see Chapter 10, p. 233). With this in mind, in the case-control study of Reye's syndrome in relation to antecedent analgesic use conducted by the Centers for Disease Control (Hurwitz et al., 1985), only cases with a substantial degree of neurological impairment (stage 2 or higher) were included. The use of this criterion minimized the chances that children with diseases other than Reye's syndrome, diseases that generally would have a lesser degree of severity, would be included in the case group. It also was intended to serve as protection against selective misclassification of Reye's syndrome based on knowledge of a child's exposure status, since the hypothesis that aspirin was associated with Reye's syndrome was well known by the time the study took place. Conceivably, the knowledge that the child had consumed aspirin could have led some physicians to diagnose Reye's syndrome in cases with an atypical illness.

CONTROL DEFINITION

Occasionally, the proportion of ill persons who have had a specific exposure is so high, unequivocally more than would be expected in the population they were derived from, that the presence of an association (though not its magnitude) can be surmised from a case series alone (Cummings and Weiss, 1998). For example, when it was learned that all cases of a form of pneumonia that was epidemic in Spain in 1981 had ingested adulterated rapeseed oil, a causal inference was drawn, leading to efforts to eliminate further use of that oil. This action was taken before any formal comparison of cases with controls was made (Tabuenca, 1981).

In the vast majority of instances, however, an explicit control group is needed to estimate the frequency and degree of exposure that would have taken place among cases in the absence of an exposure–disease association. An ideal control group would be one that consists of individuals:

1. selected from a population whose distribution of exposure is that of the population the cases arose from;
2. who are identical to the cases with respect to their distribution of all characteristics
   (a) that influence the likelihood and/or degree of exposure, and
   (b) that, independent of their relationship to exposure, are also related to the occurrence of the illness under study or to its recognition; and
3. in whom the presence of the exposure can be measured accurately and in a manner that is identical to that used for cases.

If the criteria above are not met in a particular study, then selection bias, confounding, or information bias, respectively, may be present.

Minimizing Selection Bias

If the cases identified in the study are all or a representative sample of those that occurred in a defined population, one can seek to achieve comparability by choosing persons sampled from the same population as controls. For geographically defined populations, a number of different methods of sampling have been used, including random-digit dialing of telephone numbers, area sampling, neighborhood sampling, voters' lists, population registers, motor vehicle licenses, and birth certificates, among others. When cases are members of a prepaid health care plan who develop an illness or injury, a sample of persons who were members of the health plan when the illness or injury occurred can serve as controls. When cases are sick or injured members of an employed population, controls can be selected from the same group of employees.

In some studies, cases have not been selected from a definable population at risk for the disease, but rather from persons treated for a particular illness at one or a few hospitals or clinics. Selection bias may be present in such studies if: (a) controls are not chosen from persons who, had they developed the illness under study, would have received care at these hospitals or clinics; and (b) persons who do and do not receive care from these sources differ with regard to their frequency or level of exposure.

Therefore, when cases are chosen from a narrow range of providers of health care, often controls are chosen from other ill persons treated by these providers. Such ill controls may also be used if, irrespective of the source of cases, there is no feasible way to sample from the population at large, or if sampling from the population at large would be likely to result in a substantial level of non-response or information bias (see below). For these reasons, in some studies of fatal illness, exposures in persons with a given cause of death are compared to exposures in a sample of persons who died for other reasons (Gordis, 1982).

But the choice of sick or deceased controls can itself give rise to selection bias if the illnesses (or causes of death) represented in the control group are in some way associated with the exposure of interest. For example, ill or recently deceased persons tend to have been smokers of cigarettes more often than other people (McLaughlin et al., 1985), since smoking is associated with a variety of causes of illness and death. Because smoking histories of ill persons overstate the cigarette consumption of the population from which the cases arose (even if that population cannot be defined), the odds ratio associated with smoking based on the use of ill persons as controls will be spuriously low.

To minimize selection bias related to having chosen sick or deceased controls, an attempt can be made to omit potential controls with conditions known to be related (positively or negatively) to the exposure. For example, in the analysis of a hospital-based case-control study of bladder cancer in relation to prior use of artificial sweeteners, the investigators excluded from their control group persons who were hospitalized for obesity-related diseases (Silverman et al., 1983). They showed that without this restriction, the control group would have a spuriously high proportion of users of artificial sweeteners relative to the population from which their cases actually had come. This approach will succeed to the extent that one judges correctly which conditions truly are exposure-related, and how accurately the presence of those conditions can be determined. For many exposures, this may pose little problem, and judicious exclusion will yield a control group capable of providing an unbiased result. For others, such as cigarette smoking or alcohol drinking, it has been shown that admitting diagnoses or statements of cause of death are incapable of identifying all persons with illnesses related to these exposures (McLaughlin et al., 1985).

Occasionally, controls are chosen from individuals who are tested for the presence of the disease under study and are found not to have it. For example, persons demonstrated to have coronary artery occlusion on coronary angiography have been compared to angiography patients without occlusion with regard to potential risk factors (Thom et al., 1992). As another example, the prior use of oral contraceptives was compared between women diagnosed with venous thromboembolism and women seen at the same institution for suspected venous thromboembolism who turned out not to have this condition (Bloemenkamp et al., 1999). It may be relatively inexpensive to select controls from persons who receive the same diagnostic evaluation as do cases, and it is also possible to achieve case-control comparability with regard to the choice of a health-care provider (and the correlates of that choice). This approach can have an impact on the study's validity when the frequency or degree of exposure differs between otherwise-comparable members of a population who do and do not receive the test:

1. It will increase the study's validity if the disease being investigated is generally asymptomatic, and so would not be detected in the absence of testing. Thus, the relationship of the use of oral contraceptives to the incidence of in situ cancer of the cervix is best studied in women who have received cervical screening, by comparing oral contraceptive use between cases of in situ cancer and women with a negative screen. This is because:

   (a) In most societies, screening is more commonly administered to women who use oral contraceptives than women who do not; and

   (b) In situ cancers are asymptomatic and will not be identified in the absence of cervical screening.

   Therefore, if controls are chosen from women in general, who may or may not have received cervical screening, an apparent excess of oral contraceptive users would be present among cases of in situ cancer even if no true association were present.

2. The choice of test-negative controls, however, will detract from a study's validity if the large majority of persons who develop the disease soon would get diagnosed whether or not the test was administered. There was a controversy in the late 1970s regarding the suitability, in case-control studies of postmenopausal estrogen use and endometrial cancer, of a control group restricted to women with no evidence of cancer on endometrial biopsy. Among women without endometrial cancer, estrogen use differs greatly between those who have undergone biopsy and those who have not, because estrogen use predisposes to uterine bleeding of nonmalignant causes that often leads to endometrial biopsy. Investigators who believed that there was a great prevalence of occult endometrial cancer in the population suggested that the optimal control group ought to be women undergoing endometrial biopsy and found not to have cancer (Horwitz and Feinstein, 1978). The majority of investigators, however, believed that no such large pool of prevalent, occult disease existed, and that choosing biopsy-negative controls would lead to a spuriously high estimate of

estrogen use in the population at risk, and thus a spuriously low odds ratio (Shapiro et al., 1985).

No matter how controls are defined in a case-control study, selection bias may be introduced to the extent that exposure information is not obtained on all who have been selected to take part. The magnitude of the bias will increase in relation to the frequency of missing data and the degree to which exposure frequencies or levels differ between study subjects for whom exposure status is and is not known. The problem of incomplete ascertainment of exposure on study subjects is particularly common in interview- or questionnaire-based case-control studies. Strategies for minimizing the degree of non-response in case-control studies are discussed in detail elsewhere (Armstrong et al., 1992).

Minimizing Information Bias

In case-control studies in which information on exposure status is sought through an interview or questionnaire, the chief safeguards against information bias entail asking questions about events that are salient to the respondent, that are framed in an unambiguous way, and that are presented identically to both cases and controls. Employment of these safeguards, however, will not prevent differential accuracy of reporting between cases and controls in all circumstances. Some past exposures or events will simply be more salient to persons with an illness, who might have dwelled on possible reasons that it occurred, than to persons without that illness. Other exposures may be viewed as socially undesirable, and there may be a difference between cases and healthy controls in their willingness to admit to them. If the anticipated difference in the quality of information between cases and otherwise-appropriate controls is too great, a control group that is less than ideal in other respects may be selected instead to minimize the potential for information bias. For example, some studies of prenatal risk factors for a particular congenital malformation that utilize maternal interviews as the source of exposure data have selected as controls infants with other malformations (Rosenberg et al., 1983). This control group will provide a more valid result than a control group that consists of infants in general if: mothers of malformed and mothers of normal infants report prenatal exposures to a different degree even in the absence of an association, and if the exposure in question is not associated with the occurrence of the malformations present in control infants. [For some exposures, such as use of multivitamin supplements during pregnancy, there is an association with a broad range of malformation types (Werler et al., 1999), making it difficult or impossible to define a subgroup of malformed infants as controls that would yield an unbiased result.]

Similar reasoning led Daling et al. (1987), when conducting their case-control study of anal cancer in relation to a history of anal intercourse, to eschew the geographic population their cases had arisen from as a sampling frame for controls. They feared that interviews that sought information about prior anal intercourse might be more complete among men with cancer than men in the population at large. Thus, they chose as controls men with a cancer of a different site (colon). They had reason to believe that colon cancer was unlikely to have been etiologically related to prior anal intercourse, and suspected that in terms of their willingness to answer sensitive questions reliably, men with colon cancer would be more similar to men with anal cancer than would be men selected at random.

When the measurement of the exposure under consideration is inherently imprecise, or when there is a large subjective component involved, it may be difficult or impossible to identify a control group that will provide information comparable to that provided by cases. An instructive example comes from a case-control study of Down's syndrome (Stott, 1958) conducted shortly before the chromosomal basis for the etiology of this condition had been learned. The study sought to determine whether emotional "shocks" during pregnancy might be a risk factor. The author interviewed mothers of children with Down's syndrome about any occurrence of a "situation or event [that would be] stress- or shock-producing . . . in an emotionally stable woman." Identical interviews were administered to mothers of normal children, but also to mothers of retarded children who did not have Down's syndrome. Even though it is not possible that an emotional shock in pregnancy could play any etiologic role in a condition already determined at conception, a far higher proportion of mothers of cases of Down's syndrome reported an emotional shock than did mothers of normal controls (odds ratio estimated from the data = 17.0). The use of other retarded children as controls only partially reduced the spuriously high odds ratio, to a value of 4.3.

When conducting an interview-based study of a rapidly fatal disease, or a disease that impairs a person's ability to provide valid interview data, it is necessary to obtain information from at least some surrogate respondents. Typically, these respondents are close relatives of the cases. For purposes of comparability, similar information generally ought to be obtained from surrogates of controls, even though the control would be expected to provide more accurate data.

Example: In their case-control study of vigorous exercise as a possible precipitant of primary cardiac arrest, Siscovick et al. (1984) compared information obtained from the wives of men in whom an arrest had occurred with that obtained from wives of men identified at random (controls) in the same community. (Though it would have been feasible to interview the control men themselves, the large majority of the cases had died.) The investigators were willing to accept the likely greater degree of exposure misclassification arising from the use of interviews with spouses of controls at the price of achieving a higher degree of case-control comparability of exposure data.

Results of case-control studies based on exposure information provided by surrogate respondents need to be interpreted with particular caution. Though by no means present in every instance (Nelson et al., 1990), there can be a large difference in the validity of the responses given by case and control surrogates. For example, Greenberg et al. (1985) investigated the basis for an apparently strong association between cancer mortality and "nuclear" work among employees of a naval shipyard that had been found in a comparison of work histories provided by surrogates of men who died from cancer and of those who died of other conditions. They observed that, regarding work in the nuclear part of the industry, surrogates of the cases generally provided information similar to that contained in employment records of the shipyard. In contrast, the surrogates of controls substantially misclassified the nature of their relatives' jobs as not involving radiation. Using the more accurate data provided by employment records, which included individual radiation dosimetry (Rinsky et al., 1981), little or no association was present between cancer mortality and radiation exposure received at the shipyard.

What was undoubtedly a spuriously negative association was found in a case-control study of lung cancer and passive cigarette smoking that used, for one analysis, information obtained from surrogate respondents (Janerich et al., 1990). In this analysis, the relative risk of lung cancer among nonsmokers associated with a spouse's having smoked—0.33 (i.e., a 67% reduction in risk)—would seem almost certainly due to a spurious minimization or denial of smoking by spouses of cases, who may have feared their habit caused their spouse to develop lung cancer.

Differentially accurate assessment of exposure status between cases and controls is not confined to interview- or questionnaire-based studies. Most laboratory-based studies seek to prevent this by testing samples blind to case/control status. If feasible, it is desirable to do this blinding as well in studies in which exposure is to be determined from medical or other records. There are instances, however, in which the nature of the information available in records has already been influenced by whether the subject is a case or a control. For example, it was found that among 100 infertile women who underwent laparoscopy (Strathy et al., 1982), 21 had endometriosis. Only two percent of 200 women undergoing laparoscopy for another indication, tubal ligation, were noted in the records of their procedure to have endometriosis. Taken at face value, these data would suggest that the presence of endometriosis predisposes to infertility. But the interpretation of this association is not straightforward, since the means of identification and recording of endometriosis in cases and controls (women undergoing tubal ligation) may well have not been comparable—only in the infertile women was the laparoscopy expressly done as a diagnostic tool to investigate the possible presence of conditions such as endometriosis.

Additional delineation of the rationale underlying control definition and selection can be found in Wacholder et al. (1992a, b, c).

CONTROL OF CONFOUNDING IN CASE-CONTROL STUDIES

Characteristics of Confounding Variables in Case-Control Studies

Confounding is present when the estimate of the relationship between an exposure and disease is distorted by the influence of another factor. In any study design, confounding generally will occur to the extent that the other factor is associated both with an exposure (though not as a result of the exposure) and with the occurrence of the disease or its recognition. In case-control studies alone, a factor may confound even if it is not associated with an altered risk of disease, if the proportions of cases and controls vary across levels or categories of the factor. For example, in a collaborative study of ovarian cancer in relation to use of oral contraceptives (Weiss et al., 1981), an attempt was made to identify and interview all incident cases during a several-year period in two U.S. populations. In one of the populations (western Washington State), several controls per case were interviewed, whereas the control/case ratio in the other (Utah) was 1.0. Thus, the design created an association between study population and disease status among persons actually studied. Since oral contraceptive use was more common in Washington women than in Utah women, failure to take into account the state of residence in the analysis (e.g., by adjustment) would have led to a spuriously high estimate of the frequency of oral contraceptive use in controls relative to that in cases.

Means of Controlling for Confounding

One straightforward way of preventing confounding is to restrict cases and controls to a single category or level of the potentially confounding variable. For example, in their study of physical activity in relation to primary cardiac arrest, Siscovick et al. (1982) excluded persons with conditions, such as clinically recognized heart disease, that could both predispose to cardiac arrest and might be expected to alter someone's level of activity. A second way is to obtain information on exposures or characteristics that may differ between cases and controls, and then make statistical adjustments for those that also are found to be related to the exposure or characteristic under investigation (see Chapter 11).

Alternatively, it is possible to match controls to cases (either to individual cases, or to groups of cases with a shared characteristic) on the category or level of a potentially confounding factor. It should be kept in mind, though, that in case-control studies, matching alone is not sufficient to eliminate a variable's confounding influence, and that failure to consider a matching variable in the analysis of the study can lead to a biased result (Rothman and Greenland, 1998). It is appropriate to match if:

- The variable is expected to be strongly related both to exposure and to disease. Thus, in a case-control study of breast cancer in relation to use of hair dye, it would make sense to match on gender (if the study had not already been restricted to women) since: *(a)* in most cultures, use of hair dye is more common in women than in men; and *(b)* in the absence of matching, the case-to-control ratio would be very uneven between women and men. While confounding by gender could be prevented even without matching by adjustment in the analysis, the statistical precision of the unmatched study would be substantially less than that of a case-control study having a more similar proportion of female cases and controls.
- Information on possible matching variables can be obtained inexpensively. There are some means of control selection in which information regarding some confounders can be obtained at no cost. For example, from voters' lists or prepaid health plan membership records, it would generally be possible to directly choose one or more controls who were nearly identical to a given case's age. On the other hand, if a population-sampling scheme such as random-digit dialing were being employed, the age of the respondent would not be known in advance of approaching her or him. Rather than omitting already contacted controls who did not match a particular case's age, the matching can be done much more broadly. Additional control for finer categories of age can be accomplished in the data analysis.
- Information on exposure status cannot be obtained inexpensively. The higher the cost of exposure ascertainment, the greater the incentive to limit the number of control subjects to the number of cases. Differences between cases and controls regarding confounding factors will particularly reduce the statistical power of a study that does not have a surplus of controls. Enriching the group of controls selected with persons more similar to the cases with regard to confounding factors (i.e., matching) can prevent this loss of statistical power.

In case-control studies of genetic characteristics as possible etiologic factors, some investigators have used a matched design in which a specified type of relative (such as a parent, sibling, or cousin) is chosen as a control for each case

(Yang and Khoury, 1997; Witte et al., 1999). This approach has the advantage of minimizing potential confounding by other genetic characteristics with which the one of interest is associated. It has a disadvantage, though: the exclusion of a possibly large fraction of cases for whom there is no relative available of the type needed to provide a sample for genetic analysis.

Analyses of studies that have matched controls to cases on a given characteristic can adjust for that characteristic as if no matching had taken place. Alternatively, these analyses can explicitly consider cases and controls as matched sets. In the instance of matched case-control pairs and a dichotomous exposure variable, the following table could be constructed:

	Control	
CASE	EXPOSED	NON-EXPOSED
Exposed	a	b
Non-exposed	c	d

Only the b pairs in which the case was exposed but not the matched control, and the c pairs in which the reverse was true, would enter the analysis. The odds ratio would be calculated as b/c. When there is more than one control per case, or an uneven number of controls per case, an odds ratio that accounts for the matching can be calculated as well (Breslow and Day, 1980; Hosmer and Lemeshow, 2000).

CASE-CONTROL STUDIES THAT DIRECTLY COMPARE DISEASE OR EXPOSURE SUBGROUPS

Imagine that an ordinary case-control study has been conducted in which ill and well persons are to be compared in terms of the proportion who have received a given exposure. If the sick individuals can be subdivided on the basis of a manifestation of their illness (e.g., histological type of cancer, or hemorrhagic versus thrombotic stroke), it is straightforward to compare separately each of the subgroups of cases to the controls. Similarly, when comparing a single case group to controls for the presence of an exposure with multiple categories (e.g., type of oral contraceptive, brand of cellular phone), odds ratios can be calculated for each type of exposure subcategory, using non-exposed persons as a common referent category.

For a variety of reasons, primarily relating to feasibility, some case-control studies do not include a group of nondiseased individuals. Others include, among both cases or controls, only persons who sustained a broadly defined exposure, within which a particular exposure subcategory is of interest. Under what circumstances can these studies provide useful information?

Example: In a study of oropharyngeal cancer, Gillison et al. (2000) compared the smoking and drinking habits of persons whose tumors were positive for human papillomavirus type 16 (HPV16) and those whose tumors were negative. All but one of the 25 persons with a tumor that was HPV16-negative had smoked cigarettes, as opposed to 27 of 34 of those with an HPV16-positive tumor. Similarly, half of the HPV16-negative patients consumed 100 grams or more of alcohol per week prior to diagnosis, in contrast to just 5 of the 34 persons whose tumor was HPV16-positive.

Since the study did not include men and women without cancer as a basis for comparison, from these data alone it is impossible to distinguish the two possible interpretations of these results (we will also assume that neither chance nor bias is an explanation): *(a)* smoking and drinking particularly predispose to the occurrence of HPV16-negative oropharyngeal tumors; or *(b)* smoking and drinking protect against the occurrence of HPV16-positive tumors. But there are ample data from other studies (Blot et al., 1996) that did include controls without cancer to indicate that smoking and drinking are strongly positively associated with the incidence of oropharyngeal cancer in general. (These studies were conducted before it was possible to assess a tumor's HPV status.) Thus, the most plausible explanation is *(a)* above: smoking and drinking predispose to the incidence of oropharyngeal cancer through a causal pathway that does not require the presence of an infection with HPV16. The hypothesis that smoking and drinking also predispose to oropharyngeal cancer when HPV infection is present, but simply to a relatively smaller degree, could be tested in a case-control study only by including controls without oropharyngeal cancer.

Example: *Helicobacter pylori (H. pylori)* is a heterogeneous bacterial species. A number of studies (summarized by Spechler et al., 2000) have examined the possibility that *H. pylori* strains that express cytoxin-associated gene A (cagA) are particularly virulent in terms of their ability to produce gastric pathology. These studies have compared the presence of serum antibodies to the cagA protein among patients with gastric disease (e.g., ulcer or carcinoma) and healthy individuals (e.g., blood donors), with both cases and controls being serologically positive for *H. pylori* infection. Most (though not all) such studies observed a higher proportion of *H. pylori* infections to be cagA-positive in cases than in controls.

The exclusion of *H. pylori*-negative persons in the analysis of data from these studies, strictly speaking, limits the interpretation of the results. Examined in isolation, the data are equally compatible with the hypothesis that *H. pylori* strains that express cagA predispose to gastric pathology as they are with the hypothesis that cagA-negative strains lead to a reduced risk (relative to the absence of *H. pylori* infection).

Here is another, older, example in which the restriction of the study population to "exposed" individuals alone prevented an appreciation of the impact of each of the exposure subgroups on disease risk.

Example: In 1975, a study was conducted on 20 women under 40 years of age in the U.S. who developed endometrial cancer and who had a history of oral contraceptive use (Silverberg and Makowski, 1975). Thirteen (65%) of these women had taken a sequential preparation (almost all of which was the brand Oracon), substantially more than the eight percent expected based on U.S. national sales of oral contraceptives. This observation is compatible with the hypothesis that use of Oracon predisposes to endometrial cancer, but it is equally compatible with the hypothesis that use of other types of oral contraceptives protects against this disease. In fact, both hypotheses turned out to be correct: When a case-control study was done that was not restricted to users of oral contraceptives (Weiss and Sayvetz, 1980), Oracon users were observed to have about a seven-fold increased risk of endometrial cancer, and users of non-sequential oral contraceptives ("combination" pills) a 50% *lower* risk, relative to women who had not taken oral contraceptives.

CASE-CONTROL STUDIES: ANSWERS TO QUESTIONS OF DISEASE ETIOLOGY?

Randomized trials will not be able to answer all of our questions about the reasons diseases occur. Many potential disease-causing or disease-preventing exposures cannot be manipulated, either at all—e.g., most genetic characteristics—or in any practical way for purposes of a study. For many exposure–disease relationships, either the disease is too uncommon or the induction period is too long to conduct a randomized trial that is not infeasibly large in size or long in duration. Finally, it generally will not be possible to conduct separate randomized trials to measure the impact of all potential types, amounts, and durations of a class of exposure.

For many of the same reasons, it is not possible to rely solely on cohort studies for answers. Just as with randomized trials, the disease outcome being studied may be too rare to allow a cohort approach to be useful. This explains why the etiologies of vaginal adenocarcinoma and Reye's syndrome, for example, have been evaluated exclusively by case-control studies—these diseases are simply too rare for most cohort studies to generate any cases, even in "exposed" individuals. Prospective cohort studies are also of limited use when the induction period for the exposure–disease relationship is either very short or very long. If the induction period is very short, and the exposure status of an individual varies over time, a cohort study would need to assess exposure status repeatedly among cohort members. For this reason, studies of alcohol consumption in relation to the occurrence of injuries typically are case-control in nature (Holcomb, 1938). Similarly, unless information on exposure status can be ascertained retrospectively at the time the cohort is formed, it would rarely be feasible to initiate a cohort study of a suspected etiologic relationship that requires several decades to manifest itself.

While case-control studies may be of particular value in evaluating the etiology of uncommon diseases, they may have difficulty obtaining statistically precise results if the frequency of the exposure in the population under study is either extremely common or extremely uncommon (Crombie, 1981). Thus, only an association as strong as the one between cigarette smoking and lung cancer could have emerged reliably from case-control studies of several hundred British men conducted in the late 1940s (Doll and Hill, 1950), given that well over 90% of that population were cigarette smokers. For very uncommon exposures—e.g., occupational exposure to a specific substance suspected of posing a risk to health, or an infrequently prescribed drug—unless there truly is a strong association and there is a large number of subjects available, even the best-designed case-control study can offer no more than a suggestion of an association with the occurrence of a given illness.

EXERCISES

1. A study of bladder cancer in relation to occupation among women was conducted in Southern California (Anton-Culver et al., 1992). For women diagnosed with this condition during 1984–1988, current occupation was ascertained from medical records. As a basis for comparison, interviews were conducted with a random sample of similar-aged women who resided in the same counties as the cases. A far greater proportion of cases than controls were categorized as "homemakers": Compared to women who had a professional, technical, or managerial occupation, homemakers were estimated to have about a fivefold increase in the risk of bladder cancer (95% confidence interval of the relative risk = 2.4–12.0). The authors hypothesized that the hobbies and household tasks of the homemakers might expose them to carcinogenic agents to a

Table 15–1. Hip and Forearm Fractures in Relation to
Duration of Unopposed Estrogen Use among Female
Residents of King County, Washington

DURATION OF UNOPPOSED ESTROGEN USE	CASES	CONTROLS
None	210	272
1–5 years	60	108
6+ years	50	187
Total	320	567

greater extent than other women. What is a (possibly more plausible) noncausal explanation for the association?

2. The following data were obtained in an epidemiologic study of hip and forearm fracture. Female residents of King County, Washington, ages 50–74 years, who were treated for either of these conditions during a two-year period by one of 59 orthopedists in the county ($n = 320$) were identified and interviewed regarding prior receipt of postmenopausal unopposed estrogen therapy. Similar information was obtained from a sample of King County women of the same ages ($n = 567$). The results are shown in Table 15–1.

   (a) Relative to the risk of hip or forearm fracture in estrogen non-users, what is the risk in women who used unopposed estrogens for 1–5 years? For 6+ years?

   (b) Assume that long-term unopposed estrogen use (e.g., 6+ years) truly protects against the occurrence of fracture of the hip and forearm. From the data provided, can you determine the amount by which the rate of hip or forearm fracture is reduced in women who have used unopposed estrogens for 6+ years? If yes, what is that amount? If no, why not?

3. During the mid-1980s several epidemiologists conducted a case-control study of childhood cancer in relation to birth weight. Cases were all children under two years of age in King County, Washington, who developed cancer during 1974–1982. Controls were selected from this county's birth certificates, and were matched to the cases on the basis of year of birth and sex. The results of the study are summarized in Table 15–2.

   The study was criticized for having included in the analysis children with birth weights <2500 grams, because of the relatively high mortality of this group during the first days and weeks of life.

   (a) Does this criticism have some merit? If yes, why? If no, why not?

Table 15–2. Birth Weight Distribution of Children Diagnosed with Cancer Prior
to Age 2 Years, and of Controls

| | Birth Weight (Grams) | | | | | |
	<2500	2501–3500	3501–4000	4001–4500	>4500	ALL
Cases (%)	5.6	44.9	27.0	16.9	5.6	100.0
Controls (%)	6.1	53.2	29.6	9.1	1.9	100.0

(b) Should this criticism influence the conclusion that high birth weight (i.e. >4000 grams) was associated with cancer incidence in the first two years of life? If yes, why? If no, why not?

4. While primary pulmonary hypertension can be a fatal disease, it may be present in a relatively mild form, at least temporarily. Therefore, some people may not seek medical attention for symptoms of primary pulmonary hypertension in its early stages, or their physician may fail to diagnose the condition.

Some time ago, data became available to suggest strongly that a particular appetite-suppressant agent, aminorex, could predispose to the development of primary pulmonary hypertension. Years later, a case-control study of primary pulmonary hypertension (Abenhaim et al., 1996) observed an elevated odds ratio associated with use (before the onset of symptoms) of several newer appetite-suppressant drugs. The odds ratio was particularly high in the analysis pertaining to patients with moderate and severe symptoms and signs, but was only slightly elevated when restricted to cases with less-serious illness. Does this pattern of results suggest that the association between use of the newer appetite-suppressant drugs and primary pulmonary hypertension is not genuine, but rather is due to differential recognition of pulmonary hypertension according to prior use of these drugs?

5. One of the early studies of the possible association between the use of oral contraceptives and the risk of myocardial infarction (MI) was conducted in Great Britain. During 1973, investigators identified and obtained information on all cases of MI in women under the age of 40 years who resided in a portion of that country, and in 50 percent of the women ages 40–44. Controls were selected from patient rosters of general practitioners. The data from the study are shown in Table 15–3.

(a) Without adjusting for age, estimate the risk of myocardial infarction in current users of oral contraceptives relative to that in women who were not current users. Now estimate the corresponding relative risk adjusted for age. Why do the two estimates differ? Which one do you believe more

Table 15–3. Oral Contraceptive Use in Myocardial Infarction Cases
and Controls, by Age

CURRENT ORAL CONTRACEPTIVE USE	<40 years		40–44 years	
	CASES	CONTROLS	CASES	CONTROLS
Yes	21	17	8	2
No	26	59	44	50
	47	76	52	52

accurately reflects the size of the association between oral contraceptive use and the incidence of myocardial infarction?

(b) On the basis of these and other data you have concluded that the current use of the oral contraceptives available in 1973 was a cause of myocardial infarction, and to roughly the same relative degree across age groups. By what percentage do you estimate the incidence rate of this disease would have fallen in British women under 45 years of age if oral contraceptives had no longer been used?

6. The following is a hypothetical abstract from an article reporting results of a case-control study of testicular cancer in relation to occupation: "The men with testicular cancer ($n = 18$) were much more likely to be plastics workers (33%) than controls (11% of 159 men). Occupational histories showing exposure to agent X for five out of six cases known to have been plastics workers further support a causal association between agent X and testicular cancer."

Do you agree that a causal association between exposure to agent X and testicular cancer is strengthened by the observation that exposure to agent X had occurred among five of six cases known to be plastics workers? If yes, why? If no, why not?

7. The following is excerpted from the abstract of an article that appeared in the *Lancet* (Meier et al., 1998):

Background: There is growing interest in the role of infections in the etiology of acute myocardial infarction (MI). We undertook a large, population-based study to explore the association between risk of MI and recent acute respiratory-tract infection.

Methods: We used data from general practices in the UK (General Practice Research Database). Potential cases were people aged 75 years or younger, with no history of clinical risk factors, who had a first-time diagnosis of MI between January 1, 1994, and October 31, 1996. Four controls were matched to each case on age, sex, the practice attended, and the absence of clinical risk factors for MI.

The date of the MI in the case was defined as the index date. For both cases and controls the date of the last respiratory-tract infection before the index date was identified.

Findings: In the case-control analysis of 1922 cases and 7649 matched controls, significantly more cases than controls had an acute respiratory-tract infection in the 10 days before the index date [54 (2.8%) vs. 72 (0.9%)]. The odds ratios adjusted for smoking and body-mass index, for first-time MI in association with an acute respiratory-tract infection 1–5, 6–10, 11–15, or 16–30 days before the index date (compared with participants who had no such infection during the preceding year) were 3.6 [95% CI 2.2–5.7, 2.3 (1–4.2), 1.8 (1.0–3.3), and 1.0 (0.7–1.6)] (test for trend $p < 0.01$).

Interpretation: Our findings suggest that in people without a history of clinical risk factors for MI, acute respiratory tract infections are associated with an increased risk of MI for a period of about two weeks.

Because this study was conducted within the U.K. General Practice Research Database, controls could be readily selected from the defined population from which each case came; i.e., the patients of an individual general practitioner.

In the U.S., where many physicians do not have such a well-defined group of patients who necessarily would seek primary care from them, a different case-control design might be considered. Imagine that in a U.S. study of this question, for each case that developed an MI, four controls (matched for age and sex) could be selected from among those who visited the case's primary care physician on the day of the case's MI. Would you expect this latter design to produce a biased estimate of the relation of recent acute respiratory tract infections to the incidence of MI? If yes, why, and in which direction? If no, why not?

ANSWERS

1. Given the very different means by which current occupation was assessed in cases and controls—medical records and interviews, respectively—it seems that a large degree of information bias could have been present in this study. In their Discussion, the authors acknowledge that "traditionally, one would use similar methodology to interview both cases and controls, to determine with the same degree of accuracy and completeness the risk factor of occupation. Alternatively, this study, which used previously collected data from two different sources, required no additional resources for data collection." Earlier (Chapter 6) we commented that epidemiologists often are data scavengers, and that the analysis of previously collected data often can yield valid and useful information. Nonetheless, there are situations in which this is not so. We recommend that the "tradition" of case-control comparability regarding exposure ascertainment should be respected!

2. (a) The two relative risks can be estimated by means of the respective odds ratios. For 1–5 years' use relative to never-use, $OR = 60/210 \div 108/272 = 0.72$. For $\geq$ 6 years' use relative to never-use, $OR = 50/210 \div 187/272 = 0.35$.

   (b) The amount by which estrogen use reduces risk of fracture cannot be estimated from these data alone. What would be required in addition is the *rate* of fracture in one of the three categories of women or in the 50–74 year old female population as a whole.

3. The study was criticized for having included in the analysis children with birth weights <2500 grams, because of the relatively high mortality of this group during the first days and weeks of life.

   (a) The criticism is valid. Proportionately fewer children who live to develop cancer will have low birth weights than a matched sample of newborns. Thus, even if there were no association between birth weight and cancer in early childhood, with this design the risk of cancer in high birth weight babies relative to that in low birth weight babies would be expected to slightly exceed 1.0.

   (b) Compared to infants of average birth weight (e.g., 2501–3500 g.), the cancer risk in those of high birth weight was also elevated, as shown in Table 15–4.

   Thus, assuming that among infants who weigh >2500 g. at birth there is no increase in infant mortality with decreasing birth weight, the authors' conclusion is valid.

4. Bias can arise in a non-randomized study when some persons with a disease go undiagnosed, and when there is reason to believe that exposed persons (e.g., to appetite-suppressant drugs) are relatively less likely to go undiagnosed. In the present example, it might be true that some physicians, aware of the association between use of aminorex and the incidence of pulmonary hypertension were more alert to the presence of this condition in patients taking appetite-suppressant drugs, or had a lower threshold for making a diagnosis of pulmonary hypertension in users of these other appetite-suppressant drugs.

Table 15–4. Odds Ratio for Cancer in Relation to Birth Weight

BIRTH WEIGHT	CASE	CONTROL	ODDS RATIO
>4000 g.	22.5	11.0	2.23
≤2500 g.	5.6	6.1	1
>4000 g.	22.5	11.0	2.42
2501–3500 g.	44.9	53.2	1

In such a situation it might be expected that, unlike persons with mild pulmonary hypertension, those with a more severe form of the disease would be recognized as having it irrespective of exposure status. If this were true, the most valid assessment of an association with the exposure of concern would be restricted to them. Since the association between primary pulmonary hypertension and the use of appetite-suppressant drugs was particularly great once the milder cases had been excluded from the analysis, this bias does not appear to be present here.

5. (a) Age is a confounder, in that: (1) current OC use was more common in younger than in older women; and (2) the ratio of cases/controls differed (by design) in the two age categories.

$$\text{Crude } OR(= RR) = \frac{29/70}{19/109} = 2.38$$

$$\text{Adjusted } OR(= RR) = \frac{(21 \times 59 \div 123) + (8 \times 50 \div 104)}{(17 \times 26 \div 123) + (44 \times 2 \div 104)}$$

$$= 3.14$$

(b)
$$PAR\% = \frac{RR - 1}{RR}(P_c) \times 100\%$$

$$= \frac{3.14 - 1}{3.14}(P_c) \times 100\%$$

Since only half the deaths in women ages 40–44 were included, as opposed to all deaths in women under 40,

$$P_c = \frac{21 + 2(8)}{47 + 2(52)} = .245$$

$$PAR\% = \frac{RR - 1}{RR}(P_c) \times 100\%$$

$$= \frac{3.14 - 1}{3.14}(.245) \times 100\%$$

$$= 16.7\%$$

6. The observation would only support an association if, among men *without* testicular cancer who had been workers, fewer than 5/6 had been exposed to agent X. Note the difference in the interpretation of the top and bottom panels in Table 15–5.

Table 15–5. Two Sets of Hypothetical Results in a Case-Control Study
of Testicular Cancer

PLASTICS WORKER	EXPOSED TO AGENT X	CASES	CONTROLS	ODDS RATIO
No	—	12	141	1.0
Yes	—	6	18	3.9
	Yes	5	9	6.5
	No	1	9	1.3
No	—	12	141	1.0
Yes	—	6	18	3.9
	Yes	5	15	3.9
	No	1	3	3.9

Only the data in the upper table, in which the proportion of plastics workers exposed to agent X differs between cases (83%) and controls (50%), support the hypothesis of there being a subgroup of plastics workers at particularly high risk of testicular cancer.

7. Yes, the results would be biased, because respiratory infections are a common reason for visiting a doctor. An atypically high proportion of controls chosen in this manner would be expected to have a respiratory infection on the index date, leading to a falsely low estimate of the association between recent respiratory infection and the incidence of the MI.

REFERENCES

Abenhaim L, Moride Y, Brenot F, Rich S, Benichou J, Kurz X, et al. Appetite-suppressant drugs and the risk of primary pulmonary hypertension. International Primary Pulmonary Hypertension Study Group. N Engl J Med 1996; 335:609–16.

Anton-Culver H, Lee-Feldstein A, Taylor TH. Occupation and bladder cancer risk. Am J Epidemiol 1992; 136:89–94.

Armstrong BK, White E, Saracci R. Principles of exposure measurement in epidemiology, Chapters 6 and 7. New York: Oxford, 1992.

Bloemenkamp KW, Rosendaal FR, Buller HR, Helmerhorst FM, Colly LP, Vandenbroucke JP. Risk of venous thrombosis with use of current low-dose oral contraceptives is not explained by diagnostic suspicion and referral bias. Arch Intern Med 1999; 159:65–70.

Blot WJ, McLaughlin JK, Devesa S, et al. "Cancers of the oral cavity and pharynx." In: Schottenfeld D, Fraumeni JF (eds.). Cancer epidemiology and prevention (2nd ed.). New York: Oxford, 1996.

Breslow NE, Day NE. Statistical methods in cancer research. Volume I: The analysis of case-control studies. Lyon, France: International Agency for Research on Cancer, 1980.

Crombie IK. The limitations of case-control studies in the detection of environmental carcinogens. J Epidemiol Community Health 1981; 35:281–87.

Cummings P, Weiss NS. Case series and exposure series: the role of studies without controls in providing information about the etiology of injury or disease. Inj Prev 1998; 4:34–57.

Daling JR, Weiss NS, Hislop TG, Maden C, Coates RJ, Sherman KJ, et al. Sexual practices, sexually transmitted diseases, and the incidence of anal cancer. N Engl J Med 1987; 317:973–77.

Daling JR, Weiss NS, Klopfenstein LL, Cochran LE, Chow WH, Daifuku R. Correlates of homosexual behavior and the incidence of anal cancer. JAMA 1982; 247:1988–90.

Doll R, Hill AB. Smoking and carcinoma of the lung. BMJ 1950; 2:739–48.

Gillison ML, Koch WM, Capone RB, Spafford M, Westra WH, Wu L, et al. Evidence for a causal association between human papillomavirus and a subset of head and neck cancers. J Natl Cancer Inst 2000; 92:709–20.

Gordis L. Should dead cases be matched to dead controls? Am J Epidemiol 1982; 115:1–5.

Green LM, Miller AB, Agnew DA, Greenberg ML, Li J, Villeneuve PJ, et al. Childhood leukemia and personal monitoring of residential exposures to electric and magnetic fields in Ontario, Canada. Cancer Causes Control 1999; 10:233–43.

Greenberg ER, Rosner B, Hennekens C, Rinsky R, Colton T. An investigation of bias in a study of nuclear shipyard workers. Am J Epidemiol 1985; 121:301–8.

Greenwald P, Barlow JJ, Nasca PC, Burnett WS. Vaginal cancer after maternal treatment with synthetic estrogens. N Engl J Med 1971; 285:390–92.

Herbst AL, Ulfelder H, Poskanzer DC. Adenocarcinoma of the vagina: association of maternal stilbestrol therapy with tumor appearance in young women. N Engl J Med 1971; 284:878–81.

Holcomb RL. Alcohol in relation to traffic accidents. JAMA 1938; 111:1076–85.

Horwitz RI, Feinstein AR. Alternative analytic methods for case-control studies of estrogens and endometrial cancer. N Engl J Med 1978; 299:1089–94.

Hosmer DW, Lemeshow S. Applied logistic regression (2nd ed.). New York: John Wiley & Sons, 2000.

Hurwitz ES, Barrett MJ, Bregman D, Gunn WJ, Schonberger LB, Fairweather WR, et al. Public Health Service study on Reye's syndrome and medications. Report of the pilot phase. N Engl J Med 1985; 313:849–57.

Janerich DT, Thompson WD, Varela LR, Greenwald P, Chorost S, Tucci C, et al. Lung cancer and exposure to tobacco smoke in the household. N Engl J Med 1990; 323:632–36.

McLaughlin JK, Blot WJ, Mehl ES, Mandel JS. Problems in the use of dead controls in case-control studies. II. Effect of excluding certain causes of death. Am J Epidemiol 1985; 122:485–94.

Meier CR, Jick SS, Derby LE, Vasilakis C, Jick H. Acute respiratory-tract infections and risk of first-time acute myocardial infarction. Lancet 1998; 351:1467–71.

Needleman HL, Schell A, Bellinger D, Leviton A, Allred EN. The long-term effects of exposure to low doses of lead in childhood. An 11-year follow-up report. N Engl J Med 1990; 322:83–88.

Nelson LM, Longstreth WT Jr, Koepsell TD, van Belle G. Proxy respondents in epidemiologic research. Epidemiol Rev 1990; 12:71–86.

Rinsky RA, Zumwalde RD, Waxweiler RJ, Murray WE Jr, Bierbaum PJ, Landrigan PJ, et al. Cancer mortality at a Naval Nuclear Shipyard. Lancet 1981; 1:231–35.

Rodrigues LC, Smith PG. Use of the case-control approach in vaccine evaluation: Efficacy and adverse effects. Epidemiol Rev 1999; 21:56–72.

Rosenberg L, Mitchell AA, Parsells JL, Pashayan H, Louik C, Shapiro S. Lack of relation of oral clefts to diazepam use during pregnancy. N Engl J Med 1983; 309:1282–85.

Rothman KJ, Greenland S. Modern epidemiology (2nd ed.). Philadelphia: Lippincott-Raven, 1998.

Selby JV. Case-control evaluations of treatment and program efficacy. Epidemiol Rev 1994; 46:91–101.

Shapiro S, Kelly JP, Rosenberg L, Kaufman DW, Helmrich SP, Rosenshein NB, et al. Risk of localized and widespread endometrial cancer in relation to recent and discontinued use of conjugated estrogens. N Engl J Med 1985; 313:969–72.

Silverberg SG, Makowski MD. Endometrial carcinoma in young women taking oral contraceptive agents. J Obstet Gynecol 1975; 46:503–6.

Silverman DT, Hoover RN, Swanson GM. Artificial sweeteners and lower urinary tract cancer: hospital vs. population controls. Am J Epidemiol 1983; 117:326–34.

Siscovick DS, Weiss NS, Fletcher RH, Lasky T. The incidence of primary cardiac arrest during vigorous exercise. N Engl J Med 1984; 311:874–77.

Siscovick DS, Weiss NS, Hallstrom AP, Inui TS, Peterson DR. Physical activity and primary cardiac arrest. JAMA 1982; 248:3113–17.

Spechler SJ, Fischbach L, Feldman M. Clinical aspects of genetic variability in helicobacter pylori. JAMA 2000; 283:1264–66.

Stallones RA. A review of the epidemiologic studies of toxic shock syndrome. Ann Intern Med 1982; 96:917–20.

Stott DH. Some psychosomatic aspects of casualty in reproduction. J Psychosomatic Res 1958; 3:42–55.

Strathy JH, Molgaard CA, Coulam CB, Melton LJ 3d. Endometriosis and infertility: a laparoscopic study of endometriosis among fertile and infertile women. Fertil Steril 1982; 38:667–72.

Tabuenca JM. Toxic-allergic syndrome caused by ingestion of rapeseed oil denatured with aniline. Lancet 1981; 2:567–68.

Thom DH, Grayston JT, Siscovick DS, Wang SP, Weiss NS, Daling JR. Association of prior infection with Chlamydia pneumoniae and angiographically demonstrated coronary artery disease. JAMA 1992; 268:68–72.

Ulfelder H, Robboy SJ. The embryologic development of the human vagina. Am J Obstet Gynecol 1976; 126:769–76.

Victora CG, Smith PG, Vaughan JP, Nobre LC, Lombardi C, Teixeira AM, et al. Infant feeding and deaths due to diarrhea. A case-control study. Am J Epidemiol 1989; 129:1032–41.

Wacholder S. Practical considerations in choosing between the case-cohort and nested case-control designs. Epidemiology 1991; 2:155–58.

Wacholder S, McLaughlin JK, Silverman DT, Mandel JS. Selection of controls in case-control studies. I. Principles. Am J Epidemiol 1992a; 135:1019–28.

Wacholder S, Silverman DT, McLaughlin JK, Mandel JS. Selection of controls in case-control studies. II. Types of controls. Am J Epidemiol 1992b; 135:1029–41.

Wacholder S, Silverman DT, McLaughlin JK, Mandel JS. Selection of controls in case-control studies. III. Design options. Am J Epidemiol 1992c; 135:1042–50.

Weinmann S, Glass AG, Weiss NS, Psaty BM, Siscovick DS, White E. Use of diuretics and other antihypertensive medications in relation to the risk of renal cell cancer. Am J Epidemiol 1994; 140:792–804.

Weiss NS. Application of the case-control method in the evaluation of screening. Epidemiol Rev 1994; 16:102–8.

Weiss NS, Lyon JL, Liff JM, Vollmer WM, Daling JR. Incidence of ovarian cancer in relation to the use of oral contraceptives. Int J Cancer 1981; 28:669–71.

Weiss NS, Sayvetz TA. Incidence of endometrial cancer in relation to the use of oral contraceptives. N Engl J Med 1980; 302:551–54.

Werler MM, Hayes C, Louik C, Shapiro S, Mitchell AA. Multivitamin supplementation and risk of birth defects. Am J Epidemiol 1999; 150:675–82.

Witte JS, Gauderman WJ, Thomas DC. Asymptotic bias and efficiency in case-control studies of candidate genes and gene-environment interactions: Basic family designs. Am J Epidemiol 1999; 149:693–705.

Yang Q, Khoury MJ. Evolving methods in genetic epidemiology. III. Gene-environment interaction in epidemiologic research. Epidemiol Rev 1997; 19:33–42.

16

INDUCTION PERIODS AND LATENT PERIODS

Knowledge of an etiology of a disease is a first step towards being able to prevent some cases of that disease. Alternatively, this knowledge may be useful in targeting people at high risk for efforts at detecting the disease at an early stage. Achieving these goals, however, may require not only an understanding of the presence and magnitude of an association of the disease with a given exposure, but also having the answers to one or more of the following questions: How soon can disease result after the exposure has first been incurred? To what extent does the size of the altered risk depend on the duration of exposure? Once the exposure has ceased, does the alteration in risk disappear? If so, how quickly?

For example, while postmenopausal women who receive oral estrogen therapy for an extended duration (e.g., more than five years) probably have some increase in the risk of breast cancer, shorter-term use appears not to be associated with an increase in risk (Collaborative Group on Hormonal Factors in Breast Cancer, 1997). When weighing the risks against the benefits of hormone use of less than five years' duration, these data suggest that an altered incidence of breast cancer need not be considered. As another example, it is commonly recommended that postmenopausal women with an intact uterus who take estrogens unopposed by a progestogen, and who therefore are at a substantially increased risk of endometrial cancer, be regularly screened (by means of vaginal ultrasound or endometrial biopsy) for the presence of endometrial cancer. Once a woman has stopped taking these hormones, can the screening stop as well? If not immediately, then when? The answers to these questions would be based heavily on the results of studies that documented the incidence of endometrial cancer in women who have discontinued estrogens. [These show a decline in risk relative to continuing users, but are divided as to whether the risk ultimately returns to that of a postmenopausal woman who never used hormones (Cook and Weiss, 2000).] Finally, it is recommended that hepatitis A immune globulin be given within two weeks to persons following exposure to hepatitis A infection, but not thereafter, as a means of reducing the risk of later contracting clinical hepatitis (Krugman et al., 1960). Apparently, the time course of the progression of infection to disease is such that, unless given relatively early, this therapy has little or no efficacy.

An important goal of epidemiologic studies is to provide information that bears on disease prevention. Therefore, persons conducting epidemiologic studies that deal with exposures that vary over time must consider, in both their design and analysis, the likely temporal relationship between exposure and disease occurrence. Studies of aspirin use in relation to the incidence of acute myocardial infarction have focused on the initial hours-to-weeks after the most recent dose was taken, since aspirin could have a relatively transient influence by means of its anticoagulant properties. In contrast, studies of aspirin use in relation to the incidence of colon cancer typically concern themselves with long-term use or use years earlier, given the long preclinical duration of most colon tumors and of the polyps from which many of these tumors arise.

Example: As described in Chapter 13, 22,071 U.S. physicians were assigned at random to receive aspirin, 325 mg. every other day, or a placebo for a period of five years (Gann et al., 1993). A reduction in the incidence of myocardial infarction among the group assigned to aspirin led to the termination of the study at that time. Because a number of earlier non-randomized studies had observed a reduced risk of colorectal cancer associated with long-term aspirin use, an analysis of the accumulated data was done for colorectal cancer as well. No difference was found between members of the aspirin and placebo groups for this outcome (relative risk = 1.15, 95% confidence interval = 0.8–1.7). It is possible that truly no association is present between aspirin use and colorectal cancer, that the earlier observational studies were flawed in some way, and that a randomized study was needed to obtain an unbiased result. But it seems more likely that five years is too short a period to determine the effect of aspirin on the incidence of this disease; even a substantial decrease in risk might not start to be evident until more than a decade from the onset of regular aspirin use. Indeed, the authors of the physicians' study concluded that "prevention trials with longer follow-up of randomized participants" were needed (Gann et al., 1993).

Some illnesses have features that signal a period of time during which the etiologic agent(s) must have been acting. Bunin et al. (1989) exploited this phenomenon in their case-control study of environmental exposures in relation to the development of retinoblastoma. First, they excluded children in whom the disease had already occurred in a first- or second-degree relative, since (for this disease) no further nongenetic basis for its occurrence need be considered. They further divided the remaining cases into two groups:

1. Children with a constitutional deletion on chromosome 13q (i.e., a deletion present in all cells of the body) and those with bilateral disease (in whom

a constitutional genetic abnormality is believed to be present in every case.)

2. Children with unilateral disease and no constitutional chromosome 13q deletion.

In the first group of cases and their controls, interviews with parents focused on exposures that took place prior to conception (e.g., gonadal irradiation), since only exposures prior to conception could have given rise to the genetic abnormality that predisposed to retinoblastoma in these cases. In contrast, parents of cases in the second group and parents of their controls were queried about exposures that took place after conception (e.g., multivitamin use during pregnancy), since earlier exposures were unlikely to have played an etiologic role.

Failure to take into account the relevant period of time during which an exposure is capable of causing disease can dull the ability of an epidemiologic study to document an exposure–disease association. For example, Hertz-Picciotto et al. (1996) have illustrated how the influence of exposures that act during only a part of pregnancy to give rise to adverse outcomes can be underestimated in non-randomized studies if data on their presence are not collected and analyzed during the appropriate window of time during the pregnancy. Considerations of temporality can be important when planning a randomized study as well:

Example: In order to test the hypothesis that replacement of dairy fat with vegetable fat in the diet can lead to a lower incidence of coronary heart disease, changes were made in the kitchen of one of two Finnish hospitals providing long-term care for patients with mental illness (Miettinen et al., 1983). The incidence of coronary disease among patients 44 to 64 years old was monitored for a six-year period, after which the policies of the two kitchens were reversed—the one that had switched to vegetable fats reverted to dairy fats, while the other now began to use vegetable fats—and the residents of the two hospitals were observed for another six years. About one-third of the residents of each institution during the first follow-up period also were residents of that institution during the second, and so would have had a diet that, during different periods of time, would have been high in dairy fat and in vegetable fat. Since the influence of diet on the incidence of coronary heart disease is not likely to be immediate—the arteriosclerotic changes that diet may modify take time to develop—the authors' primary comparison of incidence rates before and after the dietary change at the six-year point within each hospital probably substantially underestimates the true size of the association between type of dietary fat and the incidence of coronary heart disease.

INDUCTION AND LATENT PERIODS

For etiologic exposures of brief duration, such as eating food contaminated with the hepatitis A virus or being subjected to a single, intense dose of ionizing radiation, the *induction period* in a given sick person is the interval between receipt of the exposure and the first presence of the disease. (When the exposure in question is an infectious agent, an alternative term—the *incubation period*—is also commonly used.) The time between the disease's first presence and its recognition is the *latent period.* Since the first presence of disease can almost never be observed, what is measured in specific individuals is the sum of the induction and latent periods (Rothman, 1981). Most epidemiologists, being economical (or lazy!) with language, simply refer to this sum either as the induction or as the latent period. We will refer to it, clumsily, as the *induction/latent period.*

The distribution of the length of time required for an exposure to give rise to disease can be estimated by examining the relative risk associated with that exposure over successive periods of time after it was sustained. Figure 16–1 depicts the risk of leukemia and other forms of cancer in survivors of the atomic bomb detonations in Hiroshima and Nagasaki, relative to that of Japanese who were not exposed, in relation to the time since their exposure to the detonations in 1945.

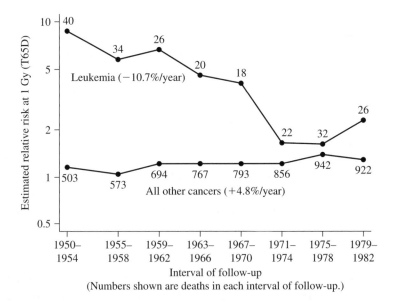

Figure 16–1. Relative Risk of Mortality from Leukemia and All Other Cancers Other Than Leukemia in A-Bomb Survivors, 1950–1982, in Relation to Time after Irradiation (adapted from Figure 5–2 in Committee on the Biological Effects of Ionizing Radiations, 1990).

For leukemia, the pronounced increase in the relative risk during the 1950s suggests that the induction/latent period associated with this intensity of radiation could be as short as 5 to 10 years (or even shorter, since there are no data provided for 1945–1950). The persistence of at least a small increase in the risk of leukemia through the late 1970s is compatible with a maximum period for induction/latency associated with radiation exposure of at least 30 years.

In some circumstances, nearly all cases of disease among exposed individuals are due to the exposure (i.e., the attributable risk percent is close to 100%). For example, the association between *in utero* DES exposure and vaginal adenocarcinoma is so strong that almost no cases arising in a given cohort exposed to DES would be expected had DES not been used (Herbst et al., 1971). In this circumstance, the distribution of the length of the induction/latent periods after DES exposure can be assessed simply by enumerating the times when cases occur following exposure. Since the period of exposure was restricted to the nine months prior to birth, the range of incubation/latent periods following exposure can be gleaned, approximately, from the age distribution of the cases at the time of their diagnosis.

Occasionally, an examination of variations in disease occurrence across populations, or within a population over time, can offer strong clues to the minimum duration of the induction/latent period associated with a particular exposure.

Example: Infection with hepatitis B virus is a strong risk factor for hepatocellular carcinoma (HCC). In Taiwan, mass immunization in newborns against hepatitis B infection began in July, 1984, because of the extensive transmission of the virus at that time of life. To evaluate the possible early impact of this program on the incidence of HCC, Chang et al. (1997) analyzed data from the records of the Taiwan Cancer Registry through 1994. They identified three cases of HCC among the cohort of 6 to 9-year-old children who had been born between July 1984 and June 1986, a cohort in which 85% to 90% of the children had been vaccinated. Based on the rates in 6 to 9-year-old children born during July 1974 and June 1984 (nearly all of whom would not have been vaccinated), 12 cases would have been expected among children in the later cohort (relative risk = 0.25). This dramatic reduction suggests not only that the vaccine has been effective, but that the induction/latent period for liver cancer after hepatitis B infection in the perinatal period can be as short as 6 to 9 years.

For etiologic exposures that are prolonged (e.g., aflatoxin consumption, cigarette smoking), there is no known point in time that can be specified as being the one at which the accumulated exposure is first able to cause disease, and after which additional exposure does not continue to add to the risk. Studies of these agents in relation to disease occurrence can examine the variation in relative risk as a function of time since first exposure, cognizant that the range of time periods during which elevations are present may well not correspond to the range of induction periods following a cumulative dose of an exposure that is adequate to give rise to disease.

INFLUENCE OF THE SUSPECTED INDUCTION/LATENT PERIOD ON STUDY DESIGN

Short Induction/Latent Periods

In many instances, the close connection in time between an exposure and the development of a rare illness makes possible the identification of an association between them. For example, because anaphylaxis has been observed to follow so soon after the administration of parenteral penicillin therapy, a causal relationship has been inferred despite the absence of contemporaneous data on the incidence of anaphylaxis in a nonexposed group. The incidence of such dramatic and unusual symptoms in any short period of time is presumed to be vanishingly small in the absence of a recent injection of penicillin (or some other drug).

When there are many causal pathways that can lead to a given illness, including some that do not involve the exposure in question, we need formal epidemiologic studies that include an explicit basis of comparison to document the presence and magnitude of an association. The presence of a very short induction period can pose problems in this regard, however. For example, it is plausible on toxicological grounds that consumption of a large quantity of alcohol could predispose acutely to the occurrence of a myocardial infarction. A cohort study could not be expected to examine this issue, since it would not be feasible to identify the very large number of inebriated persons necessary to observe any appreciable number of infarctions during the few hours they remain inebriated. Similarly, a study that compared blood alcohol levels between cases and controls would be unlikely to provide a valid result: Even if it were possible to obtain a blood sample by which to estimate recent alcohol consumption in each case, the generally available means of recruiting controls—which require making appointments in advance and obtaining informed consent—would almost certainly result in a group in which the proportion of inebriated persons would be atypically low.

Exposures that rapidly give rise to disease can sometimes be identified in case-control studies that obtain exposure information by means of interviews. For example, Siscovick et al. (1984) found that of 133 Seattle-area residents ages 25 to 75 years who sustained a primary cardiac arrest during a 14-month period, nine were engaged in vigorous physical activity at the time (based on reports of spouses or other bystanders). This proportion—9/133—was some 50 times greater than expected based on the proportion of time a sample of demographically similar persons was reported (by spouses) to be typically engaged in vigorous physical activity. Just as for case-control studies in general, however:

- The validity of studies investigating possible short-term effects rests on the comparability of exposure ascertainment between cases and controls. In the above example, there probably was some non-comparability of reporting of vigorous exercise by witnesses of a cardiac arrest, on one hand, and persons reporting the usual patterns of vigorous activity of their spouses, on the other. Thus, while a 50-fold case-control difference almost certainly must be attributable to more than differences in the means of exposure ascertainment, a much more modest difference could be entirely explained on that basis.
- The power of a case-control study to evaluate a short-term etiologic relationship is often low, due to the rarity of the relevant exposure. For example, if it is hypothesized that it is only the initiation of a pharmacological therapy that is associated with an increased risk (e.g., new use of a product containing phenylpropanolamine and hemorrhagic stroke [Kernan et al., 2000]), or the recent cessation of such a therapy (e.g., discontinuation of beta blocker use in relation to the incidence of coronary heart disease [Psaty et al., 1990]), then only moderate or large associations can be reliably identified in even the largest case-control studies.

Close relatives of case-control studies, *case-crossover* studies, also are used to assess the influence of some short-term risk factors (Maclure, 1991). These studies compare a case's exposure status at the time of the onset of his/her illness to that person's expected exposure status, based on his/her past history, obviating the need for a separate control group. For example, among persons who had recently sustained a myocardial infarction, one could contrast their alcohol consumption during the hour or two prior to the event and that predicted based upon their usual pattern of consumption. Such a study would be feasible if exposure status, both recent and usual, could be ascertained accurately by means of an interview or questionnaire. It would not be feasible in situations where only recent status could be ascertained; e.g., if one were estimating alcohol intake from levels in blood drawn at the time of the infarction.

Considerations pertaining to the design, analysis, and interpretation of case-crossover studies have been discussed in detail by Redelmeier and Tibshirani (1997). Briefly, the analysis of these studies proceeds like that of a matched case-control study (see Chapter 15), in which each study subject acts as her/his own control. The interpretation of the results will be influenced by the ways questions such as the following are answered:

- How much misclassification of exposure status may have occurred from incorrectly judging the length of the relevant "window" of exposure prior to disease onset? For example, what if heavy alcohol consumption predisposed to myocardial infarction not just during the several hours when blood alcohol levels were above a certain threshold, but for several more hours or days (as a result of some delayed physiological response)? An analysis that labeled as "exposed" only the subjects with heavy consumption immediately before the infarction would mis-assign exposure status of some subjects, reducing the study's ability to detect an association.
- To what extent was the confounding influence of other exposures taken into account? By having a person serve as his/her own control, confounding by factors that do not vary to any appreciable extent over short periods of time (e.g., demographic characteristics) is reduced or eliminated. But there remains the possibility of confounding by risk factors that do vary over time in relation to the exposure. For example, if heavy alcohol consumption were always accompanied by cigarette smoking, and the latter acutely predisposed to myocardial infarction, a spurious association between alcohol and myocardial infarction could be induced.

Long Induction/Latent Periods

As indicated in the earlier example of aspirin consumption in relation to the incidence of colorectal cancer, many randomized trials are not designed to extend over a long enough period to be able to identify a delayed impact of an exposure. Facing the same problem are cohort studies of newly exposed persons that initiate follow-up around the time the exposure has taken place. Alternatively, if an exposure sustained in the past can be ascertained by means of interviews or records, then it is feasible for both case-control studies and cohort studies that use these sources of information to address the possible long-term impact of the exposure. If a study subject's exposure status cannot be ascertained in retrospect however—as would be likely to happen, for example, in a cohort or case-control study among middle-aged women that wished to investigate whether breast-cancer risk is associated with levels of endogenous sex hormones during puberty—then there are no attractive options. One tries either to: (a) identify correlates of the exposure that can be measured retrospectively (in this case, perhaps, a weak correlate such as age at menarche); (b) identify a valid "surrogate" outcome, a condition that strongly predicts the later appearance of the disease of interest (for breast cancer, no such surrogate outcome has yet been identified; for a condition such as colon cancer, however, the surrogate might be the occurrence of an adenomatous polyp); or (c) conduct a very long (and thus very expensive) cohort study with prospective follow-up.

Example: Efforts to assess the potential role of micronutrient deficiencies in the etiology of stomach cancer have been hindered, in case-control studies, by difficulties in measuring exposure status: Recall of past diet does not provide accurate information regarding intake of most micronutrients, and measurement of serum micronutrient levels in cases after a diagnosis of stomach cancer may not yield values indicative of those present during the genesis of the cancer. In order to overcome these problems, You et al. (2000) conducted a cohort study in Linqu County, China. At baseline in 1989–1990, serum was drawn for determination of micronutrient levels, and an endoscopy was performed in which a biopsy specimen was obtained. The latter procedure was repeated in 1994. The presence of gastric dysplasia at baseline was a strong risk factor for the development of gastric cancer: Persons with dysplasia had some 30 times the risk of those with normal mucosa or with lesions no worse than superficial gastritis or chronic atrophic gastritis. Therefore, the investigators felt justified in considering the development of dysplasia during the follow-up period as a relevant endpoint, in addition to the development of gastric cancer per se. In the approximately 400 subjects on whom micronutrient levels had been measured at baseline and in whom gastric dysplasia had not been present at that time, gastric biopsies revealed that 60 had progressed either to dysplasia or to cancer by 1994. Had the authors restricted the analysis to the incidence of cancer alone, only a handful of cases (less than 10) would have been present from which to draw any inferences.

As much as lengthy induction/latent periods can be a challenge and frustration to the researcher, they can be a blessing to those who are trying to prevent disease. Whatever exposures in early reproductive life are involved in the etiology of breast cancer, they do not usually give rise to the disease until two or more decades later. This delay allows time to attempt interventions (e.g., administration of tamoxifen to women judged to be at high risk) that have the potential to block the causal influence of those earlier exposures.

EXERCISES

1. Phenylpropanolamine (PPA) is a sympathimometic agent that, until November, 2000, was a component of a number of over-the-counter decongestant medications sold in the U.S. for the treatment of cough and flu symptoms. Based on

the pattern of events described in some case reports submitted to the Food and Drug Administration, it was hypothesized that in rare individuals, initiation of use of a PPA-containing medication could promptly (within one day) give rise to a hemorrhagic stroke.

Let's say that during the time PPA was being used in decongestants, the manufacturers of these drugs approached you to design a study to test the above hypothesis. Because immense resources would have been required to conduct a randomized trial or a cohort study of a rare event such as hemorrhagic stroke—rare during a given one-day period—you believe that a case-control study is the only feasible approach. And, there being no practical alternative, you decide that information regarding newly initiated PPA use would come from the survivors who were able to provide an interview. You would like to choose controls from persons demographically similar to the cases. In the population in which the study is to be done, such controls can be identified and recruited by means of random-digit dialing of telephone numbers. An in-person interview would be conducted as soon as possible among those willing to participate, and (to reduce recall bias) these persons would be asked questions about their use of PPA-containing medications in the day prior to interview.

When you propose this design to the manufacturers, they (gently) suggest that because a substantial fraction of potential controls asked to participate in fact do not do so, and because others delay the interview for reasons of illness, a spuriously high odds ratio associated with recent initiation of a PPA-containing medication might be obtained. Why is their concern likely to be a valid one?

2. In their article, "Carcinogenicity of lipid lowering drugs," Newman and Hulley (1996) contend that "All members of the two most popular classes of lipid-lowering drugs (the fibrates and the statins) cause cancer in rodents, in some cases at levels of animal exposure close to those prescribed to humans. Evidence of carcinogenicity of lipid-lowering drugs from clinical trials in humans is inconclusive, [however]."

The results of clinical trials published by mid-1996 indicated that the incidence of cancer (overall) was nearly identical after five years of follow-up in users of simvastatin and placebo (Scandinavian Simvastatin Survival Study Group, 1994) and in users of pravastatin and placebo (Shepherd et al., 1995), respectively. By "inconclusive," Newman and Hulley no doubt were referring to the relatively small number of cancer cases identified in these studies (collectively, only about 200 in users of a statin), and especially to the much smaller number of cancers of individual sites. What do you believe was another important reason for their reluctance to accept the results of these well-done trials as assurance of no increased risk of cancer associated with long-term statin prophylaxis?

ANSWERS

1. The purpose of the control group in this study is to estimate the proportion of the underlying population at risk who began to use a PPA-containing medication during any given recent one-day period. Persons with symptoms towards which these medications are directed (colds, flu) might be more inclined to decline to participate than other persons and, if they agreed to participate, might choose to postpone the interview until they expected to recover. For these reasons, the proportion of the interviewed controls reporting very recent initiation of medications containing PPA would probably be smaller than the proportion in the population they had been sampled from. Since this same source of bias cannot exist for the cases—they are recalling a one-day period prior to a fixed point in time; i.e., the time the first symptoms of their stroke occurred—a falsely high odds ratio will ensue.

   To reduce bias from this source, the information from the controls can refer to an earlier one-day period. For example, when studying this question, Kernan et al. (2000) chose a period ending up to one week prior to the interview. Even though the latter choice runs the risk of a greater degree of incomplete recall by controls than would asking about the day immediately prior to the interview, overall it would seem to produce a more valid estimate of the frequency of new use of PPA in the population.

2. It may require more than five years of statin use to produce an increase in the risk of one or more forms of cancer. Alternatively, it may require a period of time after even five years of use for cancers caused by such use to manifest themselves. Studies that have not followed statin users for more than five years cannot address these possibilities.

REFERENCES

Bunin GR, Meadows AT, Emanuel BS, Buckley JD, Woods WG, Hammond GD. Pre- and postconception factors associated with sporadic heritable and nonheritable retinoblastoma. Cancer Res 1989; 49:5730–35.

Chang MH, Chen CJ, Lai MS, Hsu HM, Wu TC, Kong MS, et al. Universal hepatitis B vaccination in Taiwan and the incidence of hepatocellular carcinoma in children. Taiwan Childhood Hepatoma Study Group. N Engl J Med 1997; 336:1855–59.

Collaborative Group on Hormonal Factors in Breast Cancer. Breast cancer and hormone replacement therapy: collaborative reanalysis of data from 51 epidemiological studies of 52,705 women with breast cancer and 108,411 women without breast cancer. Lancet 1997; 350:1047–59.

Committee on the Biological Effects of Ionizing Radiations. Health effects of exposure to low levels of ionizing radiation: BEIR V. Washington, D.C.: National Academy Press, 1990.

Cook LS, Weiss NS. "Endometrial cancer." In Goldman MB, Hatch MC (eds.). Women and health. San Diego: Academic Press, 2000.

Gann PH, Manson JE, Glynn RJ, Buring JE, Hennekens CH. Low-dose aspirin and incidence of colorectal tumors in a randomized trial. J Natl Cancer Inst 1993; 85:1220–24.

Herbst AL, Ulfelder H, Poskanzer DC. Adenocarcinoma of the vagina. Association of maternal stillbestrol therapy with tumor appearance in young women. N Engl J Med 1971; 284:878–81.

Hertz-Picciotto I, Pastore LM, Beaumont JJ. Timing and patterns of exposures during pregnancy and their implications for study methods. Am J Epidemiol 1996; 143:597–607.

Kernan WN, Viscoli CM, Brass LM, Broderick JP, Brott T, Feldmann E, et al. Phenyl-propanolamine and the risk of hemorrhagic stroke. N Engl J Med 2000; 343:1826–32.

Krugman S, Ward R, Giles JP, et al. Infectious hepatitis, study on effect of gamma globulin and on the incidence of apparent infection. JAMA 1960; 174:823–30.

Maclure M. The case-crossover design: A method for studying transient effects on the risk of acute events. Am J Epidemiol 1991; 133:144–53.

Miettinen M, Turpeinen O, Karvonen MJ, Pekkarinen M, Paavilainen E, Elosuo R. Dietary prevention of coronary heart disease in women: the Finnish mental hospital study. Int J Epidemiol 1983; 12:17–25.

Newman TB, Hulley SB. Carcinogenicity of lipid-lowering drugs. JAMA 1996; 275:55–60.

Psaty BM, Koepsell TD, Wagner EH, LoGerfo JP, Inui TS. The relative risk of incident coronary heart disease associated with recently stopping the use of beta-blockers. JAMA 1990; 263:1653–57.

Redelmeier DA, Tibshirani RJ. Interpretation and bias in case-crossover studies. J Clin Epidemiol 1997; 50:1281–17.

Rothman KJ. Induction and latent periods. Am J Epidemiol 1981; 114:253–59.

Scandinavian Simvastatin Survival Study Group. Randomised trial of cholesterol lowering in 4444 patients with coronary heart disease: the Scandinavian Simvastatin Survival Study (4S). Lancet 1994; 344:1383–89.

Shepherd J, Cobbe SM, Ford I, Isles CG, Lorimer AR, MacFarlane PW, et al. Prevention of coronary heart disease with pravastatin in men with hypercholesterolemia. West of Scotland Coronary Prevention Study Group. N Engl J Med 1995; 333:1301–7.

Siscovick DS, Weiss NS, Fletcher RH, Lasky T. The incidence of primary cardiac arrest during vigorous exercise. N Engl J Med 1984; 311:874–77.

You W, Zhang L, Gail MH, Chang Y, Liu W, Ma J, et al. Gastric dysplasia and gastric cancer: helicobacter pylori, serum vitamin C, and other risk factors. J Natl Cancer Inst 2000; 92:1607–12.

17

IMPROVING THE SENSITIVITY
OF EPIDEMIOLOGIC STUDIES

If an exposure truly has the capacity to cause a disease, at least in a portion of exposed individuals, a sensitive epidemiologic study is one that will observe an association between that exposure and the disease. If an epidemiologic study is large enough to render chance an unlikely explanation for that association, the study is deemed to have a high level of statistical power. In this chapter we restrict our attention to strategies that can enhance sensitivity, irrespective of the size of the available study population. These strategies include:

I. Disaggregation of categories of the exposure of concern that are hetero-geneous with respect to their impact on disease occurrence
II. Disaggregation of disease entities that are heterogeneous with respect to their association with the exposure of concern
III. Disaggregation of study subjects who, because of the presence of one or more other exposures or characteristics, are not affected to the same degree by the exposure of concern

I. DISAGGREGATION OF HETEROGENEOUS EXPOSURES

The dose or duration of a hazardous exposure received by an individual often is critical in determining his/her chances of developing a disease that the exposure is capable of producing. Smoking one pack of cigarettes per day for 30 years has a substantial influence on a person's chances of developing lung cancer. In contrast, smoking one pack of cigarettes per day for just one month, or just one cigarette per day for 10 years, probably has little impact on the risk of this disease. All of us inhale asbestos fibers, but only if we are exposed to the high concentrations found in some workplaces will we have more than an infinitesimal chance of developing mesothelioma.

Some epidemiologic studies fail to obtain information on the dose, duration, recency, or other features of a particular exposure; others fail to use that information in the analysis of the data that have been collected. Either of these shortcomings

Table 17–1. Incidence of Endometrial Cancer in Relation to Type
of Exogenous Hormone

TYPE/PATTERN OF USE OF EXOGENOUS FEMALE HORMONES	INFLUENCE ON RISK OF ENDOMETRIAL CANCER[a]
Contraceptive estrogens	Decrease
Non-contraceptive estrogens	
"Unopposed"	
Short duration (e.g., <1 year)	None
Longer duration	Large increase
"Opposed" by a progestogen	
Progestogen < 10 days/month, cyclic administration, long duration	Moderate increase
Progestogen ≥ 10 days/month, cyclic administration, long duration	None, or small increase
Progestogen daily administration, long duration	Probable decrease

[a]Relative to women who have never taken hormones.
[*Source:* Based on Cook and Weiss (2000); Weiderpass et al. (1999).]

can prevent the recognition of an altered risk of disease associated with a particular exposure dose, duration, recency, etc.

Exposures that have some properties in common often are lumped together in analyses of epidemiologic studies, but sometimes these common properties may not be the ones that are relevant to disease occurrence. Aspirin and acetaminophen both are anti-pyretic agents, but only the former has an adverse effect on the incidence of Reye's syndrome. Female hormones are formulated and prescribed in a variety of ways and, despite some shared endocrinologic features of each regimen, their impact on the incidence of endometrial cancer differs substantially from one to the next (see Table 17–1). In an epidemiologic study of endometrial cancer, if an effort is not expended to gather and analyze information at the level of detail shown in Table 17–1, then:

1. Particularly high or low risks associated with the use of certain types of hormones will not be identified; and
2. The aggregate results obtained will not apply to women in any individual category of hormone use.

Gathering information detailed enough to separate individuals with a common exposure from among a larger group of individuals with heterogeneous exposures is often beyond the resources of even the best-intentioned investigators.

Example: Blair et al. (1990) conducted a retrospective cohort mortality study of members of a dry cleaning union in the U.S. One of the goals of the study was to evaluate the hypothesis that various chemicals used in dry cleaning—in particular perchloroethylene, which was the major solvent in use when the study results were reported—were related to mortality from certain types of cancer. Unfortunately, though the intensity of solvent exposure could be approximated by the job category listed for each subject, and the duration of exposure by the length of union membership, the records contained no information on the type of solvent used in the individual establishments. As a consequence, it was unclear whether it was exposure to perchloroethylene or to a different agent that was responsible for several large positive associations observed in that study.

II. DISAGGREGATION OF HETEROGENEOUS DISEASE ENTITIES

William Farr, the Registrar General of England and Wales during the middle of the nineteenth century, was trying to determine a sensible means of forming a classification of causes of death. He approached the task in a systematic way, first asking, Just what is the goal of any classification scheme? His answer: A "classification that brings together in groups diseases that have considerable affinity ... is likely to facilitate the deduction of general principles" (Eyler, 1979). He recognized that in order for lessons to be learned from the conditions that caused people to die, these conditions would have to be grouped in some way. A secure basis for any sort of generalization would have to come from the experience of a number of persons, not from deaths considered one at a time.

Farr went on to discuss possible bases for a classification of causes of death (Eyler, 1979), and acknowledged that there were several that could "be used with advantage; and the physician, the pathologist or the jurist, each from his own point of view, may legitimately classify ... the causes of death in the way he thinks best adapted to facilitate his inquiries. The medical practitioner may found his main division of diseases on their treatment as medical or surgical; the pathologist, on the nature of the morbid action or product; the medical jurist on the suddenness or slowness of the death; and all their points well deserve attention in a statistical classification." Farr realized that there is no "natural" way of categorizing ill or deceased persons. Rather, he (and his successors) were obliged to make up the rules by which this would be done. A scheme that met the needs of the medical practitioner, another that met the needs of the pathologist, or a third for the medical jurist—none of them was inherently better than any of the others, except insofar as a different priority was given to each of these needs.

Farr decided that priority be given to the goal of using information on cause of death to understand etiology:

> In casting about for a classification, it struck me that it should have special reference to the causation and prevention of death; and that would be most effectually accomplished by making the three distinct groups of *(1)* deaths by epidemic, endemic, and contagious diseases; *(2)* deaths by sporadic diseases; and *(3)* deaths by evident external causes. This classification was framed and used in forming the abstracts of causes of death.

In broad terms, Farr's approach to creating a classification of the proximate causes of death and illness is the approach we take to this day. In the current Revision of the International Classification of Disease, the first group of entries is for such entities as cholera and tuberculosis; i.e., "epidemic, endemic, and contagious diseases." The second group—"sporadic diseases"—includes conditions such as malignant neoplasms and diabetes. The final group comprises transportation accidents, homicides, etc.; i.e., "evident external causes."

The specific categories within the classification scheme have changed, of course, since the nineteenth century. Nonetheless, the underlying motivation behind the changes has been related to Farr's notion of having a scheme that is most relevant "to the causation and prevention of death." As subcategories of a broader disease entity are identified—often on the basis of their distinctive etiologies—they are split out to constitute categories of their own. For example, Table 17–2 lists

Table 17–2. International Classification of Diseases (ICD), 1900 and 1992

Some presently defined conditions that would have been included under the term used in 1900, "Acute yellow atrophy of the liver":

CONDITION	ICD CODE, 10TH REVISION 1992
Alcoholic liver disease	K70
Toxic liver disease	K71
Viral hepatitis	B15–19
Liver disorders in other infectious and parasitic diseases, e.g.:	
Schistosomiasis	B65
Toxoplasmosis	B58.1
Syphilis	A52.7
Other inflammatory liver diseases (e.g., liver abscess)	K75
Other diseases of liver (e.g., portal hypertension, hepatorenal syndrome)	K76

the conditions in the 10th Revision of the International Classification of Disease—developed in 1992—that would have been included in a single category from the first ICD of 1900, "Acute yellow atrophy of the liver." Most of the categories were formed on the basis of a known etiologic factor's having been present to account for the liver pathology; e.g., alcohol abuse or infection with one of the hepatitis viruses.

Had we not been able to subdivide the broad category "Acute yellow atrophy of the liver" into some etiologically heterogeneous components, studies of the existence of the etiologies of liver disease would be hindered substantially. For example, studies of the effect of long-term alcohol abuse on the incidence of "acute yellow atrophy" would include as cases persons whose disease was caused by infection with Leptospira, in which the alcohol abuse probably played no role at all. This would result in the association between alcohol and liver disease (considered in aggregate) being smaller than the one that would have been seen had it been possible to eliminate these other cases.

Epidemiologic study of injuries also depends on being able to distinguish between injuries that may be anatomically and pathologically similar but that arise by quite different mechanisms. For example, fracture of a thoracic vertebra (ICD-10 code S22.0) could result from a fall, a sports injury, a motor-vehicle collision, or by other mechanisms. Fortunately, current versions of the ICD also provide codes for "external causes of morbidity and mortality," which are to be used in addition to codes that describe the anatomical location and pathological type of injury. For example, code V47 is used for "Car occupant injured in collision with fixed or stationary object." Such a code could also be used to group injuries to different parts of the body that all resulted from a similar type of motor-vehicle crash.

Sometimes, pathophysiological processes underlying a broadly defined disease entity can be identified, and cases can be separated on that basis. For example, persons can sustain a stroke from an arterial thrombus, a hemorrhage, or an embolus. In other instances, there is variation in the manner in which a broadly defined disease entity manifests itself; e.g., as in the various histologic categories of a given site of cancer. By subdividing groups of ill persons according to the type of pathophysiology or manifestation, epidemiologic studies can increase their chances of identifying an association between a given exposure and just one of the types when one truly exists.

Example: Assume there is an exposure, X, that is present in half the persons in a given community who sustain a thrombotic stroke, and is associated with a fourfold increase in risk. The data from a case-control study of thrombotic stroke conducted in that community might look like this:

X EXPOSURE	THROMBOTIC STROKE	CONTROLS	ODDS RATIO
Yes	50%	20%	4
No	50%	80%	

But let's say that in studying this association: (a) we are unable to sort out thrombotic from other types of stroke; (b) of 200 total stroke cases, only 120 actually had a thrombotic stroke; and (c) the occurrence of the remaining 80 stroke cases is uninfluenced by X exposure. If there were also 200 controls included in the study, the following results would be obtained:

X EXPOSURE	ALL STROKES	CONTROLS
Yes	60 + 16	40
No	60 + 64	160
	120 + 80	200

In this study, the exposed cases would comprise: 50% of the 120 with thrombotic stroke, and 20% of the 80 other cases (since X exposure in them is just as common as in controls). The odds ratio now would be only:

$$\frac{76}{124} \div \frac{40}{160} = 2.5,$$

quite a bit less than had it been possible to focus the analysis on the subgroup of cases with a thrombotic stroke.

One of the great strengths of many studies investigating the source of a disease-producing infectious agent is their ability to subdivide persons who are ill and infected according to the narrowly defined type of infectious agent:

Example: Among the strains of *Mycobacterium tuberculosis,* there is one that has a particular pattern of antibiotic resistance (defined by its characteristic DNA "fingerprint"). Though the organism was responsible for large numbers of cases of tuberculosis in New York State during the 1990s, the identification of this particular organism in eight cases in South Carolina in 1996 was anomalous (Agerton et al., 1997). One of the cases had lived in New York for some time and had returned to South Carolina in 1993. Three of the other cases were relatives of that person (two shared his household), and one additional case had been his next-door neighbor. The remaining three cases, however, had no known contact with any of the first five or with one another. A detailed medical history revealed that, though these persons were diagnosed with tuberculosis six months apart, all three had been admitted to the same hospital for other reasons prior to their diagnosis within the same three-week period. One of the ill family members of the original case also had been hospitalized there shortly before the others. This patient had undergone a bronchoscopy at that time as part of the management of his tuberculosis. Each of the other three persons also had undergone bronchoscopy during their earlier hospitalization (to evaluate an unrelated condition), at which time cultures for *M. tuberculosis* had been negative (that is, they did not already have tuberculosis when the bronchoscopy had been done).

Though there was no formal control group employed in this study, it is extraordinarily improbable that all three additional cases of tuberculosis would have had bronchoscopy within a three-week period and in the same location as the first case to undergo bronchoscopy, had there not been some etiologic link. The investigators evaluated the hospital's procedures for cleaning and disinfecting endoscopic equipment, and found several features that "did not follow the hospital's guidelines or the published guidelines" which could have been responsible for transmitting the infectious agent from one patient to another.

There are many potential sources of tuberculosis transmission in South Carolina other than a contaminated bronchoscope. But the investigators' ability to identify that particular source was made possible by their being able to restrict attention to the cases of tuberculosis who shared a common infecting strain. Inclusion of tuberculosis cases caused by other strains would almost certainly have obscured the association with a prior history of bronchoscopy in one place and at (approximately) one point in time.

III. DISAGGREGATION OF EXPOSED SUBJECTS WHO ARE NOT AFFECTED TO THE SAME DEGREE

It is commonly stated that diseases have multiple causes. There are at least two distinct ideas contained in such a statement:

1. A disease can have more than one separate causal pathway leading to it. For example, a child can acquire hepatitis B infection from her/his infected mother, but so can an adult by sharing a needle or a syringe with a person who is infected with this virus. The overall incidence of hepatitis B infection in a population would reflect the sum of the separate incidence

rates due to the operation of these two pathways (along with others). As another example, mental retardation can be caused by the access of a young child to lead in his/her environment and also by prematurity even in the absence of harmful levels of lead. Assuming there is no influence of lead exposure on the risk of prematurity, the occurrence of retardation due to these two pathways would sum, and would be responsible for a portion of a population's total incidence of mental retardation.

2. Two or more exposures are capable of causing disease only by acting together in a single causal pathway. For example, a genetic abnormality, deficiency of the enzyme glucose-6-phosphate dehydrogenase (G6PD), is a cause of hemolytic anemia only if a person with this genotype is exposed to quinidine, sulfonamides, naphthalene, infection, or some other oxidative stress.

When two exposures act through separate means to produce a disease, the relative impact of either of them is greater in that segment of the population in which the other exposure is absent. For example, assume that the prevalence of mental retardation in five-year-old children who had been born full-term is four per 100, whereas in those born prematurely it is 14 per 100 (Table 17–3). Assume that in a group of five-year-olds there were children with enough lead exposure to produce an additional frequency of mental retardation of two per 100, both in those who were and in those who were not premature. In children who had not been born prematurely, the prevalence of mental retardation in lead-exposed children would be six per 100, representing a 1.5-fold increase in risk associated with lead exposure. In premature children, however, the prevalence would be increased from 14 to 16 per 100, just a 1.14-fold increase.

Recognition of the presence of alternate pathways leading to an illness can facilitate the detection of an outbreak of that illness, and also can help identify the

Table 17–3. Relative Influence of Exposure in Early Childhood
on the Prevalence of Mental Retardation—Hypothetical Data

RISK FACTOR(S) FOR RETARDATION	PREVALENCE OF RETARDATION (PER 100 CHILDREN)	RELATIVE PREVALENCE
None	4	
		$6/4 = 1.5$
Lead only	6	
Prematurity only	14	
		$16/14 = 1.14$
Both lead and prematurity	16	

cause of the outbreak.

Example: Between December, 1991, and April, 1992, Abulrahi et al. (1997) identified 41 cases of acute *Plasmodium falciparum* malaria in children admitted to a hospital in Riyadh, Saudi Arabia. The vectors of malaria, anopheline mosquitoes, are not present anywhere near Riyadh, so the first step in understanding the causes of the illness in these children was to determine if any of them had traveled to areas where malaria was endemic. Twenty of the 41 children indeed had been in such an area during the month prior to the onset of fever that signaled the presence of malaria. A case-control study was done to determine the source of the infection in the other 21 children.

The study obtained a striking result: 20 of the 21 children (95%) with locally acquired malaria (LAM); i.e., those who had not traveled to endemic areas for malaria, had been hospitalized at some point during the month prior to admission for their malaria, in contrast to 15 of 61 control children (25%). (Strictly speaking, any potential control who had traveled to an endemic area for malaria during the prior month should have been excluded from this analysis. But the number of such children was probably so small that little bias would be present had they inadvertently been included.) Also, only five of the 20 cases of "imported" malaria had been hospitalized during the month prior to the onset of their fever. The odds ratio for LAM associated with hospitalization during the prior month was:

$$\frac{20}{1} \div \frac{15}{46} = 61.3.$$

This finding led the investigators to evaluate practices in the hospital that could have allowed for transmission of the infection from one patient to the next. They discovered that the nursing staff were routinely using heparin locks on multiple patients, allowing for hematologic spread of *P. falciparum* from infected patients to uninfected patients.

In the design and analysis of the case-control study, Abulrahi et al. exploited the fact that most of the 41 cases of malaria were attributable to two distinct causal pathways: One involved mosquito-borne transmission in an endemic area; the other, some local factor(s). If the local factor were operating independently to cause malaria—i.e., it did not require an exposure to an infected mosquito to produce the disease—then the incidence of malaria in Riyadh simply would be the sum of the separate incidences resulting from the two pathways.

What if Abulrahi et al. had not recognized the presence of the imported malaria pathway, or had not bothered to assess a history of foreign travel in the children with malaria? They would have observed 20 LAM cases + 5 imported cases = 25 total cases with a history of hospitalization in the prior month, and $1 + 15 = 16$ cases without such a hospitalization. The odds ratio, based on all malaria cases in the study,

$$\frac{25}{16} \div \frac{15}{46},$$

would have been only 4.8, very much smaller than the value of 61.3 when the analysis was restricted to the LAM cases. In this instance, the recognition that recent hospitalization played an etiologic role in the transmission of malaria in Riyadh was facilitated by the recognition of the likely presence of a second causal pathway that could lead to malaria, and by the subsequent effort to confine one analysis to the individuals (without the history of foreign travel) in whom the impact of any local factor identified would be *relatively* high.

In some instances, the investigation of a particular exposure as a possible cause of disease is enhanced by the recognition of more than just one alternative causal pathway, and once again by the subsequent exclusion of subjects who have been exposed to a component of those other pathways.

Example: In a medical record–based study, Grether and Nelson (1997) tested the hypothesis that maternal infection predisposes to spastic cerebral palsy (CP). The presence of infection was defined as a notation of one of a variety of prespecified events and conditions in the record, including maternal fever, chorioamnionitis, urinary tract infection, and histological evidence of placental infection. From the medical record, the investigators also were able to identify children with CP who had one of several other conditions whose presence was likely to have been responsible for their CP even had no maternal infection been present. These were conditions such as a destructive lesion or malformation of the brain, or a syndrome that typically includes spasticity as a feature. The table below summarizes the history of infection during pregnancy in the "explained" cases of CP, along with that in the remaining "unexplained" cases and in a control group of term infants without CP:

| | Cases | | | |
	"EXPLAINED" CP	"UNEXPLAINED" CP	TOTAL CP	CONTROLS
Evidence of infection	1 (3.3%)	10 (21.7%)	11 (14.4%)	11 (2.9%)
No infection	29	36	65	367
Total	30	46	76	378

Evidence of maternal or placental infection was present in 10 (21.7 percent) of "unexplained" CP cases, but only in 11 (2.9 percent) of controls, and the odds ratio was

$$\frac{10}{36} \div \frac{11}{367} = 9.3.$$

Yet, because infection had occurred in the "explained" CP cases just about as often as in controls, the association between "total" CP and infection would have been less strong: the odds ratio would have been

$$\frac{11}{65} \div \frac{11}{367} = 5.6.$$

By identifying conditions that strongly predispose to CP independent of maternal infection, and by restricting the analysis to persons in whom these other conditions were not present, the investigators were able to focus their attention on the children in whom the relative contribution of infection to CP occurrence was the greatest.

If two factors have the capacity to act together in a single causal pathway leading to disease, the incidence of that disease in persons in whom both factors are present would be more than the sum of the two rates produced by either factor's presence alone. For example, during epidemics of Reye's syndrome in the United States during the late 1970s and early 1980s, the disease would typically occur in a child who had recently had a bout of chickenpox or influenza who had taken aspirin during the course of that illness. The incidence of Reye's syndrome in children with both the prior infection and aspirin use was far higher than that predicted from the sum of the near-zero incidence rates in children who (a) had chickenpox or flu but did not receive aspirin, or (b) took aspirin for reasons other than chickenpox or flu. Similarly, the neurological manifestations of phenylketonuria (PKU) occur in children born with a defective or absent enzyme, phenylalanine hydroxylase, who also consume a typical quantity of the amino acid phenylalanine. Phenylalanine hydroxylase converts phenylalanine to another amino acid, tyrosine, thus not permitting the accumulation of phenylalanine in tissues. The prevalence of neurological damage characteristic of PKU is far higher in children with phenylalanine hydroxylase deficiency who consume a normal diet than would be predicted by the sum of the prevalence of this type of damage in children (a) who have the genetic abnormality but, having been screened for PKU, consume a diet extremely low in phenylalanine content; or (b) who possess a normal gene and have no dietary restriction (Table 17–4).

If aspirin use only predisposes to the incidence of Reye's syndrome when chickenpox or flu are present, then of course only in children with these infections

Table 17–4. Interplay of Heredity and Diet in the Etiology of the
Neurological Damage Characteristic of PKU

PHENYLALANINE HYDROXYLASE DEFICIENCY	PHENYLALANINE INTAKE	CLINICAL EVIDENCE OF NEUROLOGICAL DAMAGE CHARACTERISTIC OF PKU
Yes	Normal	Yes
Yes	Low	No
No	Normal	No
No	Low	No

will the relative risk associated with aspirin use be above one. To the extent that there are Reye's syndrome cases that occur without one of these antecedent infections, an analysis that adds them to cases who have been infected will obtain a relative risk associated with aspirin that is intermediate between the value of 1.0 (the RR of persons with no prior infection) and that of 10-40 that has been observed in most studies of Reye's syndrome based on children who did have chickenpox or flu. A more sensitive analysis—i.e., one that has a greater chance of determining whether aspirin use has any deleterious effect with respect to the incidence of Reye's syndrome—would be to obtain data on a history of prior infection on all study subjects and examine the association with aspirin use separately in children with and without such a history.

VARIATION IN THE SIZE OF RELATIVE RISK ACROSS SUBGROUPS

So far, we have discussed ways of increasing the sensitivity of an epidemiologic study by identifying a subgroup of the population in whom the relative impact of exposure on disease incidence is particularly large. It is the size of the relative risk that we use as one guideline for inferring the presence of a causal relationship between an exposure and a disease, and we do not want to overlook the possibility that, among the whole of the population, there is a segment in whom the relative risk associated with exposure is noticeably different than 1.0. It is important to keep in mind, however, that once a causal action of an exposure on a disease occurrence has been inferred, a possible difference in the importance of that association across these same subgroups—in clinical or public-health terms—can only be assessed by considering the size of the attributable risk in each of these subgroups. We saw in Chapter 8 that, for a given disease, a high relative risk associated with an exposure does not necessarily translate into an attributable risk high enough to be of clinical or public-health importance, since the size of the attributable risk is influenced heavily by the underlying incidence of that disease in the absence

Table 17–5. Age-Standardized Lung Cancer Death Rates[a] for Cigarette Smoking and/or Occupational Exposure to Asbestos Dust Compared with No Smoking and No Occupational Exposure to Asbestos Dust

GROUP	EXPOSURE TO ASBESTOS?	HISTORY OF CIGARETTE SMOKING?	DEATH RATE	MORTALITY DIFFERENCE	MORTALITY RATIO
Control	No	No	11.3	0.0	1.00
Asbestos workers	Yes	No	58.4	+47.1	5.17
Control	No	Yes	122.6	+111.3	10.85
Asbestos workers	Yes	Yes	601.6	+590.3	53.24

[a]Rate per 100,000 man-years standardized for age on the distribution of the man-years of all the asbestos workers.
[*Source:* Hammond et al. (1979).]

of the exposure. By the same token, when the incidence of the disease differs in two subgroups of individuals, defined on the basis of one exposure, then: (1) if the relative risk associated with another exposure is the same in each of the subgroups, the corresponding attributable risks will differ, possibly to an important degree; and (2) differences in the relative risk associated with an exposure between the subgroups simply may be a reflection of the exposure's adding to the risk by the same amount in each of the subgroups.

Let us consider each of these separately. As an example of (1) above, Table 17–5 shows results obtained in a cohort study of the mortality from lung cancer in men in relation to heavy occupational exposure to asbestos.

Do these data suggest that the increased risk of lung cancer associated with a history of cigarette smoking—very likely causally associated—should weigh more heavily in the decision to stop smoking by a man with a history of heavy asbestos exposure than a man without such a history? The relative risk associated with cigarette smoking is nearly the same between men with and without a history of asbestos exposure ($122.6 \div 11.3 = 10.85$ in men not exposed to asbestos, and $601.6 \div 58.4 = 10.30$ in men who were exposed to asbestos). But the AR in the latter group is higher (by more than a factor of five) than in the former ($601.6 - 58.4 = 543.2$ per 100,000 man-years in asbestos workers versus $122.6 - 11.3 = 111.3$ per 100,000 in other persons). This dissimilarity in the respective ARs, in the presence of comparability between the RRs, is due to the fact that among nonsmokers the mortality from lung cancer was higher, by more than a factor of 5, in men exposed to asbestos. Since it is the size of AR that ought to bear on decisions pertaining to health (and on the recommendations of providers of health care), the same tenfold increase in the risk of lung cancer should be given more weight by a man who has a history of heavy occupational asbestos exposure than by one who does not.

(Of course, the AR for lung cancer and for many other conditions associated with cigarette smoking is so large, even in persons without occupational exposure to asbestos, that all persons have a strong incentive to discontinue smoking.)

As an example of (2) above, some studies of endometrial cancer observed a difference in the relative risk associated with long-term use of unopposed estrogens depending on a woman's weight. In lean women and women of average weight who participated in one of these studies (Shields et al., 1999), the incidence in hormone nonusers was about 0.26 per 1000 woman-years, in contrast to a rate of about 4.45 per 1000 in long-term hormone users (relative risk = 17.1). Among heavy women in the same study (those in the upper fourth of the distribution of body mass index), the rates in hormone nonusers and users were 0.75 and 8.92 per 1000 woman-years, respectively, and the relative risk was not so strongly elevated (11.9). Based on these results it would be incorrect to conclude, however, that the adverse impact of the use of unopposed estrogens on the endometrium should bear less strongly on the decision of a heavy woman to use unopposed estrogens than on the decision of a woman who is not heavy. These data suggest that the absolute change in incidence resulting from hormone use (i.e., the attributable risk) is actually greater in heavy women—$8.92 - 0.75 = 8.17$ per 1000 woman-years—than it is in other women—$4.45 - 0.26 = 4.19$ per 1000 woman-years.

The term "effect modification" is used by epidemiologists to describe the circumstance in which the size of an association between exposure and disease differs according to the presence or level of another exposure or characteristic. But the meaning of effect-modification as applied to a particular instance may be ambiguous if the measure of association is not specified. In one example presented earlier, the relative risk of mental retardation associated with lead exposure was modified by a history of prematurity; the RR was 1.14 in children born prematurely, whereas it was 1.5 in children born full-term. But the size of the attributable risk associated with lead exposure did not depend on a history of prematurity (2 per 100 in both subgroups of gestational length). In a different example, it was the relative risk that was similar across subgroups of the additional variable—the RR for MI associated with OC use was 4.4 in women under 35 years and 4.3 in older women—whereas the attributable risk was modified by age (2.7 versus 31.0 per million women-years, respectively). Our recommendation is that whenever the term "effect-modification" is used, the criterion for its presence (i.e., variation in the size of the relative or attributable risk) should be provided.

INVESTIGATING AGE AS A POSSIBLE EFFECT MODIFIER

Age can exert a potent influence on the ability of an exposure to influence the risk of disease. For example, compared to adults, very young children are relatively refractory to the development of polio if infected with polio virus. They have much greater susceptibility than adults, however, to the occurrence of the hemolytic uremic syndrome if they ingest food containing *E. coli* O157:H7. Examining age as a potential effect-modifier generally is straightforward: as with any other variable, one looks for a difference in the presence or size of the association between the exposure of interest and disease in two or more age categories. Some investigators, however, have instead simply compared the mean (or median) ages of cases who do or do not have a particular exposure or characteristic. This practice is to be avoided, since it can give misleading results.

- A study of women with breast cancer, identified from a tumor registry in the U.S., observed that black patients tended to be younger than white patients at the time of the diagnosis (mean age 55 years vs. 60 years). The authors of the study suggested this difference may have etiologic implications. Not considered was the possibility that there was a corresponding age difference in the underlying population in which the women with breast cancer resided. If, for example, the mean age of black women in that part of the U.S. were five years less than the mean age of white women, then identical age-specific rates between the two races would produce a corresponding difference between the black and white women diagnosed with breast cancer.

- Even when the exposure in question is not related to age in the underlying population, the interpretation of a difference in age between exposed and non-exposed cases can be ambiguous. Consider the following hypothetical example of a disease with a bimodal age distribution: The mean age of "young" cases is 30 years, whereas that of "old" cases is 60 years. Assume there is a fivefold excess disease risk associated with the presence of a particular genetic marker that is confined to "young" cases (Table 17–6A). In a population whose members are distributed in terms of age and marker status as in Table 17–6A, the mean age of cases possessing this marker is 35 years. The mean age of the cases without the marker is 45 years.

  Table 17–6B displays hypothetical data from a population that is identical to that in Table 17–6A in terms of age and marker status, but in which there is no association between the genetic marker and disease risk in young persons, and a negative association in old persons. The mean ages of diseased individuals with and without the genetic marker are, once again, 35 and 45, respectively!

  In short, the interpretation of the 10-year difference in mean age at diagnosis is ambiguous, since it can be produced by completely different patterns of effect modification.

Table 17–6. Two Hypothetical Examples of Effect Modification by Age

A. Genetic Marker Associated with Increased Risk in Young Cases Only

GENETIC MARKER PRESENT?	Young (Mean = 30 Years)			Old (Mean = 60 Years)			MEAN AGE
	NO. OF CASES	PERSON-YEARS	RATE[a]	NO. OF CASES	PERSON-YEARS	RATE[a]	
Yes	50	10,000	5	10	5000	2	$\dfrac{50(30) + 10(60)}{60} = 35.0$
No	100	100,000	1	100	50,000	2	$\dfrac{100(30) + 100(60)}{200} = 45.0$

B. Genetic Marker Associated with Decreased Risk in Old Cases Only

GENETIC MARKER PRESENT?	Young (Mean = 30 Years)			Old (Mean = 60 Years)			MEAN AGE
	NO. OF CASES	PERSON-YEARS	RATE[a]	NO. OF CASES	PERSON-YEARS	RATE[a]	
Yes	10	10,000	1	2	5000	0.4	$\dfrac{10(30) + 2(60)}{12} = 35.0$
No	100	100,000	1	100	50,000	2	$\dfrac{100(30) + 100(60)}{200} = 45.0$

[a]Cases per 1,000 person-years.

DOES INCREASING THE SENSITIVITY OF EPIDEMIOLOGIC STUDIES DECREASE THEIR SPECIFICITY?

The answer to the above question is "yes." Dividing study subjects into subgroups of exposures and diseases and examining possible associations for various combinations of subgroups will make the number of "false positive" results grow. That is, an increasing number of associations will be seen in the sample of persons studied that do not represent an underlying association in the "universe" of persons from which the sample was drawn. This loss of specificity is the price we must pay to avoid missing a true association (or underestimating its magnitude) that is present for some category of exposure or disease, or in some segment of the population at risk.

Nonetheless, by being cognizant of the presence of false positive associations that a thorough analytical approach must produce, we will know to be cautious when trying to interpret those associations that do emerge in an individual study. We will tend to interpret an association restricted to (or most prominent in) a subgroup as indicating a genuine causal (or protective) relationship when it: is large; is based on a sizeable number of subjects, to minimize the role of chance; has been observed in one or more other studies; and there is a plausible explanation for the pattern of associations across subgroups that has been observed.

Example: In a randomized trial, U.S. male physicians assigned to take 325 mg. of aspirin on alternate days were observed to have a lower incidence of myocardial infarction than those assigned to take a placebo (Ridker et al., 1997). But the reduction in incidence associated with aspirin use varied according to a man's plasma level of C-reactive protein, being most prominent in those with relatively high levels and absent in men in the lower fourth of the distribution (Fig. 17–1).

The hypothesis that the efficacy of aspirin use in the prevention of myocardial infarction truly differs depending on a man's plasma level of C-reactive protein is supported by: (1) the large, graded, difference in the observed association across C-reactive protein levels; (2) the large number of observations this was based on (a total of 246 men with myocardial infarction); and (3) the fact that C-reactive protein is a marker of chronic inflammation, and that aspirin has anti-inflammatory effects. If corroborated in one or more other studies, it is likely that most observers would interpret these results as being indicative of a genuine ability of the level of C-reactive protein to predict the presence and degree of benefit (in terms of heart attack risk) that would ensue from aspirin use.

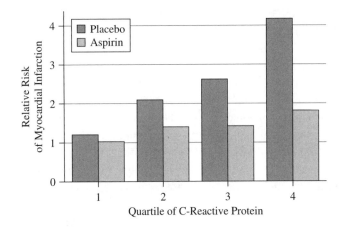

Figure 17-1. Relative Risk of Myocardial Infarction in the Physicians Health Study, by Treatment Group and Quartile of C-Reactive Protein (based on Ridker et al., 1997).

Table 17–7. Results from a Case-Control Study of Vasectomy and Testicular Cancer

RELIGIOUS PREFERENCE	HISTORY OF VASECTOMY	CASES ($n = 228$)	CONTROLS ($n = 513$)	ODDS RATIO[a]
		Numbers in Percentages		
Catholic	Yes	24.4	6.2	8.7
	No	75.6	93.8	
Other or none	Yes	23.0	19.6	1.1
	No	77.0	80.4	
All men	Yes	23.3	17.1	1.5
	No	76.7	82.9	

[a] Age-adjusted.
[*Source:* Strader et al. (1988).]

Example: An interview-based case-control study of testicular cancer was conducted to test the hypothesis that a history of vasectomy might predispose to this disease (Strader et al., 1988). Cases were identified through the records of a population-based cancer registry, while controls were enumerated from random-digit dialing of telephone numbers. The results shown in Table 17–7 were obtained.

The odds ratio associated with a history of vasectomy of 1.5 among men in general represents only a modest elevation and argues for a cautious interpretation.

The odds ratio did vary considerably between Catholic and other men (8.7 versus 1.1), but it seems implausible that religious preference could somehow bear on the ability of a vasectomy to predispose to the incidence of testicular cancer. Rather, it seems more likely that the ascertainment of a history of vasectomy was relatively incomplete among Catholic controls: Vasectomy is proscribed by the Catholic religion, and it is possible that some Catholic men chosen at random from the community to serve as a member of a comparison group in a study of cancer may have been reluctant to admit to having had this procedure.

If the ascertainment of vasectomy had been relatively more complete among Catholic cases—perhaps they felt more of an obligation than controls to acknowledge a proscribed behavior, because of their relatively greater interest in helping to understand the causes of testicular cancer—the resulting differential misclassification could have produced a spuriously elevated odds ratio.

Example: Beresford et al. (1997) conducted a case-control study to assess the impact of long-term "sequential" hormone replacement therapy (HRT)—daily estrogens plus cyclic use of a progestogen each month—on the risk of endometrial cancer among postmenopausal women.

Among women who had not previously taken unopposed estrogens, those who had used HRT for more than five years had 2.6 times the risk of women who had not taken any hormones (95% CI = 1.3–5.5) (McKnight et al., 1998). In contrast, the risk associated with more than five years' use of HRT was but 0.21 (95% CI = 0.07–0.66) in women who had earlier taken unopposed estrogens (and 0.6 if non-HRT users also were restricted to women whose last use of unopposed estrogens was at least five years earlier).

It is plausible that there is a true difference in the influence of sequential HRT on risk of endometrial cancer between the two groups of women:—perhaps the earlier "priming" of the endometrium to a hyperplastic state by unopposed estrogen renders it particularly susceptible to the beneficial differentiating influence of the progestogen component of HRT. Other studies that observe the same phenomenon will be needed before the difference can be accepted as true, and indeed a subsequent Swedish study (Weiderpass et al., 1999) has not observed prior use of unopposed estrogens to modify the association between sequential HRT and risk of endometrial cancer. Nonetheless, without the examination of the two subgroups separately, the possibility of an effect of long-term use of HRT may not have surfaced: the relative risk associated with such use among women as a whole in the study of Beresford et al. was 1.0 (95% confidence interval = 0.54–1.7).

When considering whether an association between exposure and disease is indicative of a causal relationship between the two, we ask if that association has been observed consistently from study to study. We are looking for that same consistency before concluding that the variation observed in the direction or size of an exposure–disease association across strata of another exposure or characteristic is indicative of genuine effect-modification. For example, because studies have observed repeatedly that being overweight is associated with an increased risk of breast cancer in postmenopausal women and yet a decreased risk in premenopausal women (van den Brandt et al., 2000), the modifying influence of menopausal status on this association between weight and breast cancer is widely accepted. Yet, when evaluating the consistency of inter-stratum variation of this sort from study to study, it is necessary not to lose sight of the studies of the overall association that have *not* presented data relevant to the possibility of effect modification.

Example: Green et al. (2000) reviewed the results of 21 studies that examined the association between N-acetyltransferase 2 (NAT2) genotype or activity and the incidence of bladder cancer. NAT2 is an enzyme involved in the inactivation of arylamines, carcinogens present in cigarette smoke. The NAT2 gene that directs the synthesis of this enzyme is polymorphic, and as a result all persons are either "fast" or "slow" acetylators. It was hypothesized that being a slow acetylator might be a particularly strong risk factor for bladder cancer in persons with a high level of exposure to arylamines, e.g., by means of cigarette smoking. Results from five (of the 21) studies reviewed by Green et al. that addressed this question supported the hypothesis: The pooled odds ratio relating slow acetylation status to bladder cancer was 1.6 in cigarette smokers but only 1.0 in nonsmokers. As pointed out by Green et al., however, the failure of the large majority of studies to report data on the possible modifying influence of smoking status on this association severely limits the interpretation of the difference between these two odds ratios. Specifically, it is all too likely that the authors of some of the other 16 studies examined their data for the presence of effect modification, found it *not* to be there, and simply omitted a presentation of these results from their manuscript.

The example above describes a form of "publication" bias: that is, a distortion of the truth by the appearance in the medical literature of a skewed sample of results. Publication bias can be present when one seeks to summarize the overall association between an exposure and disease across studies, of course. We suspect its frequency and magnitude are greater when one is summarizing studies for the possibility of effect modification, since we believe it is more likely for an analysis that fails to suggest an interaction to be kept out of a manuscript, than for a manuscript as a whole with a null result to be kept from publication.

EXERCISES

1. David et al. (1976) wished to determine "... the quantitative extent of the relationship between lead and mental retardation," since at the time the study was done it remained "to be determined whether a smaller amount of lead—i.e., raised but non-encephalopathic concentrations in the blood—can be an etiological factor in mental retardation." From patients attending a developmental evaluation clinic, they obtained a blood sample for lead determination from 64 children with an IQ of 55 to 84. Of these, 33 had a probable explanation for being retarded, such as prematurity, maternal eclampsia, meningitis, or microcephaly. From a pediatric clinic in the same medical center, blood samples were obtained in 30 control children and also were tested for lead levels. The results are shown in the following table:

BLOOD LEAD CONCENTRATION (mcg/dl)	Mental Retardation		CONTROLS
	ETIOLOGY PROBABLY KNOWN	ETIOLOGY UNKNOWN	
<15	8	2	12
15–24	20	14	11
25–34	4	10	6
≥35	1	5	1

(a) Estimate the risk of mental retardation of unknown etiology in children with lead levels ≥25 mcg/dl relative to that in children with levels <25 mcg/dl. Exclude from the calculation the data on the retarded children in whom the etiology probably was known.

(b) Had the probable etiology of some cases of mental retardation not been known, the 31 children with no known etiology would have been combined with the 33 other retarded children to form a single case group. Using these 64 cases and the same control group, and the ≥25 versus <25 dichotomy, what is the risk ratio associated with high blood lead levels for this broader category of mental retardation? Why does it differ from the previous one?

(c) Relative to children with blood lead levels of <15 mcg/dl, what is the risk of mental retardation with no known etiology in children with levels of:
- 15–24 mcg/dl
- 25–34 mcg/dl
- ≥35 mcg/dl

Was there any advantage to having been able to measure blood lead more precisely than simply "greater or less than 25 mcg/dl"?

2. A study of chronic pancreatitis sought to determine whether persons with this disease have a mutation of the cystic fibrosis transmembrane conductance regulator (CSTR) gene more often than do other persons (Sharer et al., 1998). Because alcohol consumption is a risk factor for chronic pancreatitis, the investigators separated their cases into two groups: 71 who were felt to have alcohol-related disease, and 63 "idiopathic" cases. Six of the former group had a mutation in at least one copy of the CSTR gene, while 12 of the idiopathic cases had such a mutation. The prevalence of one or more CSTR mutations in a control group of persons without pancreatitis was 5.3%. Prior studies have shown that alcohol consumption itself is unrelated to the presence of a mutation in the CSTR gene. Do the data of Sharer et al. support the hypothesis that alcohol consumption and a mutation of the CSTR gene work jointly to produce chronic pancreatitis?

3. The first exon of the androgen receptor gene contains a trinucleotide (CAG) repeat sequence, the length of which varies from person to person. A very large number of repeat sequences (e.g. ≥ 40) is associated with androgen insensitivity. It has been observed that among women who have inherited a germline mutation in the BRCA1 gene, and went on to develop breast cancer, that the mean age at diagnosis of those with ≥ 30 CAG repeats was 6.3 years earlier than that of the other women (Rebbeck et al., 1999). Assume that the difference was not due to chance. Does this necessarily mean that the presence of ≥ 30 CAG repeats in the androgen receptor gene preferentially increases risk of breast cancer in young women with a BRCA1 mutation?

4. This question pertains to the following (excerpted) abstract (Cho et al., 1996):

> The authors extend their investigation by comparing the incidence rate of stomach cancer among three ethnic groups in the state of Illinois from 1986 to 1988. The three-year age-adjusted cumulative incidence rate for immigrant Koreans (172/100,000) was approximately four- and eightfold higher, respectively, than for African Americans (41/100,000) and whites (21/100,000). The high rate of stomach cancer in immigrant Koreans compared with African Americans and white populations residing in Illinois indicates either a drastically disproportionate undercount of immigrant Koreans in the census or a profound genetic–environmental interaction.

Assume that the results presented are not due to chance or bias (including bias due to a disproportionate undercount of immigrant Koreans in the census). Apart from "a profound genetic-environmental interaction," what are some other plausible explanations for the high observed rates of stomach cancer among immigrant Koreans in Illinois?

5. Figure 17–2, taken from Danesh et al. (1999), is a summary of studies of *H. pylori* seropositivity in relation to the occurrence of coronary heart disease. (Three other retrospective studies are not included since they did not report

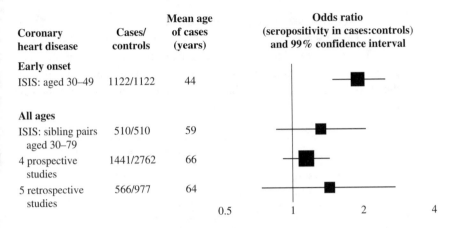

Coronary heart disease	Cases/ controls	Mean age of cases (years)	Odds ratio (seropositivity in cases:controls) and 99% confidence interval
Early onset			
ISIS: aged 30–49	1122/1122	44	
All ages			
ISIS: sibling pairs aged 30–79	510/510	59	
4 prospective studies	1441/2762	66	
5 retrospective studies	566/977	64	

Figure 17-2. Summary of Studies of *H. pylori* Seropositivity in Relation to the Occurrence of Coronary Heart Disease (from Danesh et al., 1999).

separate results for cases of myocardial infarction. Together these studies included fewer than 150 cases of myocardial infarction.) Black squares indicate odds ratio, with area of square proportional to number of cases, and horizontal lines represent confidence intervals.

From this figure, assume the most trustworthy data bearing on a possible association between *H. pylori* seropositivity and the occurrence of coronary heart disease come from:

- The ISIS study for persons 30–49 years of age; and
- The four prospective studies for persons older than this.

Also assume that the studies were done in a comparable way in the same geographic population; that *H. pylori* seropositivity is a faithful indication of *H. pylori* infection, regardless of age; and that the difference in the two odds ratios (2 vs. 1.2) is not due to chance. These results do not necessarily indicate that 30–49-year-old persons are more susceptible to the harmful influence of *H. pylori* infection on the occurrence of coronary heart disease than are persons beyond this age. Why?

ANSWERS

1. *(a)* Since this is a case-control study in which the absolute risk of retardation among children with various blood levels cannot be determined, it is necessary to estimate the relative risk by means of the odds ratio. The odds of exposure (defined here as a value ≥ 25 mcg/dl) among cases is 15/16, whereas in controls it is 7/23. The ratio of these is 3.1.

(b) The odds of exposure among all retarded children in this study is $\frac{15+5}{16+28} = 20/44$. The odds ratio when cases are defined in this way is $20/44 \div 7/23 = 1.5$. This odds ratio is lower than that calculated in part (a) because the case group now includes retarded children in whom the cause is known, and therefore in whom the relative importance of lead exposure probably was minimal.

(c)

COMPARISON	ODDS RATIO
15–24 vs. <15 mcg/dl	$14/2 \div 11/12 = 7.6$
25–34 vs. <15 mcg/dl	$10/2 \div 6/12 = 10.0$
≥35 vs. <15 mcg/dl	$5/2 \div 1/12 = 30.0$

The referent category used in the calculation of the odds ratio in (a), <25 mcg/dl, was heterogeneous with respect to its association with mental retardation. When it was subcategorized, allowing the also-high risk category of 15–24 mcg/dl to be removed, the analysis gained sensitivity in identifying the strong association between mental retardation (of no known cause) and elevated blood lead levels.

Note: Because of the way this study was designed, with measures of blood lead obtained well after the diagnosis of mental retardation, the results do not preclude the possibility that the blood lead levels observed in the participants in this study are considerably lower than those that led to the retardation. Whether "non-encephalopathic levels of blood lead (e.g., 15–34 mcg/dl) are themselves capable of causing retardation would need to be evaluated in studies that had access to blood samples (preferably at different points in time) drawn prior to the onset of retardation (Pocock et al., 1994).

2. The association between the presence of one or more mutant CSTR genes and chronic pancreatitis can be examined in the two subgroups of the disease— alcohol-related and idiopathic.

MUTANT CSTR GENE	ALCOHOL-RELATED DISEASE	IDIOPATHIC DISEASE	CONTROLS
Yes	6	12	5.3%
No	65	51	94.7%
	71	63	100.0%
Odds ratio:	$\dfrac{6/65}{5.3/94.7} = 1.6$	$\dfrac{12/51}{5.3/94.7} = 4.2$	

Because the association between a mutation of the CSTR gene and chronic pancreatitis is so much stronger (as measured by the relative risk—4.2 for idiopathic cases, as compared to 1.6 for alcohol-related cases), it seems unlikely that the abnormal gene and alcohol consumption interact to produce this disease.

Nonetheless, it should be kept in mind that the identical *attributable* risk associated with a mutation in the CSTR gene would be expected to produce a smaller *relative* risk in a high-risk subgroup—such as persons with alcohol consumption—than in other persons. Thus, it is conceivable that the impact of the CSTR mutation on the incidence of chronic pancreatitis is similar, in absolute terms, for persons with and without heavy alcohol consumption. So, while there is no support for the hypothesis of synergy, the findings do not necessarily indicate there is antagonism between these two exposures regarding the etiology of chronic pancreatitis.

3. No. The same observation—a relatively lower mean age at diagnosis in women with ≥ 30 CAG repeats—would occur if having ≥ 30 CAG repeats were associated with no alteration in risk of breast cancer in young women and a *reduced* risk in older women (see p. 428). Missing from this analysis is the distribution of CAG repeat length in controls—i.e., women with a germline BRCA1 mutation who did not develop breast cancer as of the age that the cases had done so. Information from controls would allow the following tables to be constructed:

	Younger Women Breast Cancer		Older Women Breast Cancer	
CAG REPEAT LENGTH	YES	NO	YES	NO
≥ 30	a_1	b_1	a_2	b_2
<30	c_1	d_1	c_2	d_2

An association between CAG repeat length and breast cancer that was confined to (or relatively greater in) young women is what must be observed before it could be concluded that the adverse effect of a long CAG repeat sequence in BRCA1 positive women is particularly great at younger ages.

4. • The environmental factors responsible for the high rate of cancer in Koreans—e.g., some aspect(s) of diet—differ in prevalence between Korean and other residents of Illinois.
   • The risk of stomach cancer is established by certain exposures early in life; i.e., prior to immigration to the U.S.
   • Koreans have a genetic predisposition to stomach cancer that would manifest itself in any environment.
   Data that would support a genetic–environmental interaction in the etiology of stomach cancer would be a high rate in Korean residents of Illinois relative

to the rates in Illinois residents of other races and to the rates in residents of Korea.

5. If the rate of CHD occurrence associated with *H. pylori* infection simply adds to the rate from other causes, the *relative* contribution of *H. pylori* infection will be greatest in persons in whom the rate is otherwise low. Therefore, even if 30–49-year-old and older persons had the identical susceptibility to *H. pylori* infection—as measured by the attributable risk—the odds ratio would be expected to be larger in the 30–49-year-olds because of their otherwise low incidence compared with older individuals.

REFERENCES

Abulrahi HA, Bohlega EA, Fontaine RE, al Seghayer SM, al Ruwais AA. *Plasmodium falciparum* malaria transmitted in hospital through heparin locks. Lancet 1997; 349: 23–25.

Agerton T, Valway S, Gore B, Pozsik C, Plikaytis B, Woodley C, et al. Transmission of a highly drug-resistant strain (Strain W1) of *Mycobacterium tuberculosis*. JAMA 1997; 278:1073–77.

Beresford SAA, Weiss NS, Voigt LF, McKnight B. Risk of endometrial cancer in relation to use of oestrogen combined with cyclic progestagen therapy in postmenopausal women. Lancet 1997; 349:458–61.

Blair A, Stewart PA, Tolbert PE, Grauman D, Moran FX, Vaught J, et al. Cancer and other causes of death among a cohort of dry cleaners. Br J Ind Med 1990; 47:162–68.

Cho NH, Moy CS, Davis F, Haenszel W, Ahn YO, Kim H. Ethnic variation in the incidence of stomach cancer in Illinois, 1986–1988. Am J Epidemiol 1996; 144:661–64.

Cook LS, Weiss NS. "Endometrial cancer." In: Goldman MB, Hatch MC (eds.). Women and health. San Diego: Academic Press, 2000.

Danesh J, Youngman L, Clark S, Parish S, Peto R, Collins R. *Helicobacter pylori* infection and early onset myocardial infarction: case-control and sibling pairs study. BMJ 1999; 319:1157–62.

David O, Hoffman S, McGann B, Sverd J, Clark J. Low lead levels and mental retardation. Lancet 1976; 2:1376–79.

Eyler EM. Victorian social medicine. Baltimore: Johns Hopkins University Press, 1979.

Green J, Banks E, Berrington A, Darby S, Deo H, Newton R. N-acetyltransferase 2 and bladder cancer: an overview and consideration of the evidence for gene-environment interaction. Br J Cancer 2000; 83:412–17.

Grether JK, Nelson KB. Maternal infections and cerebral palsy in infants of normal birth weight. JAMA 1997; 278:207–11.

Hammond EC, Selikoff IJ, Seidman H. Asbestos exposure, cigarette smoking and death rates. Ann N Y Acad Sci 1979; 330:473–90.

McKnight B, Voigt LF, Beresford SAA, Weiss NS. Re: Estrogen-progestin therapy and endometrial cancer. J Natl Cancer Inst 1998; 90:164–65.

Pocock SJ, Smith M, Baghurst P. Environmental lead and children's intelligence: a systematic review of the epidemiological evidence. BMJ 1994; 309:1189–97.

Rebbeck TR, Kantoff PW, Krithivas K, Neuhausen S, Blackwood MA, Godwin AK, et al. Modification of BRCA1-associated breast cancer risk by the polymorphic androgen-receptor CAG repeat. Am J Hum Genet 1999; 64:1371–77.

Ridker PM, Cushman M, Stampfer MJ, Tracy RP, Hennekens CH. Inflammation, aspirin, and the risk of cardiovascular disease in apparently healthy men. N Engl J Med 1997; 336:973–80.

Sharer N, Schwarz M, Malone G, Howarth A, Painter J, Super M, et al. Mutations of the cystic fibrosis gene in patients with chronic pancreatitis. N Engl J Med 1998; 339:645–52.

Shields TS, Weiss NS, Voigt LF, Beresford SA. The additional risk of endometrial cancer associated with unopposed estrogen use in women with other risk factors. Epidemiology 1999; 10:733–38.

Strader CH, Weiss NS, Daling JR. Vasectomy and the incidence of testicular cancer. Am J Epidemiol 1988; 128:56–63.

van den Brandt PA, Spiegelman D, Yaun SS, Adami HO, Beeson L, Folsom AR, et al. Pooled analysis of prospective cohort studies on height, weight, and breast cancer risk. Am J Epidemiol 2000; 152:514–27.

Weiderpass E, Adami HO, Baron JA, Magnusson C, Bergstrom R, Lindgren A, et al. Risk of endometrial cancer following estrogen replacement with and without progestins. J Natl Cancer Inst 1999; 91:1131–37.

18

SCREENING

Many chronic diseases evolve in an affected individual through the sequence of steps shown in Figure 18–1 unless action is taken to interrupt this progression. Cervical cancer, breast cancer, diabetes mellitus, and glaucoma are among many examples, some of which can be fatal. The amount of time that transpires from one milestone to the next can vary greatly from step to step, among diseases and among individuals.

Disease control efforts can try to thwart this progression at any of several places, often said to correspond to different *levels of prevention* (Last, 1992; U.S. Preventive Services Task Force, 1996), as shown in Figure 18–2.

- *Primary prevention* seeks to avoid the biological onset of disease. Vaccination is an example. Much epidemiologic research is aimed at creating new opportunities for primary prevention by identifying modifiable risk factors for disease.
- *Secondary prevention* seeks to minimize adverse outcomes of disease through early detection, even before symptoms develop and care is sought. Mammography for early detection of breast cancer in asymptomatic women is an example. (The term *secondary prevention* is also sometimes used to refer to reducing the risk of recurrence in someone who has already had an initial episode of disease.)
- *Tertiary prevention* seeks to reduce disability and risk of death by treating known disease cases. Antithrombotic therapy given soon after onset of a myocardial infarction is an example. Tertiary prevention is the main focus of traditional medical care.

Screening can be considered a form of secondary prevention. It has been defined as "examination of asymptomatic people in order to classify them as likely, or unlikely, to have the disease that is the object of screening" (Morrison, 1992). Screening can also be applied to detect modifiable risk factors for disease, such as high blood pressure or high serum cholesterol levels, that may not otherwise be apparent.

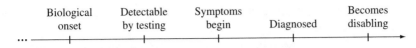

Figure 18–1. Model of Natural History for Many Chronic Diseases.

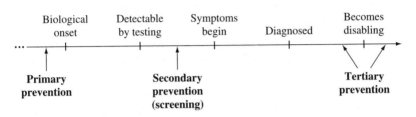

Figure 18–2. Levels of Prevention.

WHEN CAN SCREENING BE JUSTIFIED?

For a disease whose natural history generally follows the pattern depicted in Figure 18–1, it is tempting to assume that the sooner a case of such a disease is recognized, the better off the affected individual will be. Unfortunately, however, early detection does not automatically translate into better outcomes. In addition, even when early detection *is* of demonstrable benefit, screening carries costs and risks of its own—some of them rather hidden—which must be balanced against its benefits.

The decision to screen for a disease is justified to the extent that the following circumstances are present (U.S. Preventive Services Task Force, 1996; Morrison, 1992; Sackett et al., 1991):

1. *The disease is an important public health problem, in terms of its frequency and/or severity.* Resources for disease control are limited. Screening also burdens the many to benefit the few. A disease that is extremely rare, or whose effects on overall health are mild, may not warrant the burden on society of mass screening.

2. *The natural history of the disease presents a suitable "window of opportunity" for screening.* Screening focuses on the time interval between when the disease becomes detectable by a screening test and when it would be recognized anyway upon appearance of symptoms. The duration of this interval depends in part on how rapidly the disease progresses biologically, and in part on how sensitive the screening test is for early disease. If the disease progresses very rapidly through this stage, then early detection of many cases before they become symptomatic may require that the

screening test be reapplied very frequently, which may be too costly or impractical.

3. *Effective treatment is available, and capable of favorably altering the disease's natural history. Alternatively, an effective way to prevent spread to other people is at hand.* Diagnosing a condition early does the affected individual no favor if there is no good treatment. If the disease is contagious, however, early diagnosis may benefit others by preventing further transmission. In either case, effective measures must not only exist, they must actually be available for use with screenees who are found to have the disease.

4. *Treatment, or interventions to prevent spread to others, are more effective if initiated in the presymptomatic stage than when initiated in symptomatic patients.* Elaborating on requirements 2 and 3, the mere availability of effective measures for treatment or prevention of further transmission is not enough to justify screening. If these measures are just as effective once the disease has declared its presence through symptoms, then the added expense of mass screening for early detection is unnecessary and wasteful.

5. *A suitable screening test is available: reasonably inexpensive and safe, acceptable to the population screened, and able to discriminate between diseased and nondiseased persons.* The last of these factors is discussed below.

ASSESSING SCREENING TEST PERFORMANCE

Predictive Value

Sensitivity and *specificity,* as defined in Chapter 10, can be used to evaluate the performance of a screening test. To estimate them, the test is applied to a sample of individuals whose true disease status is determined by a suitable gold standard, assumed to be error-free.

Example: Allison and colleagues (1996) studied four screening tests for colorectal cancer, all designed to detect hidden traces of blood in stool. Specimen cards were mailed to several thousand enrollees aged 50 years or older in a large health maintenance organization who were scheduled for a personal health checkup. The four tests were applied to the specimens mailed back. True colorectal cancer was defined as any new pathological diagnosis of the disease within two years after screening, regardless of the mode of detection.

Table 18–1. Sensitivity, Specificity, and Predictive Value
of a Screening Test for Colorectal Cancer

| HEMESELECT RESULT | Colorectal Cancer Diagnosed Within 2 Years? | | TOTAL |
	YES	NO	
+	22	418	440
−	10	7043	7053
Total	32	7461	7493

[*Source:* Allison et al. (1996).]

Results for one of the screening tests, HemeSelect, are shown in Table 18–1. Of the 32 colorectal cancer cases, 22 tested positive on HemeSelect, for a sensitivity of $22/32 = .688$. Of the 7,461 persons who had no diagnosis of colorectal cancer, 7,043 tested negative on HemeSelect, for a specificity of $7,043/7,461 = .944$.

Sensitivity and specificity convey how likely it is that the test will yield a correct result, given presence or absence of disease. But when a test is actually used for screening, the screenee's true disease status is unknown. Instead, the task is to estimate the probability that the disease is truly present, given a certain test result. If the result is positive, how likely is it that the person tested actually has the disease? Or if the result is negative, how likely is it that he or she actually does *not* have the disease?

Answers to these questions are provided by the *predictive value* of the test. It has two forms, positive (PV_+) or negative (PV_-), depending on the test result. Both can be estimated directly from a 2×2 table that summarizes the results of applying both the screening test and a gold standard for true disease status to a sample of screenees, as shown in Table 18–2.

In the results shown in Table 18–1, the PV_+ for the HemeSelect test was $22/440 = .05$. In other words, only 5% of screenees who had a positive HemeSelect test actually had colorectal cancer. This may at first seem surprising, in view of the fact that the HemeSelect test was already found in the same data to have sensitivity $= .688$ and specificity $= .944$. The relatively low PV_+ can be explained by noting that PV_+ depends not only on sensitivity and specificity, but also on the prevalence of the disease in the population screened. In this instance, a large majority of persons in whom the HemeSelect test was used did not have colorectal cancer to begin with. Even though the test was 94.4% specific, the 5.6% of persons without colorectal cancer who had a false positive HemeSelect test

Table 18–2. Measures of Screening Test Performance

	Condition Truly Present?	
SCREENING TEST RESULT	+	−
+	a	b
−	c	d

Sensitivity $= a/(a + c)$
Specificity $= d/(b + d)$
Positive predictive value $= PV_+ = a/(a + b)$
Negative predictive value $= PV_- = d/(c + d)$

comprised a large number of people, and 95% of the positive HemeSelect tests proved to be false positives.

In mathematical terms, sensitivity, specificity, PV_+, and PV_- can all be viewed as conditional probabilities. Let C_+ denote presence of the true disease condition, C_- absence of the condition, T_+ a positive test result, and T_- a negative test result. Then

$$\text{Sensitivity} = \Pr(T_+ \mid C_+)$$

$$\text{Specificity} = \Pr(T_- \mid C_-)$$

$$PV_+ = \Pr(C_+ \mid T_+)$$

$$PV_- = \Pr(C_- \mid T_-)$$

$$\text{Prevalence} = \Pr(C_+)$$

According to Bayes' theorem (Rosner, 1995),

$$\Pr(C_+ \mid T_+) = \frac{\Pr(C_+) \cdot \Pr(T_+ \mid C_+)}{\Pr(C_+) \cdot \Pr(T_+ \mid C_+) + (1 - \Pr(C_+)) \cdot (1 - \Pr(T_- \mid C_-))}$$

$$PV_+ = \frac{\text{Prevalence} \cdot \text{Sensitivity}}{\text{Prevalence} \cdot \text{Sensitivity} + (1 - \text{Prevalence}) \cdot (1 - \text{Specificity})} \quad (18.1)$$

A similar expression can be developed for PV_- as a function of sensitivity, specificity, and prevalence but is usually of less direct interest than for PV_+.

The strong dependence of PV_+ on prevalence can be seen in Table 18–3. It shows the expected PV_+ and PV_- of the HemeSelect test when applied as a screening test in several populations with prevalence of colorectal cancer varying from 1/10,000 to 100/10,000, assuming that sensitivity and specificity remain fixed at the values calculated earlier. Even in a population with 1% prevalence of

Table 18–3. Influence of Prevalence on the Expected
Predictive Value of the HemeSelect Test, Assuming
Sensitivity = .688 and Specificity = .944

PREVALENCE OF COLORECTAL CANCER[a]	PV_+	PV_-
1	0.0012	0.99997
5	0.0061	0.99983
10	0.0121	0.99967
50	0.0581	0.99834
100	0.1104	0.99667

[a] Cases per 10,000

colorectal cancer, only about 11% of screenees with a positive HemeSelect test would turn out to have colorectal cancer; the rest would be false positives. At lower prevalences of colorectal cancer, PV_+ is still lower. In contrast, PV_- varies relatively little and usually remains quite high: with low prevalence, the probability of *not* having the disease was high to begin with, and it becomes even higher if the screening test result is negative.

The fact that the positive predictive value of a screening test can be quite low in screened populations with low disease prevalence has several implications:

- It can affect how a positive screening test result should be interpreted, and perhaps how this information is communicated to the screenee. In many situations, a positive result does *not* imply that the screenee probably has the disease.
- Persons with a positive screening test result must usually be evaluated further to determine whether the result was a true positive or a false positive. Even if it is expected in advance that a large majority will be false positives, all positives must be evaluated further in order to separate the true positives from the false positives. Any costs, discomfort, and risks involved in these follow-up evaluations must be considered a potentially important part of the overall burden of a screening program. In some instances, the costs of the follow-up evaluations can exceed the direct cost of the initial screening tests.
- It affects choice of a target population for screening. For many diseases, the prevalence of undiagnosed disease varies markedly among population subgroups. Subgroups in which prevalence is highest can yield both more cases per screening test administered and more true positives per positive screening test.

Likelihood Ratio

The *likelihood ratio (LR)* is another widely used measure of test performance, especially in clinical circles. It can be applied to both screening tests and diagnostic tests. *LR* can take on a different value for each possible test result. For a certain result, say X, the corresponding *LR* is

$$LR_X = \frac{\Pr([T = X] \mid C_+)}{\Pr([T = X] \mid C_-)}$$

In words, it is the probability of test result X when the underlying condition present, divided by the probability of test result X when the condition is absent. For a test with a binary result—positive (T_+) or negative (T_-)—the *LR* can be expressed as

$$LR_+ = \frac{\Pr(T_+ \mid C_+)}{\Pr(T_+ \mid C_-)} = \frac{\text{Sensitivity}}{1 - \text{Specificity}}$$

$$LR_- = \frac{\Pr(T_- \mid C_+)}{\Pr(T_- \mid C_-)} = \frac{1 - \text{Sensitivity}}{\text{Specificity}}$$

The *LR* provides a convenient way to update the probability that the disease is present, once a particular test result has been obtained. For example, in medical diagnosis, the clinician is concerned with the probability that a patient has a certain disease. Before a diagnostic test is done, he or she has a *prior* probability estimate in mind. That prior probability may simply be the prevalence of the disease, or it may be a subjective probability based on other information already known about the patient. After the test result becomes available, the estimated probability may be revised based on this new knowledge, and it becomes a *posterior* probability.

The *LR* enters this process as diagrammed in Figure 18–3. The steps from the prior probability to the posterior probability are:

$$\text{Prior odds} = \frac{\text{Prior probability}}{1 - \text{Prior probability}}$$

$$\text{Posterior odds} = \text{Prior odds} \times LR_X$$

$$\text{Posterior probability} = \frac{\text{Posterior odds}}{1 + \text{Posterior odds}}$$

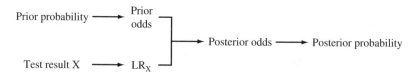

Figure 18–3. Application of Likelihood Ratio.

This process is actually just another way to apply Bayes' theorem (Rosner, 1995). Its appeal is that the arithmetic at each step is easy.

Example: Whooley and colleagues (1997) sought a rapid way to screen medical outpatients for depression, a disease that is common, disabling, treatable, and often unrecognized. They studied a combination of two questions: *(1)* "During the past month, have you often been bothered by feeling down, depressed, or hopeless?" and *(2)* "During the past month, have you often been bothered by little interest or pleasure in doing things?" Answering yes to at least one of these questions was found to be 96% sensitive and 57% specific for depression relative to a gold-standard structured psychiatric interview. Thus, $LR_+ = .96/(1 - .57) = 2.2$, and $LR_- = (1 - .96)/.57 = .07$.

Suppose that, in a certain clinic population, the prevalence of depression is thought to be about 10%. If a typical patient in this setting answers yes to one or both screening questions, the probability that he or she truly has depression can be calculated as follows, starting with .10 as the estimated prior probability:

$$\text{Prior odds} = .10/(1 - .10) = .11$$

$$\text{Posterior odds} = .11 \times 2.2 = .24$$

$$\text{Posterior probability} = .24/(1 + .24) = .19$$

Hence the probability of depression being present in such a patient is approximately doubled if a positive screening-test result is obtained. Nonetheless, this posterior probability remains less than 20% because the two-question combination has relatively low specificity. In contrast, if such a patient answers no to both questions, similar calculations using $LR_- = .07$ at the second step yield a posterior probability of only .0077, virtually ruling out the presence of depression in that person.

EVALUATING THE EFFECTIVENESS OF SCREENING

Screening for high blood pressure is commonly performed by providers of health care when they practice preventive medicine. Their basis for judging the likely benefit patients will derive, collectively, from this maneuver comes from several different sorts of research. The first documents the proportion of persons who test "positive," i.e., what fraction of them will have high blood pressure as determined by sphygmomanometer readings. The second estimates the excess risk of the conditions such as myocardial infarction and stroke to which hypertension (as measured by the sphygmomanometer) predisposes. The last type of study investigates the degree to which treatment of screen-detected high blood pressure can reduce the excess risks.

As a means of illustrating how data obtained in these studies can be put to use, let us assume that we are trying to estimate the benefit to be achieved by obtaining a blood pressure reading on an asymptomatic male patient for whom there has been no recent screening. Based on his demographic characteristics, the medical literature suggests there is a ten % likelihood that he has high blood pressure. It also suggests that, although the five-year cumulative combined incidence of myocardial infarction and stroke in normotensive men would be 30 per 1000, among those with hypertension, the corresponding incidence in the absence of treatment would be 60 per 1000. In a hypothetical group of 10,000 men just like this patient, the above assumptions would generate the observations shown in Table 18–4.

Now, assume that the results of prior research suggest that the prescription of antihypertensive therapy is associated with a 30% reduction in the risk of myocardial infarction and stroke. If this were true for men such as our patient, the five-year cumulative incidence once treatment had been instituted would be 60 per $1000 \times 0.7 = 42$ per 1000. In the group of 10,000 men, the experience would be as shown in Table 18–5.

From a comparison of Tables 18–4 and 18–5, we can see that screening for high blood pressure in 10,000 men demographically similar to our patient can be

Table 18–4. Five-Year Cumulative Incidence of Myocardial Infarction and Stroke in 10,000 Men in Whom There Is No Screening for, or Treatment of, High Blood Pressure

BLOOD PRESSURE	MYOCARDIAL INFARCTION OR STROKE	NO. OF MEN
Elevated	60	1000
Normal	270	9000
Total		10,000

Table 18–5. Five-Year Cumulative Incidence of Myocardial Infarction and Stroke in the Presence of Screening for, and Treatment of, High Blood Pressure

BLOOD PRESSURE	MYOCARDIAL INFARCTION OR STROKE	NO. OF MEN
Elevated	$60 \times 0.7 = 42$	1000
Normal	270	9000
Total		10,000

expected to lead to $60 - 42 = 18$ fewer cases of myocardial infarction over the next five years.

The positive impact of many screening tests can be gauged through a process such as the foregoing; that is, by compiling the results of studies evaluating the separate components necessary for effectiveness. The magnitude of the benefit obtained from screening people with diabetes for retinopathy (a form of ocular pathology detectable by retinal photography or ophthalmoscopy) has been estimated in this way, by taking results from separate studies that have documented:

1. The prevalence of retinopathy in people with diabetes
2. That retinal screening can identify abnormalities that are strong predictors of the development of blindness; and
3. That laser photocoagulation therapy for the changes found on screening can reduce the incidence of severe visual impairment (Early Treatment Diabetic Retinopathy Study Group, 1987).

But what is to be done if all patients who are screened as "positive" on a particular test (and, after confirmatory tests, are deemed to truly have the condition in question) happen to receive treatment? For example, persons who are screened for the presence of cancer and found to have it are almost never left untreated. Thus, while it is not difficult to determine: *(1)* the prevalence of malignancy at the time of screening, or *(2)* that a positive screening test result can predict an adverse outcome from a particular cancer, and can do so earlier than otherwise would be possible— perhaps by comparing the distribution of tumor size or stage in screened and unscreened persons diagnosed with that cancer—it is usually not possible to clearly answer the third necessary question: Does treatment given at the time of early detection lead to a more favorable outcome than treatment given when the cancer is clinically manifest? In situations such as this, it is necessary to resort to a generally more cumbersome approach: a comparison of the subsequent occurrence of untoward outcomes in screened and unscreened persons. That approach assesses the aggregate impact of the frequency of test positivity, the ability of the test result to predict an adverse outcome, and the efficacy of treatment for test-positive individuals. It will hereafter be referred to as a "one-step" design (Weiss, 1996).

The remainder of this chapter outlines the types of one-step designs available to evaluate a screening test's ability to lead to improved outcomes.

Randomized Trials and Cohort (Follow-up) Studies

It may be possible to assign study participants at random to be offered or not to be offered the test (or a program of testing). Alternatively, one can exploit (with appropriate caution when interpreting the results) the fact that in the normal course of medical or public health practice, some persons are tested while others are not, and these two groups can be monitored for the outcome(s) of interest.

Example: The first type of one-step design is illustrated by a randomized trial conducted in the state of Minnesota on the effectiveness of screening for fecal occult blood in leading to a reduction in mortality from cancer of the colon and rectum (Mandel et al., 1999). During 1976–1977, 46,551 residents of the state agreed to be assigned at random to one of three study arms: *(1)* annual screening; *(2)* biennial screening; and *(3)* usual care. The program of screening was conducted through 1982, and then again during 1986–1992. Persons who tested positive (during the course of the study they comprised approximately 20% of those assigned to be screened) received a full evaluation for colorectal cancer, including a colonoscopy. Follow-up for mortality extended for up to 18 years. For study participants who died, medical records were obtained. If the decedent had known or suspected gastrointestinal disease at the time of death, cause of death was judged by an expert panel, the members of which were blinded as to the decedent's screening assignment. The cumulative mortality from colorectal cancer per 1000 in the three groups was 9.46, 11.19, and 14.09, respectively, suggesting that a program of annual or biennial screening of this type could indeed lead to a reduction in the death rate from colon and rectal cancer.

Randomized trials have now been conducted to evaluate the efficacy of a variety of screening tests including, as examples, prenatal ultrasound exams (Ewigman et al., 1993; Bucher and Schmidt, 1993), intrapartum fetal heart rate monitoring (Mahomed et al., 1994), routine cervical evaluation during pregnancy (Buekens et al., 1994), electronic home uterine monitoring in women at high risk of premature delivery (U.S. Preventive Services Task Force, 1993), and mammography and clinical breast exam (Shapiro et al., 1982; Miller et al., 2000).

In a cohort study of a test's ability to influence the outcome of illness, Neutra et al. (1978) compared neonatal mortality among children delivered by mothers who received fetal monitoring during labor with that among children whose mothers had not been monitored. This study took place in a hospital during a period of time in which fetal monitoring was being introduced. The choice of patients to undergo monitoring was made by each woman's physician, not by the investigators (who conducted the study in retrospect through the use of the hospital's records).

Ideally, all evaluations of screening test effectiveness would be randomized: assignment of patients to screen or no-screen groups in a random way assures that the only differences between the two groups that might be relevant to the outcome in question are those that occur by chance. This is decidedly not the case in non-randomized studies, as there may be important differences that have the potential to distort (i.e., confound) the true benefit, or lack thereof, associated with use of the test. In the fetal monitoring study, for example, the investigators discovered in their review of records that a relatively higher proportion of mothers who did not receive monitoring had characteristics that predict an increased risk of mortality in the child: short gestation, breech presentation, placenta previa, and so on. Failure to have measured these characteristics, or failure to have taken them into account in the analysis, would have resulted in a comparison erroneously favorable to the monitored group and would have led to an overestimation of the benefit associated with monitoring.

Which Subjects Are to Be Compared?

In most randomized trials and cohort studies evaluating the effectiveness of screening tests, the only comparison that can be made is of the overall occurrence of the outcome in the screened versus unscreened groups. In a childhood blood-lead screening evaluation, for instance, one would compare the prevalence of retardation in children who did and did not receive screening. The lead levels in the unscreened group would never be known, so even if the investigators wished to compare outcomes in only those persons with elevated levels in each group, it would be impossible to do so.

Some conditions for which screening is done will, after a period of time, be evident even without the benefit of the test. Most cancers fall into this category, and there has been a temptation to evaluate the effectiveness of cancer screening tests by comparing mortality from the particular cancer in cases found through screening with that in other cases. Giving in to this temptation could lead to an erroneous estimate of the effectiveness of screening, primarily due to the influence of what is known as lead-time bias.

The reason for this bias is illustrated in the following example. Suppose 100 individuals are screened for cancer X, a cancer for which treatment is, in fact, ineffective. On the average, the test succeeds in identifying the cancer one year before it is clinically evident. Four persons in the group are detected as having cancer X, and the course of their illness is shown in Figure 18–4.

Two deaths occur among the four persons with cancer X in the 13 person-years that occur following screening $(3 + 4 + 2 + 4$; see Figure 18–4), and their mortality rate is 2 per 13 person-years. Had the screening not been performed, however, the same two deaths among four cases in 100 persons would occur (since no effective treatment follows early detection). But the number of person-years accruing in these cases from the time of their diagnosis (one year later than that for the screened cases) would be only 9 $(2 + 3 + 1 + 3)$ and the resulting mortality rate would be higher, 2 per 9 person-years. Since screening could not lead to improved mortality, one must conclude that there is something faulty in this method of

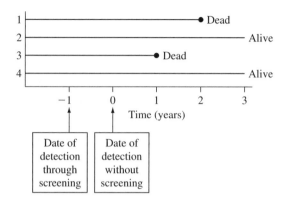

Figure 18–4. Lead Time in Studies of the Efficacy of Screening.

comparison. (If, instead of using mortality rates, the measure of outcome were n-year survival, the bias would still be present. Thus the 1.5-year survival in the cases found through screening is 100%, whereas the 1.5-year survival in the other cases is 75%, even though the two groups had, in truth, an identical survival experience.)

What is faulty, of course, is that the starting point for monitoring mortality rates is different between the screened and unscreened cases, always to the apparent detriment of the cases detected without screening. The appropriate comparison to make is the mortality experience (with respect to that cancer), not of the cases alone, but of the screened group with that of an unscreened group, *with both groups monitored from the time of screening*. In the above example, the mortality rate in the screened group is 2 deaths in 397 person-years (98 persons × 4 years, plus 1 person × 2 years, plus 1 person × 3 years). In a comparable unscreened group, the rate would be the same since the number of person-years, counted from the time the screening would have taken place had it been done, is identical to that for the screened group. Given that the natural history of this cancer is not altered by screening, this comparison of screened and unscreened groups that indicates no benefit associated with screening is clearly the preferred one.

Patients who have a long preclinical-but-detectable phase of disease are more readily found via screening than are patients with that disease whose preclinical phase is short. To the extent that the length of the preclinical phase correlates with the length of the illness once it has been detected, those whose disease was found via screening will appear to have a better survival rate, even in the absence of treatment that influences the disease's natural history. This possible artifact, due to what has been termed "length-biased sampling" (Zelen, 1976), was noted in Chapter 4 and is another reason that a comparison of survival in persons whose disease was detected by screening with that of other diseased persons will be misleading.

Other One-Step Studies of Screening Effectiveness

Ecological studies

The use of a screening test often varies widely from place to place around the world, and within one place often varies widely across periods of time. Yet because of the problems surrounding the interpretation of many ecological studies (referred to in Chapter 12), we are not often able to infer very much from correlations between population-wide screening levels and the incidence in those populations of the outcome that the screening test sought to prevent. Nonetheless, there are occasional exceptions, and it is instructive to consider what circumstances need to exist in order for an ecological study of screening effectiveness to be informative.

Example: A program of cervical screening of Icelandic women aged 25 to 59 years was begun in 1964. Whereas only occasionally would women have received screening prior to that time, by the early 1970s some 80% of the target population had been examined at the screening clinic. Some women 60 years and over were screened as well, but not in any appreciable numbers until after 1970. The mortality rate from cervical cancer during 1955–1974 is shown in Table 18–6. In 25- to 59-year-old women, a rise in mortality during 1955–1969 was reversed in 1970–1974. In women 60 to 89 years old, the group that underwent little screening, there was no systematic variation in either rate during the interval (Johannesson et al., 1978).

Table 18–6. Mortality from Cervical Cancer in Iceland, 1955–1974

AGE (YEARS)	Rate of Cervical Cancer[a]			
	1955–59	1960–64	1965–69	1970–74
25–59	11.7	16.8	26.5	12.2
60–89	27.6	33.3	28.2	34.8

[a] Rate per 100,000 person-years, age-adjusted (5-year groups) to a uniform standard.
[*Source:* Johannesson et al. (1978).]

Was it the screening that was responsible for this difference between the "populations" (i.e., the 25- to 59-year-old Icelandic women before and after the mass screening)? Features of the study's setting, design, and results that favor an affirmative answer to this question are as follows:

- The difference in the level of screening between the time periods was very great, rising from near zero before 1964 to 80% within 10 years.
- Reliable data were available on mortality from cervical cancer throughout the relevant time interval.
- The size of the population in each time period was large enough to provide enough cervical cancer deaths for meaningful analysis.
- There is evidence to indicate that in the absence of screening, the mortality rates among 25- to 59-year-old women would not have fallen: (a) Prior to the introduction of mass screening, the rates in women in this age group actually had been on the increase; and (b) in the Icelandic women who were largely unscreened—women aged 60 to 89—there was no corresponding decrease in mortality from cervical cancer during 1970–1974.
- The mortality in 1970–1974 was reduced to such a large degree that it is implausible that other, unmeasured changes during the period could have been solely responsible.

These are precisely the features that are rarely present *together* in most ecological evaluations of the efficacy of screening.

Case-control studies

These studies differ in some respects from case-control studies of etiologic factors. "Cases" are defined, not as individuals who developed a particular disease, but rather as those who have developed progressive disease or complications (such as death) that one is seeking to prevent by early detection. "Controls" are defined as persons without progression or complications who were otherwise comparable to the cases just prior to the time their disease had been detected. Thus, if the cases were persons who died of colorectal cancer, controls would be selected to be representative of the population at risk for development of colorectal cancer at the time the cases were first diagnosed. Records of the two groups would be examined to determine which persons had undergone screening—perhaps by means of a test for fecal occult blood—during a period of time prior to diagnosis in which a tumor or a detectable antecedent of a tumor plausibly could be identified by the test (or, for controls, a corresponding period). The data would be displayed as in Table 18–7.

Screening for fecal occult blood would be effective in reducing mortality in proportion to the amount by which $b/(b + d)$ exceeded $a/(a + c)$ (Weiss et al., 1992). The relative mortality from colorectal cancer associated with a history of

Table 18–7. Layout of Data for a Case-Control
Study of Fecal Occult Blood Testing for
Colorectal Cancer

SCREENING FOR FECAL OCCULT BLOOD	Death from Colorectal Cancer	
	YES	NO
Performed	a	b
Not performed	c	d

screening during this interval would equal the relative odds of screening between cases and controls; that is, $a/c \div b/d$ (see Chapter 9 for the derivation of this formula). If, perhaps, 20% of those who died of colorectal cancer had undergone screening for fecal occult blood during the two-year period ending just before diagnosis, in contrast to 30% of controls during the same interval, the relative mortality associated with screening would be $20/80 \div 30/70 = .58$.

Three features of the design and analysis of case-control studies of screening efficacy are worthy of mention:

1. Persons selected as cases should be ill or disabled to a degree that diagnosis would occur in the absence of screening (Morrison, 1982). For a disease such as cancer, the criterion for selection could be death from cancer (or possibly the presence of late-stage disease that is not believed to be curable), irrespective of the stage at which the cancer was first diagnosed.

2. Persons selected as controls should be representative of the population that generated the cases with respect to the presence and/or level of screening activity (Weiss, 1983). A control group restricted to those with earlier or less severe forms of the condition under study (e.g., early-stage cancer) is not appropriate. The fact that the condition is detected early in such persons is probably the result of their having been screened. Thus, even if screening were not followed by any effective therapy, a case-control difference would exist: the controls' level of screening would be higher than that of the population the cases arose from, falsely suggesting a benefit associated with screening. A bias of this sort is the case-control analogue of lead-time bias in follow-up studies. While the appropriate control group would not exclude persons with early or mild disease, it would include them only in proportion to their numbers in the population.

Example: In a case-control study that seeks to determine if cytological screening for cervical cancer leads to a reduction in mortality from the disease, one would not choose as controls women with in situ lesions. The presence of in situ cervical neoplasia is rarely discovered in the absence of screening, so virtually every member of the control group will have had at least one screening examination. It is unlikely that such a high level of screening activity would occur among women in the population that gave rise to the patients who died from cervical cancer. The selection of women with in situ cancer as controls would produce a finding of apparent benefit from cytological screening even if there were no effective treatment for the lesions discovered this way.

---

3. As is the case with all non-randomized strategies for assessing the effectiveness of screening, a spurious result is possible unless factors that are correlated both with the level of screening activity and with the occurrence of late-stage disease or mortality are taken into account (Weiss, 1994). Factors can be related to the occurrence of late-stage disease by virtue of their relationship to disease incidence per se, or to the likelihood of disease progression or spread. Thus, in a study of breast self-examination in relation to the occurrence of late-stage breast cancer it would be necessary to evaluate (and possibly adjust for) characteristics that are associated with breast cancer incidence (e.g., race and educational level) and that differ between cases and controls. Similarly, adjustment would have to be made if women who regularly performed breast self-examination also more commonly received the benefit of other detection methods for breast cancer (such as mammography and clinical examination), if the analysis found these other methods to have been efficacious.

EXERCISES

1. Lichtenstein and colleagues (1988) studied alternative methods for detecting hearing impairment in the elderly. One method determined whether a subject could hear a tone emitted by a handheld audioscope at a standardized frequency and loudness level. Another method asked subjects to complete a 10-item questionnaire, the Hearing Handicap Inventory for the Elderly—Screening version (HHIE-S). Each of these tests was evaluated against a gold standard, pure-tone audiometry administered at a hearing evaluation center.

    In the elderly population studied, 30% of patients proved to have impaired hearing by pure-tone audiometry. The audioscope test had sensitivity = .94

and specificity $= .72$, while the HHIE-S test (at a cutoff score of 24) had sensitivity $= .41$ and specificity $= .92$.

(a) Suppose that you are a physician in that setting, evaluating a typical elderly patient for hearing impairment. You have just obtained a positive result with the audioscope test. How likely is it that your patient actually has hearing impairment?

(b) Suppose that, to the same patient, you had administered the HHIE-S test first instead of the audioscope test, and obtained a positive HHIE-S result. How likely is it under this scenario that your patient has hearing impairment?

(c) When the audioscope test was administered to the same patients in a hearing evaluation center, its specificity was found to be significantly greater than when it had been administered in a physician's office—0.90 vs. 0.72. Why do you suppose that was?

2. The following is excerpted from a news item in the May 17, 2000, issue of the *Journal of the National Cancer Institute:*

Some Promising Biomarkers for Cancer

LPA (lysophosphatidic acid). LPA is probably the most accurate marker we have for detection of early stage ovarian cancer. A 1998 report found 9 of 10 women with stage I disease, 24 of 24 with advanced disease, and 14 of 14 with recurrent ovarian cancer had elevated blood LPA levels. In contrast, just 5 of 48 controls had elevated LPA. A growth factor, LPA is not generally present in normal ovary cells.

Based on the above information, you believe it is *un*likely that blood LPA levels will be of practical use as a screening tool for ovarian cancer. Why?

3. Several case-control studies have been conducted to estimate the degree to which mortality from breast cancer might be reduced by early detection through regular breast self-examination (BSE). In some studies, women whose cancers were diagnosed at late and early stages (i.e., cases and controls, respectively) were compared with respect to the proportion who had been performing BSE on a regular basis. Even if the information obtained on BSE practices were completely accurate, and cases and controls were comparable with regard to risk factors for late-stage breast cancer, the results of such studies could suggest a falsely great benefit associated with BSE. Why is this?

ANSWERS

1. (a) The likelihood ratio for a positive audioscope test is sensitivity/(1 − specificity) $= .94/(1 - .72) = 3.36$. Since your patient is "typical," it is

reasonable to use the overall prevalence of hearing impairment in this population, 0.3, as an estimate of the *prior* probability of hearing impairment. Once a positive audioscope test result is obtained, the *posterior* probability of hearing impairment can be calculated as follows:

$$\text{Prior odds} = \frac{\text{Prior probability}}{1 - \text{Prior probability}}$$

$$= 0.3/(1 - 0.3) = .428$$

$$\text{Posterior odds} = \text{Prior odds} \times LR_+$$

$$= .428 \times 3.36 = 1.44$$

$$\text{Posterior probability} = \frac{\text{Posterior odds}}{1 + \text{Posterior odds}}$$

$$= 1.44/(1 + 1.44) = .59$$

(b) The likelihood ratio for a positive HHIE-S test at this cutoff is $.41/(1 - .92) = 5.13$. Substituting this value for 3.36 in the above calculations gives a posterior probability of .69.

Note that a positive HHIE-S test is stronger evidence in favor of hearing impairment than is a positive audioscope test. This is because the higher specificity of the HHIE-S outweighs its lower sensitivity when calculating LR_+, resulting in a larger LR_+.

For your interest, try repeating the calculations, assuming that each test instead yields a *negative* result. You should find that a negative audioscope test is stronger evidence against hearing impairment than is a negative HHIE-S test. This is because the greater sensitivity of the audioscope test outweighs its lower specificity when LR_- is calculated.

(c) The researchers speculated that the higher ambient noise level in a physician's office may have caused more false positives in that setting. Patients may have been unable to hear the audioscope tone in the presence of other distracting sounds, which were not present in the hearing evaluation center's purposefully quiet environment. This could be a good example of how a test's specificity (or sensitivity) can depend on the specific setting and target population in which it is applied.

2. If the prevalence of ovarian cancer among screened women is low, the number of false positive tests would greatly exceed the number of true positives. For example, if the prevalence of cancer were 1/2000, and if LPA were 100%

Table 18–8. Expected Results of Applying the LPA Test to a
Hypothetical Population of 20,000 Women

| LPA | Ovarian Cancer | | TOTAL |
	YES	NO	
Positive	10	$5/48 \times 19,990 = 2082$	2092
Negative	0	$43/48 \times 19,990 = 17,908$	17,908
Total	10	19,990	20,000

sensitive in identifying ovarian cancer, Table 18–8 shows the expected results in 20,000 screened women.

The predictive value of a positive test would be just $10/2092 = 0.005$, very likely too low to warrant use of LPA for early detection. Unless a test has an extremely high level of specificity—more than $43/48$—it will not serve well for the early detection of an uncommon condition.

3. • The goal of early detection is to prevent the occurrence of late-stage disease at any time, not merely at diagnosis. Thus the criteria for selection of "cases" should not have been based solely on information available at the time of diagnosis. Cases who should have appeared (but did not) in these studies— women who only developed late-stage breast cancer at some time after the initial diagnosis of their disease—may have had early cancer found by BSE. Failure to include them in the case group would falsely inflate the measured efficacy of BSE.

   • The BSE practices of women with breast cancer diagnosed at an early stage are almost certainly not typical of those of the population of women from which the late-stage cases arose. In most instances, BSE or other early detection activity will have been responsible for the early diagnosis. Restriction of the control group to these women with higher-than-average early detection activity will cause the control-case difference in the proportion performing BSE to be falsely large, and thus the odds ratio estimating relative mortality from breast cancer in women who perform BSE to be falsely low.

Case-control studies that seek to estimate the degree of reduction in breast cancer mortality afforded by BSE need to choose, as cases, women who develop metastatic breast cancer (i.e., women who are very likely to die of the disease) during a defined period of time, irrespective of the date of diagnosis of their primary tumor. Such studies should identify as controls a representative sample of women at risk for the development of breast cancer in that population from which the cases arose.

ACKNOWLEDGMENT

Parts of this chapter were adapted from Weiss (1996).

REFERENCES

Allison JE, Tekawa IS, Ransom LJ, Adrain AL. A comparison of fecal occult-blood tests for colorectal-cancer screening. N Engl J Med 1996; 334:155–59.

Bucher HC, Schmidt J. Does routine ultrasound scanning improve outcome in pregnancy? Meta-analysis of various outcome measures. BMJ 1993; 307:13–16.

Buekens P, Alexander S, Boutsen M, Blondel B, Kaminski M, Reid M. Randomised controlled trial of routine cervical examinations in pregnancy. European Community Collaborative Study Group on Prenatal Screening. Lancet 1994; 344:841–44.

Early Treatment Diabetic Retinopathy Study Group. Treatment techniques and clinical guidelines for photocoagulation of diabetic macular edema. Ophthalmology 1987; 94:761–74.

Ewigman BG, Crane JP, Frigoletto FD, LeFevre ML, Bain RP, McNellis D. Effect of prenatal ultrasound screening on perinatal outcome. RADIUS Study Group. N Engl J Med 1993; 329:821–27.

Johannesson G, Geirsson G, Day N. The effect of mass screening in Iceland, 1965–74 on the incidence and mortality of cervical carcinoma. Int J Cancer 1978; 21:418–25.

Last JM. "Scope and methods of prevention." Chapter 1 in Last JM, Wallace RB (eds.). Maxcy-Rosenau-Last public health and preventive medicine. Norwalk, Conn.: Appleton & Lange, 1992.

Lichtenstein MJ, Bess FH, Logan SA. Validation of screening tools for identifying hearing-impaired elderly in primary care. JAMA 1988; 259:2875–78.

Mahomed K, Nyoni R, Mulambo T, Kasule J, Jacobus E. Randomised controlled trial of intrapartum fetal heart rate monitoring. BMJ 1994; 308:497–500.

Mandel JS, Church TR, Ederer F, Bond JH. Colorectal cancer mortality: Effectiveness of biennial screening for fecal occult blood. J Natl Cancer Inst 1999; 91:437–47.

Miller AB, Baines CJ, Wall C. Canadian National Breast Screening Study: 13-year results of a randomized trial in women aged 50–59 years. J Natl Cancer Inst 2000; 92:1490–99.

Morrison AS. Case definition in case-control studies of the efficacy of screening. Am J Epidemiol 1982; 115:6–8.

Morrison AS. Screening in chronic disease (2nd ed.). New York: Oxford University Press, 1992.

Neutra RR, Fienberg SE, Greenland S, Friedman EA. Effect of fetal monitoring on neonatal death rates. N Engl J Med 1978; 299:324–26.

Rosner B. Fundamentals of biostatistics (4th edition). New York: Duxbury Press, 1995.

Sackett DL, Haynes RB, Tugwell P. "Early diagnosis." Chapter 5 in Clinical epidemiology: a basic science for clinical medicine (2nd ed.). New York: Little, Brown, 1991.

Shapiro S, Venet W, Strax P, Venet L, Roeser R. Ten- to fourteen-year effect of screening on breast cancer mortality. J Natl Cancer Inst 1982; 69:349–55.

U.S. Preventive Services Task Force. Home uterine activity monitoring for preterm labor. JAMA 1993; 270:371–76.

U.S. Preventive Services Task Force. Guide to clinical preventive services: Report of the U.S. Preventive Services Task Force (2nd ed.). Baltimore: Williams and Wilkins, 1996.

Weiss NS. Control definition in case-control studies of the efficacy of screening and diagnostic testing. Am J Epidemiol 1983; 188:457–60.

Weiss NS. Application of the case-control method in the evaluation of screening. Epidemiol Rev 1994; 16:102–8.

Weiss NS. Clinical epidemiology: The study of the outcome of illness (2nd ed.). New York: Oxford, 1996.

Weiss NS, McKnight B, Stevens NG. Approaches to the analysis of case-control studies of the efficacy of screening for cancer. Am J Epidemiol 1992; 135:817–23.

Whooley MA, Avins AL, Miranda J, Browner WS. Case-finding instruments for depression. Two questions are as good as many. J Gen Intern Med 1997; 12:439–45.

Zelen M. "Theory of early detection of breast cancer in the general population." In: Hensen JC, Mattheim WH, Rozencweig M (eds.). Breast cancer: Trends in research and treatment. New York: Raven Press, 1976.

19

OUTBREAK INVESTIGATION
Jane Koehler and Jeffrey Duchin

An *outbreak* of disease occurs when the number of new disease cases observed exceeds the number expected in a defined setting over a relatively short period of time. Technically, the terms *outbreak* and *epidemic* are defined similarly and are sometimes used interchangeably among epidemiologists. The terms have different connotations, however, especially among the media and the public. Because the term *epidemic* can conjure up images of fear and vulnerability in the public mind, many epidemiologists prefer to reserve its use for larger, more widespread, and longer-term elevations in disease incidence.

Outbreak investigations can serve several purposes:

- *Limit the scope and severity of an immediate threat to public health.* There may be effective disease-control interventions, such as treatment for infected persons, vaccine or antibiotic prophylaxis for susceptibles, or withdrawal of a contaminated product from distribution. Meningococcal meningitis, hepatitis A and B, pertussis, measles, and varicella are among the common communicable diseases for which effective pharmacological interventions are available. As an example of a controllable non-infectious disease outbreak, the sudden appearance of a cluster of a rare condition, eosinophilia-myalgia syndrome among women in New Mexico in 1990, was stopped when implicated lots of an L-tryptophan supplement contaminated with an industrial lubricant were recalled (Belongia et al., 1990).
- *Prevent future outbreaks.* Once an outbreak is understood, implementing changes in products or processes can help prevent a recurrence. For example, when a sudden outbreak of the rare disease toxic shock syndrome occurred in 1980, a series of investigations was conducted. The disease was found to be associated with the use of a new "super-absorbent" brand of tampons, which fostered bacterial growth. This type of tampon was removed from the market, the outbreak ended, and further outbreaks were prevented (Shands et al., 1980). The identification of a large outbreak of *E. coli* O157:H7 due to contaminated undercooked hamburger in 1992

resulted in widespread changes in standard procedures for cooking hamburgers in the fast food industry and a subsequent decline in outbreaks from this source (Bell et al., 1994). An outbreak of salmonellosis associated with contaminated "fresh-squeezed," commercially distributed, unpasteurized orange juice in 1998 led to changes in labeling requirements for unpasteurized juice in Washington State (Centers for Disease Control and Prevention, 1999). An investigation of mesothelioma cases in Florence, Italy, led to the discovery (and subsequent cessation) of the re-use of polypropylene bags that had contained asbestos cement as baling material for fabrics (Weiss, 1991).

- *Identify new vehicles of infection.* Several outbreaks of disease due to enteric pathogens were associated with consumption of raw sprouts throughout the 1990s (Centers for Disease Control and Prevention, 2002a; Breuer et al., 2001; Mohle-Boetani et al., 2001). Subsequent research determined that seeds were often contaminated with enteric bacteria that thrived under sprouting conditions. These investigations resulted in a recommendation issued by the U. S. Department of Agriculture (USDA) and the Centers for Disease Control and Prevention (CDC) that raw sprouts not be consumed by young children, the elderly, and immunocompromised persons, who may be at increased risk for serious complications of enteric infections (U.S. Department of Health and Human Services, 1999).

- *Monitor the success of intervention programs.* The rapid emergence of *Salmonella* Enteritidis outbreaks associated with intact-shell eggs in the 1980s led to the discovery that this serotype of *Salmonella* had become adapted to the hen's ovary, and that even intact eggs could contain *S.* Enteritidis (St. Louis et al., 1988). The USDA, CDC, and the Food and Drug Administration worked with the egg industry to create programs to control exposure of laying hens to *S.* Enteritidis on the farm. The decreasing frequency with which intact-shell eggs were implicated in subsequent outbreaks of *S.* Enteritidis suggested that this intervention may have been effective in decreasing the prevalence of this pathogen in eggs (Mishu et al., 1994).

Outbreak investigations can also provide clues that good manufacturing practices or quality controls have broken down. Such a situation was revealed by the investigation of an outbreak of hyperthyroidism in a Minnesota town. A new, untrained employee at a small butcher shop decided that it was a waste to discard the thyroid glands of beef cattle and had begun adding them to his ground beef, resulting in thyrotoxicosis in consumers (Hedberg et al., 1987).

- *Identify new pathogens.* Legionnaire's disease was first described after a large outbreak of respiratory disease at an American Legion convention in

Philadelphia in 1976. Investigation of the outbreak led to the discovery of a new organism, now called *Legionella pneumophila,* in specimens obtained from outbreak cases (Fraser et al., 1977). It was found to have been transmitted in aerosols from outdoor cooling towers. Subsequently, many other cooling tower–associated outbreaks have been recognized, as well as other routes of transmission (Centers for Disease Control and Prevention, 2000; Den Boer et al., 2002). Similarly, although sporadic cases of the Acute Respiratory Distress Syndrome had been seen for years, investigation of an outbreak in the Four Corners area of the southwestern U.S. in 1993 led to the description of Hantavirus Pulmonary Syndrome and identification of a previously unrecognized etiological agent (Duchin et al., 1994). Such investigations can also reveal the mode of transmission, incubation period, spectrum of disease, and risk factors for infection. Even if the infectious agent causing illness is undetected at the time of the investigation, outbreaks often provide an opportunity to obtain historical specimens and epidemiologic data from cases that can prove valuable in later years when improved technologies for pathogen detection become available.

OUTBREAK DETECTION

The sequence of events leading up to an outbreak investigation typically begins when some kind of unusual health event in the community is detected. Sometimes the unusual event is the occurrence of even a single case of an uncommon disease that poses a clear threat to public health, such as botulism, paralytic shellfish poisoning, or anthrax. Often the unusual event is the recognition of two or more similar cases that appear to have occurred suspiciously close to each other in space or time—a *cluster* of cases—which may or may not represent an outbreak.

Common ways by which such unusual health events are detected include:

- *An astute health care worker.* Clinicians, infection control practitioners, and laboratory staff function as the eyes and ears of the public health system. In 1980, a report by an alert physician in California of an increase in the number of patients with *Pneumocystis carinii* pneumonia led to an investigation of what was originally called Gay-Related Immunodeficiency Syndrome. The disease is now known as AIDS (Centers for Disease Control and Prevention, 1981).
- *An ordinary citizen.* The borreliosis now known as Lyme disease was first recognized when the mother of a child diagnosed with rheumatoid arthritis, a condition uncommon in children, notified the local health department that she knew of at least three other cases of this disease in her neighborhood. The

subsequent investigation identified a new pathogen, *Borrelia burghdorferi,* and the tick vector responsible for the disease outbreak (Steere et al., 1977).

- *Reportable disease surveillance.* As was described in Chapter 6, each state publishes a list of communicable diseases and conditions that laboratories and health care providers are required to report to local public health authorities. Unfortunately, routine disease reports are frequently not timely or complete enough to be useful in rapidly detecting outbreaks, especially those due to common conditions. Patients may delay seeking care, appropriate specimens may not be collected or the right tests not ordered, laboratory processing and reporting of results can be delayed, and health-care providers and laboratories may not comply with reporting requirements.

  Nonetheless, frequent detailed analyses of routine surveillance data can be important in detecting smaller or geographically dispersed "hidden outbreaks" that may otherwise escape notice when total case reports remain relatively stable. For example, although overall rates of hepatitis A remained relatively stable in many areas during the 1990s, analyses of the age, sex, and geographic distribution of cases revealed an increased incidence among young men living in urban areas and led to recognition of increased transmission of hepatitis A among injecting drug users and men who have sex with men (Bell et al., 1998). In larger communities, surveillance data can even be reviewed on a daily basis, not only for unusual increases in total numbers of cases, but also for increases among subpopulations defined by age, gender, ethnicity, or geography.

- *Automated health data.* Especially for conditions that are either not reportable or for which passive surveillance is incomplete, automated data on health-care utilization inside or outside the hospital may provide information from large populations fairly efficiently. Recently there has been growing interest in surveillance using automated data for detection of outbreaks due to possible bioterrorism (Wagner et al., 2001).

VERIFYING AN OUTBREAK

What Is the Illness?

Once a suspected outbreak is identified, identifying the specific nature of the illness in question is an important early step. Usually this task involves reviewing the clinical case history and checking key laboratory results. For unusual conditions, verification may involve consulting with clinical or laboratory experts to assist with diagnosis. Even in the absence of a specific diagnosis, systematically summarizing the signs and symptoms of illness can help characterize the disease and develop a working case definition.

Is There a True Excess?

For uncommon conditions such as meningitis or rubella, or for highly contagious diseases against which effective actions to block transmission are available (such as measles or pertussis), even a single case should "raise a red flag" leading to an epidemiologic investigation. Single cases of these conditions require immediate public health investigation to attempt to identify the probable source and other persons at risk, and to formulate an intervention strategy to stop the further spread of disease. Single cases of certain noncontagious diseases, such as botulism, paralytic shellfish poisoning, and ciguatera poisoning, also require immediate investigation to allow prompt recall of contaminated food products before they are consumed by others.

In other instances, it is necessary to determine the degree to which the number of new cases or events observed truly exceeds the number expected in a given geographical area during a defined period of time. The expected number of "sporadic" cases is usually estimated from historical data. For diseases that are reportable by law to the local health department, baseline surveillance data for a comparable past time period will usually be available and can often be stratified by age, geographical location, and other variables. At other times, medical records, log books and other data will need to be reviewed. Data from health care institutions, including hospitals, microbiology laboratories and emergency departments, as well as outpatient facilities and clinicians' offices, may be useful sources with which to establish baseline incidence. For example, in investigating a cluster of cases of Legionnaire's disease, hospital records, including hospital pneumonia admissions, intensive-care-unit admissions and discharge diagnosis databases, would be good sources to identify the persons hospitalized with pneumonia during a given time interval.

Whenever possible, it is desirable to obtain comparison data from the previous weeks or months for comparison with the current figures to clearly identify the onset of the outbreak. For conditions for which data are available and may vary in incidence with time (e.g., expected seasonal variation), it is helpful to look at comparable time periods from recent years to establish baseline rates. Other potential sources of baseline data include cause of death from death certificates available through vital-statistics offices and disease registries. In the absence of standardized data sources, surveys of health-care providers may help in judging whether an increase in cases is occurring.

An apparent excess in the number of cases does not necessarily mean that an outbreak is in progress. Other possibilities to consider are:

- *Change in the population at risk.* As noted in Chapter 3, a simple case count can be adequate to compare incidence between time periods if it is safe to assume that the underlying population at risk is relatively constant. In some situations, however, this assumption is untenable—for example, in a community that has had rapid population growth or that experiences marked seasonal changes in population, such as tourist centers. To avoid this source of error, comparisons should be based on *rates,* not just case counts, whenever possible.

- *Change in case ascertainment.* Caution must be used when disease rates obtained from active or enhanced surveillance activities are compared with rates calculated using baseline or passively collected data. For example, conditions that routinely go under-reported will seem to increase when active or enhanced surveillance is used, but the increase in reports can simply reflect better ascertainment and not a true increase in disease incidence (Glatzel et al., 2002; Centers for Disease Control and Prevention, 1995). A common phenomenon during outbreaks is that more thorough and widespread diagnostic testing for the condition under question occurs, uncovering both outbreak-associated and sporadic cases that would otherwise go undiagnosed and unreported. As noted below, laboratory methods for characterizing relatedness of organisms ("molecular epidemiology") can also help distinguish outbreak-associated from unrelated background cases.

    Even when evaluating clusters of notifiable diseases in the absence of enhanced surveillance, it is important to consider whether some element of the reporting system has changed. The availability of a new laboratory test, changes in interpretation of test results (Weinbaum et al., 1998), heightened awareness of a new disease, a new physician in the community with particular expertise in a disease, improved disease-reporting by a new hospital infection-control practitioner, or changes in patient referral patterns among health-care providers can all produce apparent changes in incidence in the absence of any real change in disease occurrence (Centers for Disease Control and Prevention, 1997b; Adderson et al., 2000; Joce et al., 1995).

Are the Cases Related?

Besides being more numerous than expected, the cases in an outbreak are assumed to be related in some way. Sometimes links between them may not become apparent until after an investigation is in progress. But speciation, serotyping, serogrouping, and other subtyping data are informative laboratory-based epidemiologic tools that can help in judging whether a set of cases of illness due to an infectious agent may be connected or are simply a chance collection of sporadic cases (Centers for Disease Control and Prevention, 2002b).

For example, knowing only that an observed number of *Shigella* isolates in a given period of time exceeds the average number reported may not give the investigator much useful information. Examining the data by serogroup or species, however, can allow detection of increases in uncommon strains and additional investigation of clusters when appropriate. Similarly, careful monitoring and analysis of serogroup data from *Salmonella* isolates as soon as they are available can help an investigator detect an outbreak far earlier than waiting for results of the more time-consuming testing for serotype. If the majority of *Salmonella* cases are usually serogroups B, C1, and D, and suddenly three cases with *Salmonella* serogroup M are reported, an unusual event has almost certainly occurred, and an investigation can proceed even before the serotyping information on all cases is complete. Antibiotic sensitivity patterns are often readily available and can sometimes be used to help suggest or refute potential relatedness of strains isolated from cases.

Increasingly sophisticated molecular laboratory techniques make it possible to detect small clusters of cases as well as outbreaks due to related strains of common serotypes that would otherwise go unnoticed. For example, routine, rapid molecular typing of *Salmonella* and *E. coli* O157:H7 isolates by pulsed field gel electrophoresis (PFGE) or restriction fragment length polymorphism (RFLP) can detect clusters of related strains even when the total number of cases remains stable (Bender et al., 2001, 1997). A new CDC-sponsored surveillance tool for enteric disease pathogens, called PulseNet, enables laboratories across the country to compare PFGE patterns of local cases with isolates from other participating regions via the Internet (Swaminathan et al., 2001). This surveillance network can identify nationwide outbreaks that would have otherwise gone undetected, with only a few cases occurring in any single health jurisdiction. Application of molecular typing tools has also demonstrated that small, apparently unrelated clusters of *Salmonella* infection are often caused by related strains, suggesting that small "mini-outbreaks" may occur more frequently than previously identified.

INVESTIGATING AN OUTBREAK

The decision about whether to dedicate resources to the investigation of a cluster of illnesses depends on many factors. Outbreaks of a severe illness or outbreaks involving many cases normally prompt an investigation, as do those involving an unusual or newly recognized illness. Some investigations are conducted simply because the public, perceiving an "outbreak," demands that the situation be evaluated. The epidemiologist must anticipate and evaluate the needs of the community, the resources available, whether an effective public-health intervention exists, and the potential social and political consequences of the investigation (or of the failure to conduct one).

Overview of Steps

Although no two outbreaks evolve in exactly the same way, the steps commonly involved in investigating an outbreak are:

- Establish a case definition
- Enhance surveillance
- Describe occurrence of cases according to time, place, and person
- Develop hypotheses about the nature of exposure
- Conduct analytic studies, if appropriate
- Implement disease-control interventions
- Communicate results of the investigation

Each step is described below. Sometimes the pace of events is rapid, and the outbreak epidemiologist may need to anticipate and prepare for later steps before the results of earlier steps are complete.

A structured approach to managing outbreak investigations is desirable. The team leader(s) and other members of the outbreak investigation and response team should be identified and specific roles and responsibilities assigned. For large or complicated investigations, separate teams and leaders may be needed for surveillance, analytic epidemiologic studies, clinical investigation, environmental investigation, response activities and communication.

Establish a Case Definition

Collecting as much information as feasible on all potential cases early in the investigation can often help characterize the full spectrum of disease, save time in the long run, and help maximize the sample size available for later analysis. Once the disease symptomatology and laboratory findings have been established, an explicit working case definition is developed and applied consistently to all potential cases (Centers for Disease Control and Prevention, 1997a). As noted in Chapter 2, case definitions can include several clinical and/or laboratory criteria. A fairly loose case definition is useful early in an outbreak investigation to include as many potential cases as possible, while collecting enough specific information to enable refinement of the definition as the investigation progresses. Early cases are often categorized as *confirmed, probable,* or *possible,* depending on the extent to which a clinically compatible illness and laboratory confirmation are present.

Obtaining appropriate biological specimens for laboratory testing can be important to document potential cases as "confirmed," and also to identify otherwise obscure etiologic agents. For example, at the start of an investigation of a cluster of suspected salmonellosis cases in a nursing home that occurred over two weeks, one might initially consider anyone in the nursing home with a diarrheal illness during that two-week period as a possible case. Collecting additional information about the signs and symptoms of the clinical illness, such as presence of fever, duration of illness, and laboratory data including serogroup of salmonella isolates, allows further narrowing and refinement of the case definition. Later in the investigation, the case definition might thus become "any resident of the nursing home with culture-confirmed *Salmonella* Newport infection with onset between June 4 and June 16."

The goal of the case definition is to include all true cases and as few non-cases as possible. Inclusion of non-cases as cases, or of subclinical cases in the control group, results in misclassification, which weakens the ability to detect an association with the relevant risk factor(s) (see Chapter 10). For large outbreaks with many cases and high statistical power, misclassification may be less of a concern because it may still be possible to detect an attenuated association. If laboratory testing of each possible case is not feasible, a case definition can be created using a constellation of symptoms exhibited by the laboratory-confirmed cases. Refinement of case definitions can also be useful during the analysis of data.

Enhance Surveillance

When it is suspected that an outbreak is occurring, enhanced surveillance can be useful in identifying additional cases. Enhanced surveillance may involve both heightening awareness to increase passive case reports and implementing active surveillance. Techniques include contacting health-care providers and clinical laboratories by phone, fax, or e-mail, or implementing new reporting channels such as Internet-based reporting. For outbreaks requiring widespread notification of the health care community, a "broadcast fax" to area health-care providers, hospitals, emergency departments, laboratories, and other relevant groups can be employed. The message should contain current information about the outbreak, inform clinicians about the syndrome or case definition under surveillance, describe how reporting should be done, and provide contact numbers and resources for questions or additional information. Health department Web pages and

Internet-based communication methods such as LISTSERVs and message boards can also be effective ways to get information to the community rapidly.

For large outbreaks or public health emergencies, press releases and the print, radio, and television media can also be employed. Outbreak epidemiologists should therefore have a good working relationship with their department's public information officer, designated spokesperson, or media liaison. Using the news media allows communication directly to the public for identifying cases in persons who may not have sought medical attention and for disseminating disease control recommendations.

Describe Occurrence of Cases According to Time, Place, and Person

Descriptive analysis reveals useful information about the basic features of the cases, the population affected, the geographical scope of the problem, and the pace at which the outbreak is evolving. Early descriptive analyses can also suggest potential etiological agents, risk factors for acquisition, and mechanisms of transmission of infection. These clues can be a fertile source of hypotheses that can then be tested with analytic study designs, as described below.

To begin, a *line listing* of the cases is prepared, as illustrated in Table 19–1. It shows demographic characteristics and other key descriptors, including components of the case definition and laboratory test results. This format allows quick examination for obvious common features or unusual values. The line listing can be created by hand initially or for small outbreaks, or using computerized data management programs or spreadsheets to allow easy viewing of multiple variables.

Data in the line listing can be analyzed using simple descriptive statistics, such as percentages, means, and standard deviations. Characteristics of the illness can be summarized, and the most frequent signs and symptoms may suggest a likely differential diagnosis if the agent has not yet been identified.

If the disease has been definitively diagnosed, hypotheses regarding source of exposure and transmission can be developed based on known risk factors, incubation period, and known vehicles for that disease. For example, an outbreak of invasive *Listeria* infections among pregnant Hispanic women suggested a possible foodborne source, later found to be a home-produced unpasteurized Mexican cheese (Centers for Disease Control and Prevention, 2001). An outbreak of vomiting and diarrhea of 24 hours' duration among residents of a nursing home in January suggests that an outbreak of Norwalk-like virus might be occurring.

Plotting the location where cases reside, work, or engage in recreational activities on *spot maps* or using geographic information system (GIS) software can assist in identifying potential sources of exposure or routes of transmission.

Table 19–1. Example of a Line Listing of Data on Hepatitis A Cases

CASE #	INITIALS	DATE OF REPORT	DATE OF ONSET	MD Dx	Diagnostic Signs and Symptoms*						Lab HA IgM	Lab OTHER	AGE	SEX
					N	V	A	F	DU	J				
1	JG	10/12	10/6	Hep A	+	+	+	+	+	+	+	AST↑	37	M
2	BC	10/12	10/5	Hep A	+	−	+	+	+	+	+	ALT↑	62	F
3	HP	10/13	10/4	Hep A	±	−	+	+	+	S†	+	AST↑	30	F
4	MC	10/15	10/4	Hep A	−	−	+	+	?	−	+	HbSAg −	17	F
5	NG	10/15	10/9	NA	−	−	+	−	+	+	NA	NA	32	F
6	RD	10/15	10/8	Hep A	+	+	+	+	+	+	+		38	M
7	KR	10/16	10/13	Hep A	±	−	+	+	+	+	+	AST↑	43	M
8	DM	10/16	10/12	Hep A	−	−	+	+	+	−	+		57	M
9	PA	10/18	10/7	Hep A	±	−	+	±	+	+	+		52	F

*KEY:

S† = scleral   F = fever
N = nausea   DU = dark urine
V = vomiting   J = jaundice
A = anorexia   HA IgM = hepatitis A IgM antibody test

[*Source*: Adapted from Dicker (1998).]

John Snow used spot maps such as the one shown in Figure 7–7 in his investigations of the 1854 cholera epidemic in central London to illustrate the distribution of cholera cases in Golden Square, showing that cholera deaths were strikingly common around the Broad Street water pump (Snow, 1936).

Spot maps may be useful when the source of infection is unknown, in order to search for clustering of cases by location of home, work, or recreational activities. They can later be used to show important spatial or geographic relationships once the source or mode of transmission has been identified. Examples include outbreaks caused by exposure to contaminated aerosols, such as legionellosis associated with contaminated cooling towers, decorative fountains, or other sources of aerosol transmission; enteric infections resulting from exposure to contaminated recreational water; and institutional outbreaks in which visualizing spatial relationships among infected persons and potential sources of infection (other patients, environmental reservoirs, or caregivers) may be informative. For many outbreaks in a mobile society, however, cases will have been infected in distant locations, which will not be reflected in spot maps depicting only their local activities.

The *epidemic curve* is a standard part of the descriptive epidemiologic analysis. The date (or time) of onset is shown on the X-axis, while the number of new cases with onset in each date or time category is plotted on the Y-axis. Potentially significant case data, such as laboratory findings, confirmed versus possible cases, or exposure to some suspected risk factor, can be indicated with different colors or fill patterns.

To produce the most informative epidemic curve, the scale of the X-axis should depend on the incubation period of the disease (if known) and should include the pre-outbreak period to illustrate the background incidence of the disease. For most outbreaks, a useful scale will indicate time in units approximately one-quarter the length of the incubation period. If the disease being investigated has not yet been identified, plotting the data on a variety of scales may reveal a pattern.

When the usual incubation period of the disease is known, and if most or all cases in an initial wave were exposed at about the same time, the epidemic curve can often be used to reveal the likely time of that exposure. For example, consider the epidemic curve from an outbreak of hepatitis A, as shown in Figure 19–1. The incubation period of hepatitis A averages about 28 to 30 days, ranging from 15 to 50 days between exposure and onset of symptoms [Chin J (ed.), 2000]. Suppose that all of the cases shown were suspected of having resulted from a common exposure to a single index case. The analyst would count back 15 days from the earliest case, and 28 to 30 days from the peak of cases, to focus the investigation on a narrow range of days within which the common exposure may have occurred.

The shape of the epidemic curve often provides information about the likely mode of transmission. A "point source" outbreak, in which all cases were exposed

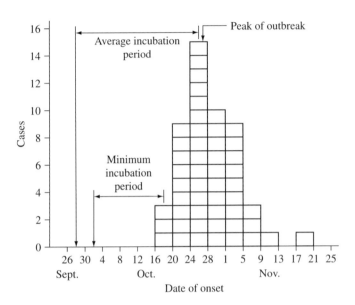

Figure 19-1. Epidemic Curve from an Outbreak of Hepatitis A (adapted from Dicker, 1998).

to a single source of infection (a common meal or highly contagious person, for example), classically exhibits a steep upswing and an early peak, followed by a gradual decline in cases (Fig. 19–1). All cases in a point source outbreak should also have onset of illness within one incubation period. Prolonged exposure of a population to a common source (such as a contaminated food product with a long shelf life) will produce a more "smeared-out" epidemic curve, in which onset of cases extends well beyond a single incubation period, reflecting a series of "mini-outbreaks." More and more such "mini-outbreaks" are being identified as molecular subtyping becomes increasingly available and rapid. In contrast, ongoing person-to-person (secondary) transmission classically produces an epidemic curve with a series of small peaks—ideally one incubation period apart, although such a regular pattern is often difficult to demonstrate.

The epidemic curve can also provide clues about the course of the outbreak: a rising curve suggests that the outbreak is in the early stages; a plateau, that transmission may be stable or decreasing; and a downward slope, that the outbreak is waning. This information is helpful in planning disease-control strategy, evaluating interventions, and communicating with local stakeholders, including elected officials and the public.

As the investigation develops and data on cases are entered into a database, more detailed and sophisticated epidemic curves can be created that convey additional information about primary and secondary cases and the timing of events and interventions.

Develop Hypotheses about the Nature of Exposure

The information needed for the initial line listing of cases and for initial descriptive analyses may be obtained through interviews with cases or medical record reviews. For most outbreaks of reportable diseases with well-recognized routes of transmission, standardized interview forms are available at local and state health departments and from the CDC. Staff of these agencies can often provide technical assistance as well.

For situations in which the clinical illness is not yet characterized, or the route or source of transmission appears to be new, an open-ended, unstructured interview with early cases and other key informants (such as family members or providers) can provide valuable information. These exploratory interviews should usually cover a wide range of potential risk factors and exposures, such as lifestyle characteristics, exposure to the outdoors, homelessness, or other factors. It is helpful if the same person can conduct these initial interviews. If the interviewer hears a similar story several times, patterns of exposure may emerge. Also, it is often worthwhile to ask the patient and family members where or how they think the illness was acquired. They may have already figured it out, and at the very least they will be more cooperative because they have been asked for their opinions. Other good sources of hypotheses can be subject-matter experts (infectious-disease specialists, public health veterinarians, laboratorians, toxicologists, industrial hygienists, water system or air handling experts, etc.) and the medical literature.

Outliers are cases that are unusual in some way—they "just don't fit in"—and these cases should be carefully scrutinized. Temporal outliers are usually easy to identify on the epidemic curve and often provide the key to understanding the basis for the outbreak. For instance, a single case occurring one incubation period before the other cases may represent an ill food-handler who contaminated a food product, or an index case who exposed a large group of susceptibles. Cases who were only in the geographic area a short time can, by their limited opportunities for exposure, also provide valuable information about means of transmission. Similarly, foodborne outbreaks in which most cases and controls ate the same food items can sometimes be solved if "dietary" outliers who consumed only one of several potentially contaminated items are identified.

Hypothesis generation will suggest a list of additional information needed, such as specific exposures, medical history, or laboratory data. This list of variables can then be used to develop more refined case investigation forms for use in collecting additional data.

Conduct Analytic Studies

Once a set of hypotheses has been developed, an analytic study—usually a case-control or cohort study—is often the appropriate next step.

Study design

Choice of a study design depends both on theoretical considerations (see Chapter 5), such as the frequency of the disease and of key exposures, and on logistics. If the outbreak occurs in a discrete, readily identified group, such as a wedding party or passengers on a cruise ship, a cohort study is the preferred option. As many members of the group as possible should be interviewed. (Cohort studies are discussed in Chapter 14.)

In contrast, if cases are few or occur among a widely scattered group, it may be more efficient to conduct a case-control study, sampling appropriate controls from the presumed population at risk. This study design is discussed at length in Chapter 15, but a few issues of special relevance to outbreak investigation will be highlighted here.

In an outbreak situation, the working case definition often limits cases in time and vicinity, and these limits should also pertain to controls. Ideally, controls should be persons who did not develop the disease but who met all other criteria that defined the cases. If the outbreak occurred among patrons of an outdoor rock festival, for example, controls should be chosen from among attendees of the festival; if at a potluck supper, from among the those who attended the supper (or unsuspecting family members who ate the leftovers).

Nonetheless, care should be taken not to match or restrict controls in such a way that exposure to a risk factor of interest is essentially predetermined. For example, consider an outbreak of shigellosis among children who visited a recreational area with a swimming pool. A reasonable control group would be children in the same age range without signs or symptoms of shigella infection who also frequented the recreational area during the incubation period of the cases. If one selected as controls only children who also swam in the pool (i.e., matched on swimming history), the analysis would not be able to determine whether exposure to the possibly contaminated water was a risk factor for infection.

Data collection

In general, the farther in time the investigation is conducted after the relevant exposure has taken place, the more difficult it is to get complete and accurate information from both cases and controls about potential risk factors of interest. In addition, with time it becomes more difficult for controls to recall events with as much certainty as cases, who were more affected. This difference can contribute to recall bias (see Chapter 15). Thus, the time spent to develop the data collection instruments must be balanced by the need for a prompt investigation. Invariably, the data instruments will appear flawed in retrospect. Outbreak investigation forms must often be created "on the fly," without the luxury of time for the methodical planning that is available in elective studies.

As in more elective analytic studies, attention should be paid to minimizing measurement error when collecting data. Helpful techniques include using pre-existing standardized questions or instruments; training field personnel to collect data in a standard way, especially if two or more of them are needed; and using visual aids such as calendars to help respondents recall the timing of events. Pilot testing of questionnaires and blinding of interviewers to disease status are desirable but often impossible in an outbreak situation.

Special care is needed in interviewing persons under the age of consent, which requires the permission of a parent or guardian. If interviews are conducted in person, the parent or guardian should be present. If interviews are by telephone, having the parent listen in on another phone line is often reassuring to the parent and can sometimes help the interviewee with recall.

It is important to collect biological specimens as soon as possible in the outbreak to establish the diagnosis, isolate the etiological agent, or further define the clinical syndrome. For presumed foodborne outbreaks, cases should be asked to retain and refrigerate any leftover suspect foods, including the original packaging when available. Outbreak investigators may need to issue recommendations to health-care providers and laboratories on appropriate diagnostic testing and handling of clinical specimens. Clinical laboratories often discard culture isolates and other diagnostic specimens after a few days unless specifically requested to do otherwise. Local laboratories should be contacted as early as possible to request that specimens be conserved or sent on to the local or state public health department laboratory.

Another reason for prompt specimen collection is that cases are never as interested in cooperating with the investigation as when they are currently or recently symptomatic. Once recovered, they soon tire of requests for additional stool specimens or blood samples, or even one more telephone interview. If specimen collection is crucial to the investigation, it is often worth the effort to send someone directly to the home or restaurant to collect appropriate specimens.

The environmental investigation is often carried out by an environmental health specialist working with the communicable disease epidemiologist, who should be explicit in specifying information needs. The first visit by the field team is the best opportunity to observe pertinent behaviors (e.g., food safety practices, hygiene, or infection control practices) and to obtain environmental samples. In foodborne outbreaks, information on suspect products and the methods of preparation may be crucial, including brand name, lot number, size of package used, expiration date, delivery date, and supplier (to assist in traceback efforts when indicated), as well as food preparation, holding, and storage conditions. Personnel (including supervisors) involved in handling and preparing implicated food items should be identified and interviewed about food preparation and handling practices and any recent illness. When possible, clinical specimens should be obtained from persons who are ill and/or are suspected of serving as a reservoir for the infectious agent.

Analysis

As data come in, they should be examined for completeness and consistency. For larger investigations, data are usually entered into a computer database. EpiInfo is a computer program developed specifically to support data management and analysis for outbreak investigations. It can be downloaded free of charge from http://www.cdc.gov/epiinfo. Preparing mock-up tables early, even before data-collection instruments are finalized, can help guide the analysis, identify gaps, and anticipate the need to reconcile data from different sources (e.g., different laboratories) onto a common scale.

Outbreaks often evolve over a short time, during which changes in the population at risk may be minor. Hence, disease frequency is often expressed in terms of the *attack rate*—technically, not a true "rate" but another term for cumulative incidence. The difference between the attack rates in persons with and without a certain exposure is thus the *attributable risk,* and the ratio of the two attack rates is the *relative risk,* as was discussed in Chapter 9. These measures of effect can be used to quantify associations, and hypotheses can be tested quickly using simple cross-tabulations (Bryan et al., 1999). In the example shown in Table 19–2, 120 persons out of 200 attendees became ill. The relative risk and the attributable risk for roast turkey both show a large positive association with illness, suggesting a possible causal relationship. Conversely, eating roast pork was negatively associated with illness, perhaps because those who chose pork avoided the turkey. The other associations are weak and do not suggest that these food items were related to becoming ill.

A second issue to consider is the fraction of cases that each exposure under consideration could account for—the population attributable risk percent—which depends on both the relative risk and the proportion of cases exposed to each item. In this example, while eating green beans was positively associated with illness ($RR = 1.18$), only 63 of the 120 ill persons recalled having eaten green beans, so that this exposure could account for only $(1.18 - 1)/1.18 \times 63/120 = .08 = 8\%$ of the cases. Roast turkey, besides being more strongly associated with illness, was eaten by 104 of the 120 ill persons and therefore could account for about $(4.35 - 1)/4.35 \times 104/120 = .67 = 67\%$ of cases.

Table 19–2. Attack Rate Table for a Hypothetical Foodborne Disease Outbreak ($N = 200$)

	Ate			Did Not Eat			ATTRIBUTABLE RISK	RELATIVE RISK
	ILL	NOT ILL	ATTACK RATE	ILL	NOT ILL	ATTACK RATE		
Roast turkey	104	15	104/119 = .87	16	65	16/81 = .20	+.67	4.35
Roast pork	15	45	15/60 = .25	105	35	105/140 = .75	−.50	0.33
Mashed potatoes	102	77	102/179 = .57	13	8	13/21 = .62	−.05	0.92
Green beans	63	34	63/97 = .65	57	46	57/103 = .55	+.10	1.18
Rolls	87	59	87/146 = .60	33	21	33/54 = .61	−.01	0.98
Apple pie	76	50	76/126 = .60	44	30	44/74 = .59	+.01	1.02

Implement Disease Control Interventions

The results of preliminary and analytic studies often implicate a particular exposure. Intervention approaches to prevent additional cases or future outbreaks depend on that exposure and on what is already known about the disease's mechanism of spread. Among many examples are recalling a contaminated food product from distribution, correcting deficient food-handling practices, and administering vaccine to susceptibles or immune globulin to those already exposed.

Communication

Effective, clear, and timely communication is a critical component of any outbreak investigation. Important target groups and forms of communication include:

- *The public.* Relevant information often includes the signs and symptoms of the disease, and recommendations for evaluation, treatment, and prevention of illness. Information can be disseminated through information hotlines with recorded messages, Web pages, press releases, or other news media channels (Covello et al., 2001; National Research Council, 1989). It is important to compose public information in clear language that is understandable by the community. Translation of materials into other languages and outreach to target specific cultural groups or hard-to-reach populations may be necessary.
- *Outbreak response team members.* Outbreak investigations often require coordinating the efforts of several people. Daily or more frequent team meetings are needed to review the status of the outbreak, share information, and update and revise the investigation and response plan. It may be useful to invite the public information officer and representatives from other affected local or state agencies to these sessions. The outbreak team leader needs to manage the overall response, anticipate where the investigation is headed, and ensure that adequate resources are available to sustain the investigation and response activities as long as necessary.
- *Public health and government officials.* It is a good idea for the outbreak epidemiologist to keep his or her supervisor aware of the status of an investigation. Health officers and elected officials often do not appreciate learning about outbreaks for the first time through inquiries from local news media. Rational and scientifically appropriate public health interventions can also be compromised when intense media attention and the resulting political considerations cause premature release of information or recommendations by elected officials before public health professionals have completed their review or investigation.

- *Local health care workers.* Local environmental health staff, infection control nurses, infectious disease experts and other medical and health care professionals are natural partners in investigations. Having pre-existing relationships and contact information readily available is very helpful.
- *Other potentially affected government agencies.* At times, what appears to be a localized outbreak or cluster of cases is actually part of a larger regional, national, or even international outbreak that is not initially recognized. If circumstances suggest that the local cases might be part of a larger outbreak (e.g., possibly involving a commercially prepared product with wide distribution, or a travel-associated outbreak), consultation with regional or national health officials is recommended, even before confirmatory laboratory test results are available. These agencies can also provide help in confirming and investigating outbreaks when local resources are not adequate. In addition, for outbreaks involving commercial products or multiple states or countries, federal agricultural or pharmaceutical agencies may need to be involved. Daily scheduled conference calls can be useful, in addition to releasing updates as needed to communicate new information. It is wise to know in advance who the relevant contacts are at local, state, and federal agencies and have methods to communicate with them after-hours.

CONCLUSION

Conducting an outbreak investigation can be a very exciting and rewarding experience for an epidemiologist. Good social and political skills can help open doors for the epidemiologist both by aiding the prompt gathering of information and by communicating results and recommendations to the public.

There are lessons to be learned from every outbreak. A formal outbreak review process or debriefing is often worthwhile after a large or complicated outbreak, to evaluate what worked and what did not. Such a review can involve representatives from many agencies and professional areas, and information from it can lead to appropriate changes in the response to future outbreaks.

Outbreak investigations can also provide an opportunity to deliver public health messages to the community. While most public health work takes place quietly behind the scenes, outbreak investigations are often the focus of intense community interest and media scrutiny. Carefully crafted communications can make a lasting impression that may favorably affect risk behavior in the population. A well-conducted outbreak investigation can also increase the public's understanding of, and appreciation for, the work that public health professionals do.

EXERCISES

1. In September, 1985, an outbreak of *E. coli* O157:H7 gastroenteritis struck 55 of 169 residents of a nursing home in southwestern Ontario, plus 18 of 137 staff (Carter et al., 1987). This microorganism can be transmitted by ingestion of contaminated food (often inadequately cooked ground beef); by person-to-person spread in such groups as families, child care centers, or custodial institutions; or by swimming in or drinking contaminated water (Chin J [ed.], 2000). The incubation period ranges from 3 to 8 days, with a median of 3 to 4 days.

   The epidemic curves for staff (top panel) and residents (bottom panel) are shown in Figure 19–2. From the information given, what would you consider to be the likeliest way(s) by which the staff and residents became infected during this outbreak and when the key exposure(s) occurred? Briefly explain your answer.

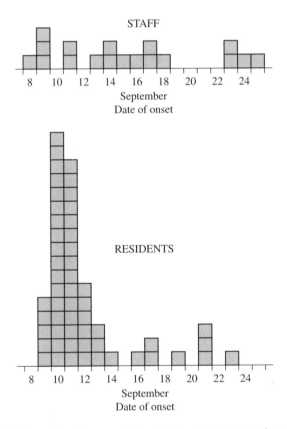

Figure 19–2. Epidemic Curve from an Outbreak of *E. coli* O157:H7 Infection in a Nursing Home (adapted from Carter et al., 1987).

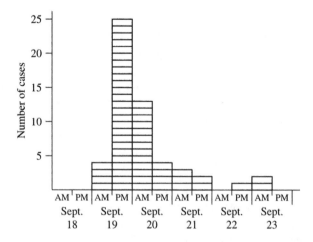

Figure 19-3. Initial Epidemic Curve from an Outbreak of Norwalk Virus among High School Football Players (adapted from Becker et al., 2000).

2. An article in the *New England Journal of Medicine* described an outbreak of Norwalk virus gastroenteritis among members and staff of a North Carolina football team in September, 1998. This illness is characterized by vomiting and diarrhea. The incubation period is 10 to 50 hours. Infection occurs by consumption of contaminated food, and person-to-person transmission can also occur from close physical contact. Figure 19–3 shows the occurrence of cases among North Carolina players and staff in each 12-hour time period over the course of several days.

   (a) Imagine that you are a field epidemiologist working on this outbreak. What period of time would you investigate most closely for a point exposure that could have initiated the epidemic?

   (b) Suggest two plausible possibilities for why the cases did not all occur within one incubation period.

ANSWERS

1. The most prominent feature is a large wave of cases among residents occurring from September 9–14, within one incubation period. This is most easily explained by a common point exposure on or about September 6. Nursing-home residents rarely go swimming in large groups, so this seems an unlikely form of exposure. Person-to-person transmission is also unlikely to explain the large initial wave, for lack of an apparent index case and because one would have to assume intimate contact between that person and a very large number of

residents over a very short period of time. A contaminated meal would be very plausible, however, as it could account for the exposure of many residents at essentially the same point in time. (In fact, a lunch on September 5 was strongly implicated.)

Early cases among staff could have represented staff who ate some of the same contaminated food as residents. Later cases in staff and in residents may well have represented person-to-person transmission from earlier cases.

2. (a) The cases did not all occur within one incubation period. But one would look especially closely at events on September 18, especially between noon and midnight that day. Given the incubation period of 10 to 50 hours, a point exposure during this time period could potentially account for the 46 cases that occurred on September 19 and 20 as part of a single "wave." Further investigation of this outbreak did indeed implicate a box lunch shared by team members on September 18.

(b) One possibility is a source of continuing exposure, such as contaminated foods or beverages consumed by team members repeatedly over a period of days. Another possibility is that later cases were infected via close contact with cases in a large initial wave. In this particular outbreak, physical combat on the football field, and contact on the sidelines between healthy teammates and others who were actively sick, were thought to be major routes of exposure for the late-occurring cases. A fuller epidemic curve is shown in Figure 19–4. Later cases, including some among members of

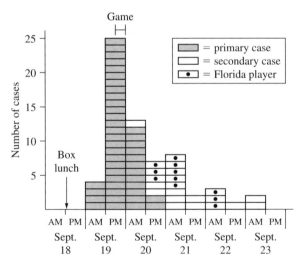

Figure 19–4. Final Epidemic Curve from an Outbreak of Norwalk Virus among High School Football Players (adapted from Becker et al., 2000).

the opposing Florida team, appeared likely to have been due to person-to-person transmission from those in the first wave who had eaten the tainted box lunch.

REFERENCES

Adderson E, Pavia A, Christenson J, Davis R, Leonard R, Carroll K. A community pseudo-outbreak of invasive *Staphylococcus aureus* infection. Diagn Microbiol Infect Dis 2000; 37:219–21.

Becker KM, Moe CL, Southwick KL, MacCormack JN. Transmission of Norwalk virus during football game. N Engl J Med 2000; 343:1223–27.

Bell BP, Goldoft M, Griffin PM, Davis MA, Gordon DC, Tarr PI, et al. A multistate outbreak of *Escherichia coli* O157:H7-associated bloody diarrhea and hemolytic uremic syndrome from hamburgers. The Washington experience. JAMA 1994; 272:1349–53.

Bell BP, Shapiro CN, Alter MJ, Moyer LA, Judson FN, Mottram K, et al. The diverse patterns of hepatitis A epidemiology in the United States—implications for vaccination strategies. J Infect Dis 1998; 178:1579–84.

Belongia EA, Hedberg CW, Gleich GJ, White KE, Mayeno AN, Loegering DA, et al. An investigation of the cause of the eosinophilia-myalgia syndrome associated with tryptophan use. N Engl J Med 1990; 323:357–65.

Bender JB, Hedberg CW, Besser JM, Boxrud DJ, MacDonald KL, Osterholm MT. Surveillance by molecular subtype for *Escherichia coli* O157:H7 infections in Minnesota by molecular subtyping. N Engl J Med 1997; 337:388–94.

Bender JB, Hedberg CW, Boxrud DJ, Besser JM, Wicklund JH, Smith KE, et al. Use of molecular subtyping in surveillance for *Salmonella enterica* serotype typhimurium. N Engl J Med 2001; 344:189–95.

Breuer T, Benkel DH, Shapiro RL, Hall WN, Winnett MM, Linn MJ, et al. A multistate outbreak of *Escherichia coli* O157:H7 infections linked to alfalfa sprouts grown from contaminated seeds. Emerg Infect Dis 2001; 7:977–82.

Bryan FL, Bartleson CA, Cook OD, et al. Procedures to investigate foodborne illness (5th ed.). Des Moines, Iowa: International Association of Milk, Food, and Environmental Sanitarians, Inc., 1999.

Carter AO, Borczyk AA, Carlson JAK, Harvey B, Hockin JC, Karmali MA, et al. A severe outbreak of *Escherichia coli* O157:H7–associated hemorrhaghic colitis in a nursing home. N Engl J Med 1987; 317:1496–500.

Centers for Disease Control and Prevention. Pneumocystis pneumonia—Los Angeles. MMWR Morb Mortal Wkly Rep 1981; 30:250–52.

Centers for Disease Control and Prevention. Enhanced detection of sporadic *Escherichia coli* O157:H7 infections—New Jersey, July 1994. MMWR Morb Mortal Wkly Rep 1995; 44:417–18.

Centers for Disease Control and Prevention. Case definitions for infectious conditions under public health surveillance. MMWR Recomm Rep 1997a; 46:1–55.

Centers for Disease Control and Prevention. Outbreaks of pseudo-infection with Cyclospora and Cryptosporidium—Florida and New York City, 1995. MMWR Morb Mortal Wkly Rep 1997b; 46:354–58.

Centers for Disease Control and Prevention. Outbreak of *Salmonella* serotype Muenchen infections associated with unpasteurized orange juice—United States and Canada, June 1999. MMWR Morb Mortal Wkly Rep 1999; 48:582–85.

Centers for Disease Control and Prevention. Legionnaires' disease associated with potting soil—California, Oregon, and Washington, May–June 2000. MMWR Morb Mortal Wkly Rep 2000; 49:777–78.

Centers for Disease Control and Prevention. Outbreak of listeriosis associated with home-made Mexican-style cheese—North Carolina, October 2000–January 2001. MMWR Morb Mortal Wkly Rep 2001; 50:560–62.

Centers for Disease Control and Prevention. Outbreak of *Salmonella* serotype Kottbus infections associated with eating alfalfa sprouts—Arizona, California, Colorado, and New Mexico, February–April 2001. MMWR Morb Mortal Wkly Rep 2002a; 51:7–9.

Centers for Disease Control and Prevention. Rashes among schoolchildren—14 states, October 4, 2001–February 27, 2002. MMWR Morb Mortal Wkly Rep 2002b; 51:161–64.

Chin J (ed). Manual of communicable disease control (17th ed.). Washington, D.C.: American Public Health Association, 2000.

Covello VT, Peters RG, Wojtecki JG, Hyde RC. Risk communication, the West Nile virus epidemic, and bioterrorism: responding to the communication challenges posed by the intentional or unintentional release of a pathogen in an urban setting. J Urban Health 2001; 78:382–91.

Den Boer JW, Yzerman EP, Schellekens J, Lettinga KD, Boshuizen HC, Van Steenbergen JE, et al. A large outbreak of Legionnaires' disease at a flower show, the Netherlands, 1999. Emerg Infect Dis 2002; 8:37–43.

Dicker R. Principles of epidemiology. An introduction to applied epidemiology and bio-statistics (2nd ed.). Atlanta, Ga.: Centers for Disease Control and Prevention, 1998.

Duchin JS, Koster FT, Peters CJ, Simpson GL, Tempest B, Zaki SR, et al. Hantavirus pulmonary syndrome: a clinical description of 17 patients with a newly recognized disease. The Hantavirus Study Group. N Engl J Med 1994; 330:949–55.

Fraser DW, Tsai TR, Orenstein W, Parkin WE, Beecham HJ, Sharrar RG, et al. Legionnaires' disease: description of an epidemic of pneumonia. N Engl J Med 1977; 297:1189–97.

Glatzel M, Rogivue C, Ghani A, Streffer JR, Amsler L, Aguzzi A. Incidence of Creutzfeldt-Jakob disease in Switzerland. Lancet 2002; 360:139–41.

Hedberg CW, Fishbein DB, Janssen RS, Meyers B, McMillen JM, MacDonald KL, et al. An outbreak of thyrotoxicosis caused by the consumption of bovine thyroid gland in ground beef. N Engl J Med 1987; 316:993–98.

Joce RE, Murphy F, Robertson MH. A pseudo-outbreak of salmonellosis. Epidemiol Infect 1995; 115:31–38.

Mishu B, Koehler J, Lee LA, Rodrigue D, Brenner FH, Blake P, et al. Outbreaks of *Salmonella enteritidis* infections in the United States, 1985–1991. J Infect Dis 1994; 169:547–52.

Mohle-Boetani JC, Farrar JA, Werner SB, Minassian D, Bryant R, Abbott S, et al. *Escherichia coli* O157 and *Salmonella* infections associated with sprouts in California, 1996–1998. Ann Intern Med 2001; 135:239–47.

National Research Council. Improving risk communication. Washington, D.C.: National Academy Press, 1989.

Shands KN, Schmid GP, Dan BB, Blum D, Guidotti RJ, Hargrett NT, et al. Toxic-shock syndrome in menstruating women: association with tampon use and *Staphylococcus aureus* and clinical features in 52 cases. N Engl J Med 1980; 303:1436–42.

Snow J. Snow on Cholera. New York: Commonwealth Fund, 1936.

St Louis ME, Morse DL, Potter ME, DeMelfi TM, Guzewich JJ, Tauxe RV, et al. The emergence of grade A eggs as a major source of *Salmonella* Enteritidis infections. New implications for the control of salmonellosis. JAMA 1988; 259:2103–7.

Steere AC, Malawista SE, Snydman DR, Shope RE, Andiman WA, Ross MR, et al. Lyme arthritis: an epidemic of oligoarticular arthritis in children and adults in three Connecticut communities. Arthritis Rheum 1977; 20:7–17.

Swaminathan B, Barrett TJ, Hunter SB, Tauxe RV. PulseNet: the molecular subtyping network for foodborne bacterial disease surveillance, United States. Emerg Infect Dis 2001; 7:382–89.

U.S. Department of Health and Human Services. Consumers advised of risks associated with raw sprouts. HHS News 1999; July 9:P9–13.

Wagner MM, Tsui FC, Espino JU, Dato VM, Sittig DF, Caruana RA, et al. The emerging science of very early detection of disease outbreaks. J Public Health Manag Pract 2001; 7:51–59.

Weinbaum CM, Bodnar UR, Schulte J, Atkinson B, Morgan MT, Caliper TE, et al. Pseudo-outbreak of tuberculosis infection due to improper skin-test reading. Clin Infect Dis 1998; 26:1235–36.

Weiss NS. Epidemiologic studies in which a necessary cause is known. Epidemiology 1991; 2:153–54.

20

EVALUATING THE EFFECTS OF POLICIES ON HEALTH

The mission of epidemiology is to understand the determinants of disease occurrence in populations. One set of potentially important determinants includes the policies that societies and organizations follow to achieve their goals. This chapter seeks to illustrate how epidemiologic study designs can be used to evaluate the health effects of such policies.

The term *policies* refers here to collective actions or strategies, such as government laws and regulations, organizational procedures, and decisions about resource allocation. Examples include whether or not screening mammography is covered under Medicare, whether smoking is prohibited in public buildings, and whether airbags are required in all new automobiles legally offered for sale in the U.S. Policies often apply broadly to a defined population, such as citizens of a geopolitical unit or members of an organization.

Policies can have many kinds of effects, extending well beyond the health arena, and evaluating them comprehensively is typically a multidisciplinary activity. Epidemiology has the most to contribute in estimating the effects of policies on population health. Some such effects may be intended, as when a new influenza-vaccination policy successfully reduces the incidence of influenza. Others may be side effects, as when economic sanctions imposed on Iraq after the Gulf War were followed by increases in infant mortality (Ali and Shah, 2000).

Under some circumstances, epidemiologic studies of individuals, which are commonly used for etiologic research, can also be applied to policy evaluation. Yet, because policies often apply to entire populations or groups, there may be insufficient variation in exposure among individuals within a target population to permit a comparative evaluation within that population. Instead, it may be necessary to study as controls separate populations or groups that are not exposed to the policies or programs of interest. For policies of very broad scope, such as federal laws, no suitable concurrent controls may exist, and inferences about the effects of such policies on health may have to depend on interpreting trends in disease occurrence over time. For these reasons, ecological and longitudinal study designs assume special importance in policy evaluation.

POLICY EVALUATION WHEN EXPOSURE VARIES
WITHIN A POPULATION

Cohort studies, case-control studies, and randomized trials of individuals generally rely on the existence of enough variation in exposure among individuals within a population to allow meaningful examination of exposure–outcome associations. These and other standard epidemiologic studies of individuals can sometimes be useful for estimating the probable impact of alternative policies, especially when a new policy being considered would be more restrictive than the current one. Occasionally a policy may actually be implemented in such a way that a natural concurrent comparison group within the target population is formed.

Cohort Studies

Example: Mortality from coronary heart disease in the United Kingdom has been among the highest in the world, and many such deaths result from sudden cardiac arrest. In 2001, British law required that ambulances be deployed in such a way as to enable a response to at least 90% of calls within 14 minutes. The National Health Service was considering reducing this target to 90% of responses within 8 minutes. Pell and colleagues (2001) sought to evaluate the impact of such a policy by examining survival to hospital discharge among cardiac-arrest victims in relation to ambulance response time. Using data on 10,554 cardiac arrests throughout Scotland, they found that after adjusting for several potential confounding factors, ambulance response time remained a strong predictor of survival to hospital discharge. They used data from this cohort to project an increase in survival from a baseline level of 6% to a new level of 8% if 90% of response times were within 8 minutes, and to 10–11% if 90% of response times were within 5 minutes.

This study could be regarded as a form of "anticipatory" policy evaluation. The policy being considered was more stringent than the policy in effect at the time of the study. The current one permitted enough variation in ambulance response times among individual cases to allow comparing their outcomes. As the investigators noted, predicting the impact of possible future policies based on current data may involve inaccuracies if other changes in patient characteristics or service delivery should occur. It also assumes that the target response times could actually be achieved.

Case-Control Studies

Example: Environmental regulations and housing codes dictate where residences may be situated in relation to power-transmission lines. Early studies raised concerns that existing policies may expose persons who live too near high-voltage power lines to increased risk of cancer or other diseases. To help determine whether living near such lines is associated with increased risk of acute lymphoblastic leukemia in children, Kleinerman and colleagues (2000) conducted a nationwide case-control study of this disease. They compared 428 cases in children under age 15 years to 428 matched control children who were identified by random-digit dialing. All participants had lived in one home for at least 3.5 of the five years before the case's diagnosis. Technicians blinded to case-control status ascertained the distance between each subjects' residence and the nearest power line, transmission line, and distribution line. No increase in risk of acute lymphoblastic leukemia was found in relation to proximity to any of these types of lines.

In this instance, relatively loose existing policies about power line placement led to variation in how close children lived to these lines. This variation could then be exploited epidemiologically to determine the potential effect of a stricter policy. Because acute lymphoblastic leukemia is rare, a case-control design was attractive for this purpose. Case-control studies, however, focus on a particular outcome (here, acute lymphoblastic leukemia), so the study could not address whether proximity to power lines might have other adverse health consequences.

Randomized Trials

Example: In 1970 and 1972, at the height of the Vietnam War, the U.S. government conducted a public lottery to determine the order in which young American men would be eligible to be drafted for military service. Each day of the year was written on a plastic ball. The balls were placed in a tumbler, mixed, and withdrawn one at a time, resulting in a random sequence of days. Men whose birthday was written on ball no. 1 were drafted first, followed by men whose birthday appeared on ball no. 2, and so on, until the military's manpower needs were met.

Years later, Hearst and colleagues (1986) recognized that the draft lottery provided an unusual opportunity to study delayed effects of military service under a policy of involuntary conscription. They examined cause-specific death rates during the postwar years from 1974 to 1983 among men who had been of draft-eligible age when the lottery was conducted. Men were divided into two groups according to whether their birth date had made them eligible to be drafted. Among men with draft-eligible birth dates, mortality from suicide was 13% higher (95% CI: 4%–23%), motor-vehicle crash mortality was 8% higher (95% CI: 1%–16%), and total mortality was 4% higher (95% CI: 0%–8%) than among men with draft-ineligible birth dates. The authors concluded that military service during the Vietnam War was likely to have caused an excess of subsequent deaths from suicide and motor-vehicle crashes.

The investigators aptly referred to this unusual study as a "randomized natural experiment." They themselves had no control over which men were draft-eligible and which were not. Yet military conscription policy had been implemented in such a way as to amount to a large randomized trial. By a formal chance mechanism, two large groups of men had been formed. Total and cause-specific death rates would be expected to be the same in both groups, apart from chance fluctuations, unless being draft-eligible affected mortality.

The effects of actual military *service* in Vietnam or elsewhere on postwar mortality would almost certainly exceed the observed difference between the two groups studied. This is because each group contained a mixture of men who ended up in military service and others who did not. The investigators retained the substantial advantages of randomization, however, by following the "intent to treat" principle. Thus the study was able to provide unusually strong evidence that the associations seen were causal.

POLICY EVALUATION USING STUDIES OF INTACT SOCIAL GROUPS

Many policies apply to entire target populations or subpopulations, and there is little or no variation in exposure among individuals within the target population to exploit. Hence, a controlled evaluation must often consider variation in policies among different populations or over time. This application of ecological studies was described briefly in Chapter 12 but merits further elaboration here. The discussion below progresses from simpler to more elaborate policy-evaluation designs. In general, the features that add complexity also render a design more resistant to certain potential sources of bias.

After-Only

Example: In 1970, the Poison Prevention Packaging Act became federal law in the U.S., requiring that most regulated prescription drugs be dispensed in a container that would resist opening by a small child, unless non–child-resistant packaging was specifically requested by the physician or patient. Once this law was in effect,

Dole and colleagues (1986) visited 60 pharmacies in the Memphis, Tennessee, area and submitted to each a prescription that should have been dispensed in a child-resistant container under the law. In 23% of cases, the drug was provided in a non–child-resistant container, indicating substantial noncompliance with the law.

After-only studies can evaluate a policy against a prespecified benchmark—in this case, 100% of test prescriptions being dispensed in child-resistant containers. But these studies provide no basis for assessing what would have been observed in the absence of the policy in question. No comparison is made to other populations that were not subject to the policy, nor is there a comparison with historically observed levels or trends in the same population. Absent such information, the benchmark level used for evaluation must often be viewed as somewhat arbitrary. Using a relatively lax benchmark may result in labelling as successful a policy that actually had no effect at all. Alternative, a policy that has had beneficial effects may be labelled unsuccessful if the target level was set high.

Before-After

Example: Attempted suicide by ingestion of the analgesic drugs paracetamol or salicylates was common in the United Kingdom, accounting for hundreds of deaths each year and over half of all cases of liver failure (Hawton et al., 2001). On September 16, 1998, a new law took effect that restricted the maximum number of paracetamol or salicylate tablets dispensed per sale to 32 tablets in pharmacies or 16 tablets in other retail outlets. A warning label was also added to packages and package inserts for paracetamol. Sales data showed sharp declines in the number of tablets per sale after the new law took effect.

Hawton and colleagues compared mortality from paracetamol or salicylate poisoning for the 24 months before and the 12 months after the new law went into effect. Poisoning deaths involving paracetamol alone declined 21% (95% confidence interval, 5%–34%), and those involving salicylates alone declined 48% (95% confidence interval, 11%–70%). Admissions to inpatient liver-disease units for paracetamol poisoning and nonfatal self-poisonings with this drug also declined.

A before-after study uses an empirical benchmark against which health outcomes after the implementation of the policy can be compared: namely, the level observed before the policy took effect. The target population is sometimes said to "serve as its own control."

Nonetheless, it may be hard to rule out the possibility that some other concurrent historical event besides the policy in question accounted for any change observed. Moreover, the change may simply be continuation of a long-term secular trend, rather than a true effect of the policy. On occasion, the policy change itself may have been triggered by perceptions that the problem had gotten worse, when in fact the high level may simply be due to random fluctuations over time. If so, then improvement after the policy takes effect may simply reflect regression to the mean (Campbell and Stanley, 1966; Cook and Campbell, 1979).

After-Only with Concurrent Controls

Example: In 1992, the age-adjusted injury mortality rate in Alaska was higher than in any other state (Landen et al., 1997). Injuries were the leading cause of death in remote parts of the state inaccessible by state roads. Landen and colleagues (1997) used death-certificate data and medical examiner records to compare injury mortality between two groups of remote villages with populations of fewer than 1,000 persons. In 78 "wet" villages, local laws did not specifically regulate availability of alcohol. In 72 "dry" villages, sale and importation of alcohol was prohibited. For the years from 1990 to 1993, the injury mortality rate was 1.6-fold greater among Alaska natives in wet villages than in dry villages. Much of the excess risk was found to be due to motor-vehicle trauma, homicide, and hypothermia.

Adoption of the alcohol policy in each village antedated the surveillance period for injury deaths, so this study qualifies as an after-only study with concurrent controls. In this instance, there were multiple villages with and without permissive alcohol policies. (Nine villages switched status during the study, and deaths and person-years at risk in those villages were divided between wet and dry accordingly.) For most villages, no "before" data were available for comparison, so the possibility that wet villages had historically always had higher injury mortality rates—perhaps reflecting greater cultural acceptance of various kinds of risky behavior—could not be ruled out.

What if only two villages, one wet and one dry, had been studied? (Injury deaths alone might have been too rare to provide a meaningful comparison, but including nonfatal injuries might have circumvented this problem.) It might still have been tempting to link any observed differences in injury occurrence to the difference in alcohol policies. But we must remember that geographical variation in disease frequency is the rule, not the exception. We could not be sure that the two villages would have had similar injury rates even if they had had similar alcohol policies. In fact, given the many ways in which communities in general can differ from each other, it would be very surprising if the true long-term incidence of injury were identical among them. Some of the differences may be due to confounding by readily measurable sociodemographic characteristics, which could be removed by suitable adjustment for these factors. But often much community-to-community variation remains unexplained (Diehr et al., 1993). A comparison of only two villages would not be able to discern how much of any observed difference in injury rates was due to differences in alcohol policy and how much was due to community-to-community variation with regard to other causes of injury.

In the study by Landen and colleagues, the number of fatal injuries and the estimated number of person-years at risk were simply pooled across all wet villages, and similarly across dry villages, to obtain two summary rates that were then compared statistically as though derived from two homogeneous populations. This method of analysis, however, assumes no community-to-community variation within the wet and dry groups. Often accounting for such variation leads to wider confidence intervals around the estimated difference (or ratio) in rates between policy categories. In this instance, the overall ratio of injury mortality between wet and dry villages was reported as 1.6 (95% confidence interval, 1.3–2.1). The confidence limits around this relative risk would probably be wider if variation among villages were incorporated into the analysis. Several techniques are now available for analysis of data from studies involving multiple clusters, such as villages (Liang and Zeger, 1993; Graubard and Korn, 1994; Neuhaus, 1992; Ashby et al., 1992).

Before-After with Concurrent Controls

Example: Before 1991, 12 U.S. states had established lower legal blood alcohol limits for drivers under age 21 years than for older drivers. Hingson and colleagues (Hingson et al., 1994) sought to evaluate the effects of these laws by studying changes in the proportion of fatal motor-vehicle crashes among drivers aged 15 to 20 years that were single-vehicle nighttime crashes, since many of these crashes are believed to be alcohol-related. The 12 states with such a law were matched to 12 nearby states without a law. In each pair of states, the pre-law period was the maximum number of years for which the required crash data were available in both states before the law took effect in one of them, and the post-law period was similarly defined. In the post-law period, the proportion of fatal crashes involving single vehicles at night fell 16% among young drivers in states with a lower blood alcohol law, while this proportion rose 1% in control states ($p < .001$).

This study design involves measuring *changes* over time in the frequency of the outcome between jurisdictions with and without the policy of interest. Possible differences in the frequency of that outcome at baseline are thus of less concern than they might be in an after-only study. In addition, studying control jurisdictions over the same time period bolsters the inference that changes in areas with the policy are not simply a reflection of widespread secular trends.

Control populations without the policy need not necessarily be geographically defined. In this example, the lower blood alcohol laws of interest applied only to drivers under the age of 21. A second kind of control group within each state that passed such a law was drivers aged 21 years or older. The proportion of fatal crashes in this age group that consisted of single-vehicle nighttime crashes declined only 1% from the pre-law to the post-law period, lending further support to the idea that little change in this proportion would be expected among younger drivers in the absence of an effect of the new law. Note, however, that these laws applied to *all* persons under age 21 and to *no* persons aged 21 years or older. Hence the study designs remains ecological in nature.

In this particular example, the frequency of fatal single-vehicle nighttime crashes was measured as a proportion of all fatal crashes, so the cautions described in Chapter 3 about interpreting proportional mortality data should also be kept in mind.

Interrupted Time Series

Example: Based on evidence that the birth prevalence of neural tube defects (NTDs) is sharply reduced if mothers consume at least 400 μg of folic acid each day, in March, 1996, the U.S. Food and Drug Administration authorized the addition of folic acid to enriched grain products sold in the U.S. Compliance became mandatory in January, 1998. To determine the extent to which this policy change produced a reduction in the birth prevalence of NTDs in the U.S., Honein and colleagues (2001) tracked the birth prevalence of NTDs in 45 states and the District of Columbia during every six-month interval from 1990 to 1999. Using statistical methods for analysis of time-series data, the 14 birth prevalence values from 1990 to 1996 were used to estimate the usual amount of variation from interval to interval. Relative to this benchmark, NTD birth prevalence was found to be significantly reduced during all three of the six-month intervals during the mandatory-supplementation period. Overall, the birth prevalence of NTDs during the combined supplementation periods was 19% lower than during the reference period.

The interrupted time series design can be thought of as an extension of the before-after design, involving multiple measurements before and after a new policy takes effect. The sequence of observations during the baseline period establishes the expected amount of variability in disease frequency among successive time intervals and/or the secular trend. These patterns provide a better basis than a single baseline observation for predicting what levels of disease frequency would have been expected in the absence of a policy effect. As in the before-after design, however, there may be other competing reasons for any change observed. In the above example, the investigators noted that they could not rule out changes over time in the completeness of reporting of NTDs on birth certificates, or in the proportion of NTD-affected pregnancies that might have been terminated before resulting in a live birth.

Interrupted Time Series with Concurrent Controls

Example: In 1988, California voters passed Proposition 99, which increased the tax on cigarettes sold in the state by 25 cents per pack. One fifth of the new tax revenues was used to fund an aggressive campaign against tobacco use. The anti-smoking media campaign was temporarily suspended in 1992 during a legal battle, and cutbacks in the program persisted thereafter. Fichtenberg and Glantz (2000), noting that surveys had suggested sharper declines in tobacco use in California than in other parts of the U.S., sought to determine the extent to which Proposition 99 may have reduced deaths from cardiovascular disease.

As shown in Figure 20–1, age-adjusted mortality rates from heart disease had been declining steadily in California and in the rest of the U.S. for some time before Proposition 99 became law. Rates in California were already below those in the rest of the U.S. The investigators hypothesized that if there were at least some short-term influence of cigarette smoking on mortality from cardiovascular disease, the effect of Proposition 99 would be to *accelerate* the downward slope in California

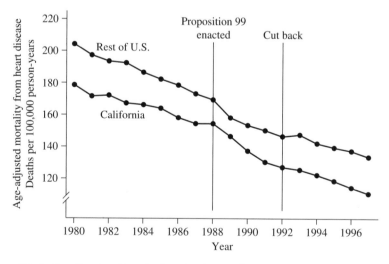

Figure 20–1. Time Trends in Mortality from Cardiovascular Disease in California and the Rest of the United States, in Relation to California Proposition 99 (based on Fichtenberg and Glantz, 2000).

relative to that in the rest of the U.S. after 1988. Moreover, the differences in slopes might be reduced after 1992 when the cutbacks took place. Multiple linear regression was used to test for these hypothesized differences in slopes during each period.

The regression results indicated that the rate of decline in mortality from heart disease in California compared to the rest of the U.S. was -2.93 deaths/100,000 person-years per year greater during 1989–1992 than before Proposition 99 had been enacted (95% CI: -3.97, -1.89). The difference in slopes was attenuated after 1992.

This design improves further on the interrupted time-series design by adding concurrently studied comparison groups. In this example, there was just one large policy-exposed group (California) and one large non-exposed group (the rest of the U.S.). Secular trends observed in the pre-policy period, as well as those in the comparison group in the post-policy period, can be used as a basis for estimating what levels of disease frequency would have been expected without the new policy. A more elaborate example is described in Chapter 12, in which Cummings et al. (1997) estimated the reduction in childhood firearm-injury deaths associated with passage of safe gun storage laws. In that example, time trends in cause-specific mortality were tracked in *multiple* states that enacted such a law and compared with trends in multiple states that did not enact such a law.

Sometimes policies are implemented intermittently, so that their effects on disease frequency would be expected to vary over time in a certain way. If the observed pattern of variation conforms closely to the hypothesized one, this can provide convincing evidence of a causal association. This situation can be considered a generalization of the interrupted time series examples considered above, now involving multiple periods with and without the policy of interest in one or more study populations.

Example: In the relatively isolated town of Barrow, Alaska, laws about possession and importation of alcohol changed several times between 1993 and 1996. The town's population composition, economic status, and local culture were in flux, in part because of the arrival of workers and money associated with the development of oil resources in nearby Prudhoe Bay. Possessing and importing alcohol in Barrow were legal until November, 1994, when a ban on both took effect following a local vote. A year later, another election was held and the ban was repealed. Balloting procedures surrounding that second election were then successfully challenged in court, and a third election was held, which led to reimposing a ban in March, 1996.

Chiu and colleagues (1997) studied the possible effects of these changes in local laws on the frequency of outpatient visits for alcohol-related conditions.

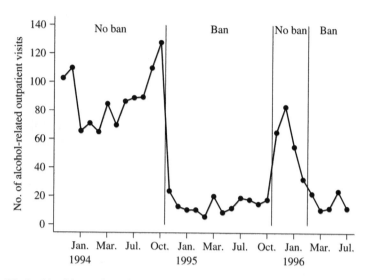

Figure 20–2. Monthly Number of Alcohol-Related Outpatient Visits in Barrow, Alaska, During Time Periods With and Without a Legal Ban on Possession and Importation of Alcohol (adapted from Chiu et al., 1997).

Computerized data were available for all outpatient visits to the only hospital in the area over a 33-month study period. Data for each visit included diagnoses and a check-off item indicating whether the diagnosis was alcohol-related, which was later checked on medical record review by physicians. As shown in Figure 20–2, the number of alcohol-related visits per month was sharply lower during periods when an alcohol ban was in effect. Analysis using an autoregressive integrated moving average (ARIMA) model found the differences in mean alcohol-related visits per month between ban and non-ban periods to be well beyond what would be expected by chance ($p < .05$).

Here, the close correspondence in time between alcohol-related visit frequency and policy changes that is visually apparent in Figure 20–2 is strongly suggestive by itself. A strength of this study was use of a statistical approach that accounted for temporal autocorrelation: that is, the possibility that the count of alcohol-related outpatient visits in a given month would be correlated with visit counts in the adjacent months before and after it. Such correlations can arise in various ways, including seasonality or other local events or trends whose effects span more than one month. To the extent that temporal autocorrelation in outcomes is present in a longitudinal study, outcome frequencies in different time intervals are not statistically independent, and special statistical methods are needed to obtain valid significance tests and confidence intervals (Nelson, 1998; Rehm and Gmel, 2001; Diggle, 1990).

CONCLUSION

In keeping with our concern with epidemiologic methods, this chapter has focused mainly on several study designs that can be useful in assessing the impact of public and institutional policies on disease frequency in populations. Except when the observed frequency of disease is to be compared only with some prespecified target, these study designs all seek to provide an empirical basis for estimating what level(s) of disease frequency would have been seen without the policy in question. These estimates may be obtained from data from one or more concurrently studied control populations or subpopulations; extrapolation of secular trends observed before a policy has taken effect; disease frequency during interspersed periods without the policy when it has been in effect intermittently; or combinations of these approaches. Each design has generic strengths and weaknesses, and choosing a design often involves balancing its susceptibility to bias against data availability, cost, and other practical considerations.

Policy evaluation can place epidemiologists in a new and sometimes unfamiliar context in which scientific considerations are only one of many sets of factors involved in decision-making. Economics, politics, and sociocultural factors are often prominent and may overshadow the scientific debate (Sommer, 2001; Brownson, 1998; Ibrahim, 1985; Deyo et al., 1997). Policy evaluation can also confront the epidemiologist with a need to make a personal choice between active advocacy and neutral objectivity. Despite these challenges, epidemiologists have an important role to play in applying the special skills and methods of our field to assessing the effects of collective decisions on population health.

EXERCISES

1. In the U.S., policies on issuance and renewal of driver's licenses are set by each state. For example, the number of years allowed between license renewals for older drivers varies from state to state, ranging from three years in some states to six years in others. How might you investigate whether shorter license-renewal intervals are associated with lower crash mortality in older drivers?
2. In 1994, the state of Tennessee changed its Medicaid program from a traditional fee-for-service system to a capitated system called TennCare. This change sought to reduce annual Medicaid costs per enrollee, enabling the state to broaden eligibility for Medicaid among low-income state residents. Because this change occurred rapidly and with some administrative confusion, there was concern that some TennCare-eligible pregnant women had trouble finding a prenatal care provider who would accept them under the new program.

Suggest a study design to assess whether TennCare had a beneficial or adverse effect on perinatal outcomes.

3. It is now widely accepted that tobacco use has many adverse health consequences. Because smoking often begins in youth and early adulthood, much effort has been devoted to reducing initiation of tobacco use among adolescents. Local policies that are intended to limit youth access to tobacco include bans on cigarette vending machines, fines levied on salespersons who sell tobacco to underage clients, bans on self-service displays of tobacco products, and periodic inspections by police to assess compliance with laws prohibiting sales of tobacco to youth.

   Would you consider it feasible to study the effects of these policies using a randomized trial? If so, how? If not, what alternative design would you consider instead?

ANSWERS

1. You could use an ecological study design, comparing crash mortality between states with long and short license-renewal intervals. In this instance, however, you might also be able to exploit the fact that some states allow relatively long intervals between renewals. Within such states, you could compare fatal crash rates among older drivers who are within, say, one year of their last renewal with rates among older drivers whose last renewal was, say, four or five years ago. Such an approach would allow you to estimate the effect of reducing the renewal interval.

2. Ray et al. (1998) studied the effects of TennCare using outcomes recorded on birth and death certificates for Tennessee for several years before and after the policy change. The analysis focused on singleton births in 1993, the year immediately preceding TennCare, and 1995, the first year during which an entire pregnancy would have been covered under the new program. Over 72,000 such births occurred to Medicaid-eligible women in each year. Several outcomes were studied, including low and very low birth weight, death in the first 60 days of life, and whether prenatal care was initiated only after the fourth month of pregnancy. The results suggested little or no change in any of these measures after the introduction of TennCare, either overall or among several subgroups of high-risk mothers, after adjustment for multiple maternal characteristics available from birth certificate data. These results provided some reassurance that administrative disruptions accompanying the switch to TennCare had not led to deterioration of prenatal care and perinatal outcomes.

3. Perhaps surprisingly, the effectiveness of a package of these local policies *has* been studied in a randomized community trial (Forster et al., 1998). Some 14 Minnesota communities were randomized to intervention or control status. The seven intervention sites took part in a 32-month effort to mobilize citizens to the cause of preventing tobacco use by youth, including changing local laws and regulations. All seven sites adopted a comprehensive anti-tobacco ordinance. (Three control communities also changed their laws, but ordinances in the control sites were weaker and less comprehensive than those in intervention sites.)

Because the frequency of smoking-related diseases was expected to be low, and because any effects on incidence could require many years to occur, the study focused on the prevalence of smoking as measured in school surveys. Although the prevalence of daily smoking among youth actually *increased* in both intervention and control communities over a three-year study period, the net increase was 4.9 percentage points greater in control sites than in intervention sites (95% confidence interval: 0.7–9.0 percentage points). Note that the intervention might thus have been judged ineffective if only a before-after study design had been used. Because of randomization of communities, the study provided unusually strong evidence that the policy changes were responsible. The comprehensive ordinances passed in intervention sites involved several provisions, however, and the study was unable to tease apart the contribution of each component.

REFERENCES

Ali MM, Shah IH. Sanctions and childhood mortality in Iraq. Lancet 2000; 355:1851–57.

Ashby M, Neuhaus JM, Hauck WW, Bacchetti P, Heilbron DC, Jewell NP, et al. An annotated bibliography of methods for analysing correlated categorical data. Stat Med 1992; 11:67–99.

Brownson RC. "Epidemiology and health policy." Chapter 12 in: Brownson RC, Petitti DB. Applied epidemiology. New York: Oxford, 1998.

Campbell DT, Stanley JC. Experimental and quasi-experimental designs for research. Chicago: Rand McNally, 1966.

Chiu AY, Perez PE, Parker RN. Impact of banning alcohol on outpatient visits in Barrow, Alaska. JAMA 1997; 278:1775–77.

Cook TD, Campbell DT. Quasi-experimentation: design and analysis issues for field settings. Boston: Houghton Mifflin, 1979.

Cummings P, Grossman DC, Rivara FP, Koepsell TD. State gun safe storage laws and child mortality due to firearms. JAMA 1997; 278:1084–86.

Deyo RA, Psaty BM, Simon G, Wagner EH, Omenn GS. The messenger under attack—intimidation of researchers by special-interest groups. N Engl J Med 1997; 336:1176–80.

Diehr P, Koepsell T, Cheadle A, Psaty BM, Wagner E, Curry S. Do communities differ in health behaviors? J Clin Epidemiol 1993; 46:1141–49.

Diggle PJ. Time series: a biostatistical introduction. New York: Oxford, 1990.

Dole EJ, Czajka PA, Rivara FP. Evaluation of pharmacists' compliance with the Poison Prevention Packaging Act. Am J Public Health 1986; 76:1335–36.

Fichtenberg CM, Glantz SA. Association of the California Tobacco Control Program with declines in cigarette consumption and mortality from heart disease. N Engl J Med 2000; 343:1772–77.

Forster JL, Murray DM, Wolfson M, Blaine TM, Wagenaar AC, Hennrikus DJ. The effects of community policies to reduce youth access to tobacco. Am J Public Health 1998; 88:1193–98.

Graubard BI, Korn EL. Regression analysis with clustered data. Stat Med 1994; 13:509–22.

Hawton K, Townsend E, Deeks J, Appleby L, Gunnell D, Bennewith O, et al. Effects of legislation restricting pack sizes of paracetamol and salicylate on self poisoning in the United Kingdom: before and after study. BMJ 2001; 322:1203–7.

Hearst N, Newman TB, Hulley SB. Delayed effects of the military draft on mortality. N Engl J Med 1986; 314:620–4.

Hingson R, Heeren T, Winter M. Lower legal blood alcohol limits for young drivers. Public Health Rep 1994; 109:738–44.

Honein MA, Paulozzi LJ, Mathews TJ, Erickson JD, Wong LC. Impact of folic acid fortification of the U.S. food supply on the occurrence of neural tube defects. JAMA 2001; 285:2981–86.

Ibrahim MA. Epidemiology and health policy. Rockville, Md.: Aspen Systems Corp., 1985.

Kleinerman RA, Kaune WT, Hatch EE, Wacholder S, Linet MS, Robison LL, et al. Are children living near high-voltage power lines at increased risk of acute lymphoblastic leukemia? Am J Epidemiol 2000; 151:512–15.

Landen MG, Beller M, Funk E, Propst M, Middaugh J, Moolenaar RL. Alcohol-related injury death and alcohol availability in remote Alaska. JAMA 1997; 278:1755–58.

Liang KY, Zeger SL. Regression analysis for correlated data. Annu Rev Public Health 1993; 14:43–68.

Nelson BK. Statistical methodology: V. Time series analysis using autoregressive integrated moving average (ARIMA) models. Acad Emerg Med 1998; 5:739–44.

Neuhaus JM. Statistical methods for longitudinal and clustered designs with binary responses. Stat Methods Med Res 1992; 1:249–73.

Pell JP, Sirel JM, Marsden AK, Ford I, Cobbe SM. Effect of reducing ambulance response times on deaths from out of hospital cardiac arrest: cohort study. BMJ 2001; 322:1385–88.

Ray WA, Gigante J, Mitchel EF, Hickson GB. Perinatal outcomes following implentationn of TennCare. JAMA 1998; 279:314–16.

Rehm J, Gmel G. Aggregate time-series regression in the field of alcohol. Addiction 2001; 96:945–54.

Sommer A. How public health policy is created: scientific process and political reality. Am J Epidemiol 2001; 154:S4–S6.

INDEX